50 Critical CANCER Answers

FRANCISCO CONTRERAS, MD
and DANIEL E. KENNEDY, MC

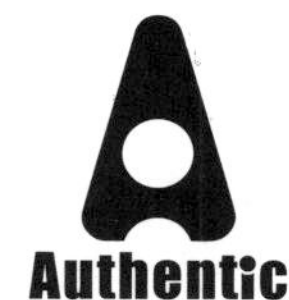

50 Critical Cancer Answers
Copyright © 2013
Francisco Contreras and Daniel E. Kennedy

Cover design by Lookout Design

The Bible text designated NIV is from the Holy Bible,
New International Version®. Copyright © 1973, 1978,
1984, 2011 by Biblica, Inc.TM Used by permission.

Scripture quotations marked NLT are taken from THE HOLY BIBLE,
NEW LIVING TRANSLATION, copyright ©1996.
Used by permission of Tyndale House Publishers, Inc.,
Wheaton, Illinois, 60189. All rights reserved.

Scripture quotations marked NKJV are taken from the NEW KING
JAMES VERSION of the Bible. Copyright © 1979, 1980, 1982
by Thomas Nelson, Inc. Used by permission. All rights reserved.

Published by Authentic Publishers
188 Front Street, Suite 116-44
Franklin, TN 37064

Authentic Publishers is a division of
Authentic Media, Inc.

Library of Congress Cataloging-in-Publication Data

Contreras, Francisco and Kennedy, Daniel E.
50 Critical Cancer Answers : Your personal battle plan for beating cancer/
Francisco Contreras and Daniel E. Kennedy p. cm.

ISBN 978-1-78078-107-5
(e-book) 978-1-78078-207-2

Printed in the United States of America

21 20 19 18 17 16 15 14 13 1 2 3 4 5 6 7 8 9 10 11 12

All rights reserved. No part of this book may be
reproduced or transmitted in any form or by any means,
electronic or mechanical, including photocopying and recording,
or by any information storage and retrieval system,
without permission in writing from the publisher.

Dedication

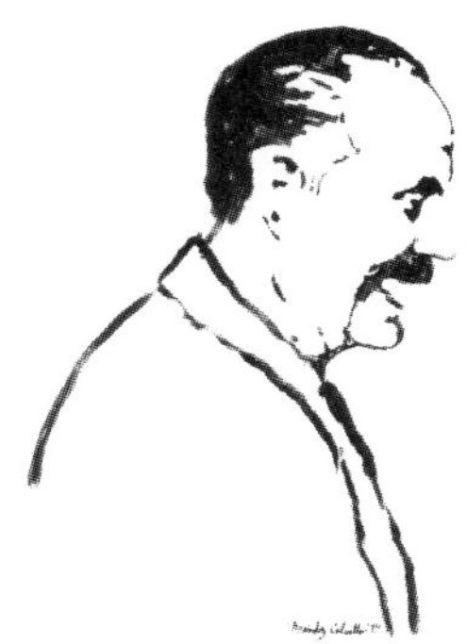

To Dr. Ernesto Contreras, Sr., founder of Oasis of Hope Hospital—

Your vision, medical expertise, and love healed tens of thousands of people around the world as they fought cancer. Your healing legacy lives on in our hearts and through our patients who receive total care for their bodies, minds, and spirits.

Francisco Contreras, MD
Founder's Son

Daniel E. Kennedy (Contreras), MC
Founder's Grandson

About the Authors

Francisco Contreras, MD, serves as director, president, and chairman of the Oasis of Hope Health Group with treatment centers in Mexico and the US. A distinguished oncologist and surgeon, he is renowned for integrating conventional and alternative cancer therapies with emotional healing and spiritual care to provide patients with treatment outcomes superior to those of conventional treatment alone.

After graduating from medical school at the Autonomous University of Mexico, Dr. Contreras specialized in surgical oncology at the University of Vienna in Austria, where he graduated with honors. He has authored or co-authored more than fifteen books on integrative therapy, including *The Hope of Living Cancer Free, The Coming Cancer Cure, Beating Cancer*, and *Dismantling Cancer*. You may enjoy following him at Twitter.com/DrContreras.

Daniel E. Kennedy, MC, is a psycho-oncology counselor and serves as Oasis of Hope's CEO and Emotional-Spiritual Life Director. He has twenty years' experience counseling and ministering to patients, holds a Master of Counseling and a Master of Business Administration, and earned a bachelor's degree in economics. He is the grandson of Dr. Ernesto Contreras, Sr., and also is pastor of the Hispanic congregation at Skyline Church in La Mesa, California (IglesiaSkyline.org). You may follow him at Twitter.com/PastorDKennedy.

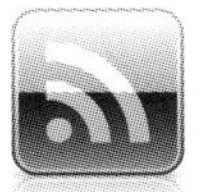

For more cancer answers, or to submit your question for Dr. Contreras and Daniel Kennedy to answer, please visit our website and listen to our podcast at:

www.yourcanceranswer.org

Acknowledgments

We would like to thank our families for their unconditional support. We're profoundly grateful to our patients who share the priceless victor tips found throughout the book; the life lessons of those who've beaten cancer are exceedingly more valid than any clinical data. Finally, we thank Kyle Duncan, Malcolm Down, and all the good people at Authentic Publishers who are taking this message of hope and empowerment around the world.

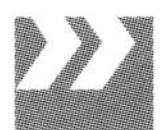

Note to the Reader

50 Critical Cancer Answers, written in the first person, expresses the thoughts and experiences of either Dr. Francisco Contreras or Daniel E. Kennedy, or both, though the book doesn't alternately identify them. Commentaries from experts in the "Cancer Q&A" podcasts and the app may not represent the views, opinions, and teachings of the authors.

All testimonials and tips submitted by Oasis of Hope cancer victors are included with their consent, and may not represent the views, opinions, and teachings of the authors.

Contents

Introduction

In a more perfect world, either no one would ever become ill, or, on the off chance that sickness should arise, a person would see the doctor, whom science would then help prescribe a curative remedy. The world of cancer is not perfect. Not only is it complex, but the associated fear of the disease and its treatment modalities also add to the chaos and confusion a person may experience when he or she hears, "We found cancer."

At the writing of this book, Oasis of Hope, the comprehensive cancer treatment center my father founded, is celebrating fifty years of providing integrative therapies to more than a hundred thousand patients from more than sixty countries. At this point it's safe to say we've learned a thing or two about how to help people become cancer victors instead of cancer victims. It is our desire to impart vital information that can be instrumental in your development of a personal plan to beat cancer. And it's our prayer that you will find blessings and life lessons that personally enrich you as you embark on your cancer journey.

Imagine you were on the Titanic and it just struck the iceberg. How crucial would it be to have critical answers to critical questions on how to survive? If you or a loved one has been diagnosed with cancer, you may feel like you're on that boat, taking on water fast. This book's purpose is to empower you to do everything you can to help your doctors help you. Some chapters provide general info on treatment, research, and the industry so you're better oriented and can know what to look for and where to find it. Some chapters speak to what doesn't help; others provide options that we have found help many people overcome cancer.

In addition to compelling topics, each chapter features three action steps to take that may make the difference you need as you face this challenge. The chapters also include a QR code that will direct your smart phone to a video commentary with Dr. Contreras or Daniel Kennedy. If you are unfamiliar with a QR (Quick Response) code, it is a code that you can scan using any smart phone, which will take you to a video linked to the topic of each chapter. (If you are like me, you may need to ask someone under 35 for help! If you don't have a smart phone or tablet, there's also a link if you prefer using a computer.)

Then there's the unique added value that may be the best part of this book for you: We've included hundreds of tips sent to us by cancer victors who've received treatment and support at Oasis of Hope. These are based not on theory but on the personal experience of those who walked the path you're on right now. And we invite you to visit www.yourcanceranswer.org to listen to our "Cancer Q&A" podcasts to hear experts comment on chapter topics. The goal of all this is to provide you with wisdom in the multitude of counsel as you gear up to win the battle.

Chapter 1

Living Cancer Free

Q: *Can I be victorious over cancer?*

A: Absolutely, yes, you can! First, cancer is not a death sentence, and second, a cure isn't necessarily the only way to win. Even if cancer is active, you may live a full life by controlling it with effective therapies.

I will never forget the consultation with a young woman who asked to see me five years after she became cancer free. She had overcome metastatic breast cancer and was able to go forward in life with her husband and three children, the eldest of whom was soon to be married.

What had such an impact on me was her response when I offered congratulations on her five-year victory. She teared up and said, "Dr. Contreras, how long do I have?"

"How long for what?" I asked.

She said, "To live. How long till it comes back?"

I gave a clinical response, explaining that her probability of ever having that cancer return after being cancer free half a decade was the same as a person who'd never been diagnosed with it. Yet I could tell from her expression that my answer was giving her no peace at all. Cancer can be so traumatic for some people that even when it has left the body it still has a residual effect on the soul.

Fear of Recurrence of Cancer (FRC)

Nearly everyone who's had it suffers from fear of recurrence of cancer (FRC), though with different levels of anxiety about the possibility of its return, even after long periods of remission. Many factors influence this worry: the intensity of the cancer, the treatment he or she went through, the recurrence statistics associated with a particular cancer, beliefs about cancer being incurable, fear of not seeing children grow up, and other issues too numerous to list.

Age is another predictor. Younger patients tend to fear a recurrence more.[1] It may be that they feel they have more to live for, or it may be that the more extensive life experience of older patients leads to better coping skills or a sense of surrender.

Fear compromises a person's ability to use logic, and, like any other type of fear, FRC isn't rational.[2] A person who gets a sore throat, someone who formerly might just have taken vitamin C and used cough drops, now, after cancer, suddenly fears it's a symptom of his cancer's return.[3] The thought that every ache and pain is related to cancer is not rational, but the fear is no less real.

In addition to fear, someone with a high level of FRC may feel depressed and have an increasingly negative outlook in general, which can keep building on negative emotions and pull her into a downward emotional spiral. Now, fears are a normal part of facing cancer, from diagnosis all the way through remission. But prolonged emotional distress compromises the immune system and provides opportunity for the disease to progress (see chapter 3). Once cancer is in remission, it's crucial to inoculate yourself emotionally from the fear that it will return.

The question is, how you can reframe FRC? The answer: Make it your goal to change from one FRC to another.

FEAR	TO	FREEDOM
Fear of	F	Forever
Recurrence of	R	Rid of
Cancer	C	Cancer

This may be confusing, but it works. . .

You must not let emotions take you wherever they will. You must be intentional about your thought life. Learn to train your mind how to live forever rid of cancer. Let me share with you the way to live fear free.

Fear vs. Faith

Fear is cancer's fuel. Much like with gasoline, even after cancer is all gone you can still smell its vapors, and you may fear they'll ignite a fire.

Faith is freedom's fuel. Faith overcomes fear. Your faith and your purpose—your reason for being—reveal the path toward peace.[4]

Sometimes discouragement tests faith. Faith is powerful—it gains power—when we allow it to lead us to surrender to the Sovereign God. Use your faith to foster peace and purpose through *all* circumstances.[5]

To truly live cancer free, you will need to build faith that overcomes fear. This isn't mental toughness; *spiritual fortitude is the key to living cancer free.* The essence of courage, of spiritual fortitude, is faith.

Scripture provides instruction on conquering fear through faith in God. Consider the following:

> Don't be afraid, for I am with you. Don't be discouraged, for I am your God. I will strengthen you and help you. I will hold you up with my victorious right hand.[6]

> "I [Jesus] have told you all this so that you may have peace in me. Here on earth you will have many trials and sorrows. But take heart, because I have overcome the world."[7]

> Hold up the shield of faith to stop the fiery arrows of the devil.[8]

Let me apply this last verse to making a prayer for you to offer now and whenever you choose:

> "God, please give me the strength
> to hold the shield of faith
> that stops fiery arrows of doubt,
> so that I can live cancer free."

The Prescription for Living Cancer Free

Earlier I spoke of people who are still slaves to the fear of cancer even after they're 100% free of physical cancer. Living cancer free is an attitude, one that's available to you now—you don't have to wait to live that way until you go into remission. Living cancer free is a function of the spirit and of the mind, putting cancer in its place. Living cancer free is surrender to the higher purpose and calling on your life. It is refusing to let cancer define who you are and determine what you do.

Embrace life and live it to the fullest. *That* is how to live cancer free. The apostle Paul wrote,

> The Lord is the Spirit, and wherever the Spirit of the Lord is, there is freedom.[9]

Live in the Spirit. Live cancer free.

Conclusion

You *can* live cancer free. Freedom comes through surrender, through faith that no matter the outcome, God will bring you through it. You can check your worries at the door when you don't put conditions on how He must answer your prayers; you begin to live free from fear by putting your faith in Him and keeping it there.

One of the most phenomenal counselors I've ever witnessed is Dr. John Huffman, the innovator of Pneumiatrics (spirit therapy). Huffman taught many ways to build faith and worked extensively with his clients in the area of faith and fear. I want to suggest three of his faith builders as action steps you can take.

ACTION STEPS

1. Read God's Word out loud.
2. Spend time with people of great faith.
3. Ask God for an increase in faith.

CANCER VICTOR TIPS

Andie Ysais, California
Breast Cancer
Victor Since 2010

1. Fear, not the cancer, is the enemy.
2. Be mindful of your *thoughts* and of *food*; in your body they are producing either life or death.
3. On the days when you feel good, take advantage—get out and do something fun, even if only for thirty minutes. Be thankful for "the good days," and enjoy life.
4. Surround yourself in positivity—with positive people, music, books, movies. . . .
5. Do not isolate from others. Allow people to be the gift they are: God's way of wrapping His arms around you. It blesses them to bless you.

Living Cancer Free
https://vimeo.com/67689808

Chapter 2

Healing Foods

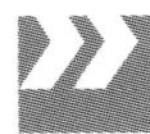

Q: *What should I be eating to help me beat cancer?*

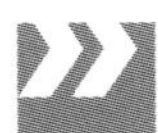

A: Eat and drink foods the way God put them on this earth—unprocessed, unadulterated, without genetic engineering, pesticide free, not radiated, un-manipulated. Consume at least five portions of fruits and vegetables a day.

Take out a pen or highlighter and underline the foods that will help you beat cancer. Then cross out the foods that will help cancer grow.

Garlic	Broccoli	Soda	Kale	French Fries
Cauliflower	Pork	Ice Cream	Pizza	Avocado
Hamburger	Cake	Lobster	Spinach	Lentils
White Bread	Cabbage	Bok Choy	Donut	Apple

I bet you got every single answer right! Odds are, you know almost exactly what to eat and what not to eat. Common sense tells us what to consume and what to avoid. The challenge isn't acquiring information; it's mustering the motivation to change habits.

Doctors apply what they learn in medical school but often ignore common sense and intuition. Through four years of pre-med, six years of medical school, and five years specializing in oncology, I realized that doctors are not health experts—we're illness specialists. We spend all our time studying how to diagnose and attack disease. We don't study health principles at all; we learn nothing about making a person healthy.

When I teach on healing foods and cancer, I use this slide:

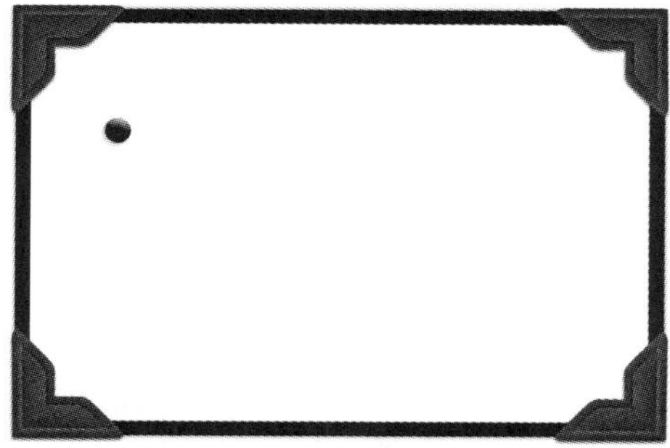

That's *it*—an empty bullet point! Most of us really don't know the first thing about nutrition. In eleven years studying medicine I received one forty-five-minute lecture on "nutrition." The class was about baby formula; we were taught that it's more nutritious than mother's milk. (I couldn't make this up if I tried.) If your doctors are ignorant on the subject, please forgive them. If you're seeing an oncologist, keep your questions focused on disease.

When it comes to cancer, oncologists' chief concern is your caloric intake. They want to ensure that you'll keep your weight on to avoid loss of muscle mass. Considering that both chemotherapy and radiation can take away the appetite, I share this legitimate concern.

However, I take issue with the notion that it doesn't matter what you eat as long as you eat. On the one hand, food can help bring about healing in the body; on the other, food can fuel cancer. I believe you already know intuitively which foods heal and which foods harm. Allow me to share why and how nutrition is a vital part of recovery.

Insulin

Many people would assume that discussing insulin level in the bloodstream is only relevant to a diabetic, but that's not true at all. The presence of two hormones—insulin and insulin-like growth factor-1 (IGF-1)—directly correlates to the incidence of some cancers. Controlling their levels is one of the most important aspects in an anticancer regimen. In fact, they have such a significant impact in this regard that every oncologist should have a diet designed to control their production integrated into every treatment program.

Researchers have conducted significant studies that help us know what foods to avoid. For example, the China Study, conducted by Cornell University, started in 1983 and spanned a period of twenty years in rural China.[1] Participants ate a primarily plant-based diet.

The study singled out the foods absolutely linked to an increased risk for cancer. It showed that risk for most cancers correlated with the proportion of dietary calories provided by animal products. What, exactly, are animal proteins, animal fats, and processed foods, along with processed sugars and white flour, doing that increases risk for cancer? A diet based largely on these "Western" staples boosts our production of insulin and "free" insulin-like growth factor-1 (IGF-1).

I've carefully examined the science that links levels of these hormones in the bloodstream to the rapid multiplication of mutated cells.[2-3] The connection is clear: these hormones block the process of cell apoptosis, the program within a cell that indicates when it's time to die and make way for a new healthy cell to take its place. It is also the process by which mutated cells, or cancers, are eliminated.

Apoptosis is the natural process God designed to help the body protect itself from cancer. Insulin and IGF-1 block apoptosis in cancerous cells, which, needless to say, allows cancer to gain a foothold within the body. So, how can diet increase or decrease the body's production of these two hormones?

Studies have determined that dietary factors in the US and other westernized nations are primarily responsible for the high levels of these hormones. We tend to consume diets high in saturated fats; we tend to carry extra weight around the abdominal area because we eat larger meals than those in more deprived countries; and we engage in a more sedentary lifestyle. All these factors increase insulin production, which stimulates the production of free IGF-1.

Let's revisit the China Study. People in rural China eat a quasi-vegan diet—almost purely vegetarian, coupled with extremely limited meat and dairy products. This diet type causes the liver to decrease production of IGF-1 and increase the production of a protein that blocks production of free IGF-1.[4-5] So, what impact do these facts have on the treatment of cancer? Let me piece it together.

Foods that increase insulin and free IGF-1 levels in the bloodstream will ultimately *stimulate* cancer's progress. These two hormones are even involved in the defense mechanism cancer uses to protect itself against chemotherapy.[6] Conversely, a diet that keeps levels of these hormones low will ultimately *inhibit* cancer's progression. It really is that simple.

What to Eat

It's critical for anyone managing chronic illness to view dietary changes in a positive light. Giving up "comfort foods" is a small price to pay to halt the growth and spread of cancer.

Ideally, it's desirable for patients to adopt a vegan or wholly plant-based diet, with one exception: The omega-3 fatty acids in fish oil present numerous benefits, and fish oil capsules do not increase insulin levels. A vegan diet is low-fat (only 15% of dietary calories should come from fats), is moderate in protein, and incorporates whole-food carbohydrate sources that are low on the glycemic index: semolina or whole-grain pastas, whole fruits, and whole-grain products like sprouted wheat breads (instead of wheat-flour breads). Further, because high-glycemic-index carbs can boost insulin levels, the diet should provide carbohydrates from sources that are low in glycemic index. For instance, as even carrot juice has quite a bit of natural sugar, we recommend green vegetable juices.

While this diet is ideal, it's difficult for some people to follow, often representing a drastic change. Patients who need a gradual change can derive modest benefit by adopting a "Mediterranean" diet, which discourages red meat and fatty dairy products, allows moderate amounts of lean white meat or fish, and encourages large amounts of fruits, vegetables, beans, and whole grains. While not as effective as a vegan diet, this is a vast improvement over the diets favored by most Americans.

A host of foods offer a range of benefits to cancer patients. For instance, cruciferous vegetables like cabbage, broccoli, cauliflower, and kale are rich in sulforaphane, while onions and garlic contain allicin. Both compounds are proven to inhibit or slow the growth of cancer cells and cause the cells to produce higher levels of antioxidants as well as enzymes that detoxify the body.[7–8] These foods also can increase the ability of healthy tissues to cope with chemotherapeutic drugs and radiotherapy. In addition, they may present post-treatment benefits by helping to block the development of additional cancers.

Another food with powerful anti-cancer properties, a must for any anticancer diet, is spirulina, a supplement produced primarily from two species of blue-green algae. Spirulina contains a phytonutrient that blocks a signal pathway that makes cancer cells more aggressive and that protects them from programmed cell death.[9–11] In addition, spirulina contains polysaccharides that boost the ability of the immune system's natural killer (NK) cells to block metastasis.[12]

Eliminating Toxins

Do you know the category of the best-selling, most self-prescribed health product in America? Not weight-loss products. *Laxatives.*

> Each year, Americans spend more than $700 million on laxatives. A recent study showed that the United States has the highest rate of laxative use compared to several other countries.[13]

To put it plainly, Americans are constipated. Many people believe it's normal to move their bowels every two to three days; actually, people need to move their bowels two to three times each day. This is especially important for cancer patients, and, unfortunately, many cancer therapies are constipating. A constipated person is not eliminating toxins. In fact, toxins, including chemotherapy, are recycled, thus exposing patients to devastating side effects again and again.

A high-fiber diet is critical to detoxing the body. Many phytonutrients found in vegetables, herbs, and fruits influence detoxification pathways, improve the liver's function, and help the bowels move. Sulforaphane, present in broccoli sprouts, specifically stimulates liver detoxification.[14]

Conclusion

In my oncology practice, I intervene simultaneously in as many ways as feasible to promote cancer cells' death and block their spread. This is the most effective way to control cancers and keep them from becoming aggressive. Using food as a cancer treatment is one such intervention.

How foolish would we be not to acknowledge the impact of nutrition in that effort? So much evidence clearly shows a range of cancer-specific benefits that can derive from a healthy diet. I'm so adamant about this that I consider the cooks at our hospital a part of the patient's healing team. That's why we provide cooking classes during treatment and send people home with recipes and recorded cooking classes on their tablets.

ACTION STEPS

1. Consult an integrative nutritionist to help you adopt a vegan diet designed to combat cancer.
2. Consider being treated at a cancer center that integrates healing foods into your treatment protocol.
3. Find a website that identifies the glycemic index of each food. Try to eat foods with a glycemic index lower than 40; avoid sugar and white bread altogether.

CANCER VICTOR TIPS

May Orr, Scotland
Stage III Breast Cancer
Victor Since 2003

1. Be very careful about what can and cannot be in your diet.
2. Stress has a profoundly negative effect on your well being.
3. Know the importance of having a good support team.
4. Remember: there are alternatives to chemotherapy and radiation.
5. You deserve the best treatment and medication available, even if you need to pay extra.

Healing Foods
https://vimeo.com/60700155

Chapter 3

Psychoendoneuro-immunology

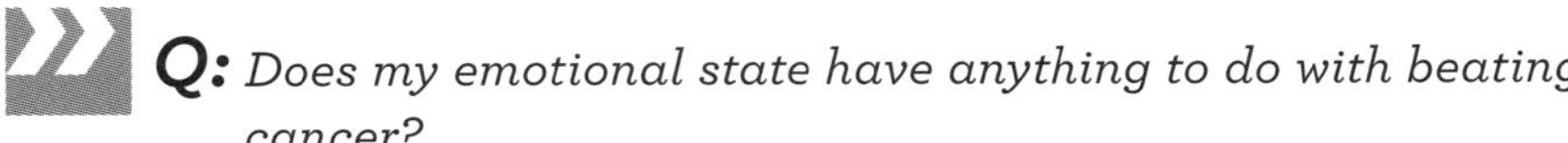

Q: *Does my emotional state have anything to do with beating cancer?*

A: A strong immune system is absolutely necessary for beating cancer, and emotions are powerful immune modulators. A positive attitude toward adversity will promote immune-stimulating emotions.

I almost didn't get my driver's license.

I was seventeen, anxious to find the freedom of the freeway, but there was this balding man in a short sleeve shirt and tie, stretch-waist brown trousers and glasses, standing between me and the thoroughfares.

Finally the behind-the-wheel test was over, and I thought I'd done everything to perfection. Yet when we pulled into a parking space back at the Department of Motor Vehicles, the evaluator looked over (and over, and over) his clipboard. Then he said, "I almost disqualified you. You did a rolling stop. You must stop *completely* behind the line. That deduction almost caused you to fail—be careful to make full stops.

"But congratulations, you passed."

• • • • • • • • • • • • •

The "California Rolling Stop" came back to haunt me two decades later. I was en route to work on a Monday morning, and seemingly there was no one around as I approached a stop sign. I slowed, almost to a full stop, but kept creeping forward while looking both ways. When I saw the intersection was clear I increased speed and continued through.

From the corner of my eye I saw a black and white car. A chill ran down my spine; my heart started pounding. Has anything ever happened to you that caused a surge like this? At that moment I was experiencing the mind-body connection, just like we all do, frequently.

• • • • • • • • • • • •

Scientists have tough-to-say names for the relationship between thoughts and physiological reactions. Every other week, at Oasis of Hope, I start the group session offering twenty-five cents to anyone who, on the first try, can correctly say *psychoneuroimmunology,* and a dollar to anyone who gets *psychoendoneuroimmunology*. I don't pay out for second and third attempts. To date, I've never doled out a penny.

The sophisticated terms are fitting, for the concept of how thoughts impact the immune system via the endocrine system is complex. Psychoneuroimmunology (PNI) and Psychoendoneuroimmunology (PENI) refer to the study of the interaction between psychological functions, the nervous system, the endocrine system, and the immune system.

Emotions, Thoughts, and Gland Stimulation

PNI is sufficiently important that we must understand what it is, how it works, and how to manage it. Your emotional state and your thoughts directly influence the stimulation of your glands to release hormones and other substances into your bloodstream. Hormones like cortisol can give you sudden bursts of energy, and while this is vital for short-term survival, it's detrimental to the immune system for the glands to be overstimulated over long periods of time.

For the person dealing with cancer, the whole topic of PNI is focused on emotional stress and its management. Negative emotions such as anxiety, fear, and anger will induce the production and release of powerful natural substances that can be harmful if the body is exposed for long periods. To better understand this, let's look at the stress response often referred to as "fight or flight."

My story about the rolling stop is a perfect example of a stress response. My negative emotion was fear, provoked by the threat of getting a ticket. Whenever you perceive a threat, synapses instantly begin to connect neurons to create pathways for signals to be delivered from the nerve cells to the adrenal glands via the amygdala, hypothalamus, and pituitary gland, all in the brain.[1] These messages travel along the hypothalamic-pituitary-adrenal axis (HPA axis).

The hypothalamus sends chemicals to the pituitary, which releases adrenocorticotropic hormone (ACTH) into the bloodstream that travels to the adrenal glands. The hypothalmus also communicates to the adrenal glands through nerve impulses that use the spinal cord as a conduit. These impulses cause the adrenals to release epinephrine, which travels throughout the body. The ACTH stimulates the production of cortisol, which is released into the bloodstream from the adrenal glands.

The epinephrine produces glucose that gives strength to the body while relaxing the bronchioles for better breathing and oxygenation. Cortisol increases blood pressure and blood sugar, and that's why we feel a rush of energy, power, and clarity. Again, for the short term, the stress response is critical for survival. But long durations of exposure to cortisol suppress the immune system,[2] and extended stress-induced activation of the HPA axis will have pathological consequences.[3]

Chronic Stress and Immune Suppression

There is no greater cancer-control agent than your own immune system. In fact, if the system is functioning perfectly, it's actually impossible for cancer to proliferate and develop into tumors. Among its many different cells with different tasks—monocytes, macrophages, dendritic cells, T cells, B cells—are natural killer (NK) cells, anti-tumor effectors that can destroy cancer cells long before tumor markers can detect them.[4] One clinical study concluded that people with long-term stress and anxiety had lower blood NK activity.[5]

A University of Kentucky study provided an ecological model to help explain the relationship between immunity and stress. Measurements were taken in a group of adults to determine how the body matches its biological resources with behavior to manage exogenous ("from outside") stressors and protect itself. The researcher, Suzanne Segerstrom, found that the body manages its finite energy by redistributing to where it's most needed for any given situation. For example, if sensing an infection, the body may produce a fever as a defense. The cost to heat the body will take away physiological resources necessary to perform other functions—e.g., the muscles receive fewer resources, like peptides, resulting in less strength and common aches. Dr. Sergerstrom found,

> Chronic stress perturbs homeostatic mechanisms in the body and results in poorer immune functions in the cellular arm, the humoral arm or both. When the fight or flight response, which was designed to meet short-term energetic demands, is prolonged, undesirable consequences ensue.[6]

If you can learn how to manage your response to stress, you will allow your immune system to improve and help you win your fight against cancer. That begs the question of what can be done to influence the HPA axis stress response, and I see two viable avenues worth pursuing: (1) biomedical engineering and (2) psycho-education.

Biomedical Engineering

With great precision, biologists, biochemists, and mathematicians have qualified and quantified what stimulates the functions of neuroendocrinology. Biomedical engineers are working to develop a mathematical predictive model to provide parameters to quantify how many nanograms of each specific substance must be secreted to achieve outcomes in the body.[7] If researchers succeed, scientists could potentially develop drug therapies and electromagnetic field devices that would stimulate the nervous and endocrine systems to secrete the right hormones in the right amounts to make the immune system work at optimal anticancer levels. But such interventions are still years away. I would put biomedical manipulation of the neuroendocrine system in the category of "interesting but not useful today."

Psycho-Education: Automatic Thoughts and Schema

Advanced psychology provides many proved interventions to manage stress and diminish the fight-or-flight's negative impact on the immune system. This is an opportunity for you. Some counselors practice psycho-education to teach techniques that could empower you to get control of your physiological stress response. At Oasis of Hope we work closely with our patients to help develop stress management skills; usually we start by demonstrating how automatic thoughts translate into fight-or-flight.

Most thoughts happen like a lightning flash, with no consideration of facts, logic, or alternatives. No process of weighing the evidence goes into the majority of what flies through our brains; the automatic is what provokes a cascade effect through the HPA axis. My automatic thought when I saw the patrol car was, "Traffic stop = traffic ticket." Automatic thoughts are rooted in *schema*.

Schema are thought patterns—part of a cognitive framework—that we all have and use to interpret what we perceive during every moment. They develop from the time of birth and are reinforced or modified through life experiences. An example I give is of a group in a room that reacts to a bearded pot-bellied man entering. One person may become instantly uncomfortable and ask to leave; his automatic thought came from a schema formed traumatically by his experience of being abused as a child by a bearded man. Another person may suddenly feel flooded with peace; her schema was based on her warm relationship with her bearded grandfather, who used to bake apple pies with her while he told stories. A third person may begin to grin as he automatically thinks of how his dad would dress like Santa Claus to pass out Christmas gifts.

Schema reflect who we are and how we became who we are. People who were nurtured as infants have lower attachment anxiety, which allows them to better cope with stress.[8] Schema about gender and sexuality, for instance, can play a significant role in how a person copes with cancer. One study showed that men suffering from prostate cancer whose schema about masculinity is inflexible have poorer health outcomes compared to those willing to adjust and adopt new beliefs about manhood.[9] A woman with a positive view of herself as a sexual being will avoid depression better when facing gynecological cancers than those with negative sexual self schema.[10]

Every aspect of life has schema that strongly influence our ability to cope with stressors. Thus it's very important that we identify automatic thoughts—they *do* directly effect negative moods.[11] Negative moods can leave a person vulnerable to chronic stress that will compromise the immune system's ability to fight off cancer. The good news is that automatic thoughts and schemas can be changed, or reprogrammed.

People facing cancer have many automatic thoughts associated with diagnosis and treatment. Two common examples are "Cancer = death" and "Chemo = nausea and hair loss." The schema behind these thoughts usually come from what a person observed in a loved one who went through cancer, and/or references from books, movies/shows, and blogs. But we can replace negative automatic thoughts with positive ones through psycho-education, psycho-oncology, and spiritual care. This will lead to generating new schema to replace old thought patterns. Elsewhere (see esp. chapters 6 and 9) I'll discuss emotional self-care techniques to help you develop a perspective, a belief system, and stress management skills that can get your immune system working for you.

Conclusion

Researchers have done remarkable work identifying how thoughts stimulate or diminish gland secretions resulting in immune suppression or activation. Much is known about the mechanics of how it takes place.

How thoughts are generated a nanosecond before cognition remains a mystery. Where do they come from? What starts the chain of events? Thoughts are birthed in the soul, where the emotions and the will come together and cause synapses to connect nerve cells into neuron chains that will transmit chemical and electrical stimuli to the glands. But what stimulates the soul?

The human spirit is the source of the raw materials needed to produce that thought. The spirit is the ultimate frontier that the most adventurous of practitioners will explore over the next hundred years.

Science is finite. The spirit is infinite.

ACTION STEPS

1. Work with a counselor to identify your automatic thoughts associated with cancer.
2. Identify your triggers for anxiety, fear, and depression.
3. Develop alternative positive thoughts to avoid negative triggers.

CANCER VICTOR TIPS

Myrna Oswill, California
Breast Cancer
Victor Since 1972

1. Consider looking for alternative and natural medicine to overcome the limitations of orthodox medicine.
2. Find information on a diet and vitamins that can make a difference in your cancer treatment.
3. Partner with the Lord for your life.
4. Go to a treatment center that will support your body, soul, and spirit; work with a spiritual counselor.
5. "Count it all joy" (see James 1:2 NKJV).

Psychoendoneuroimmunology
https://vimeo.com/60691319

Chapter 4

Cell Signal Transduction Therapy

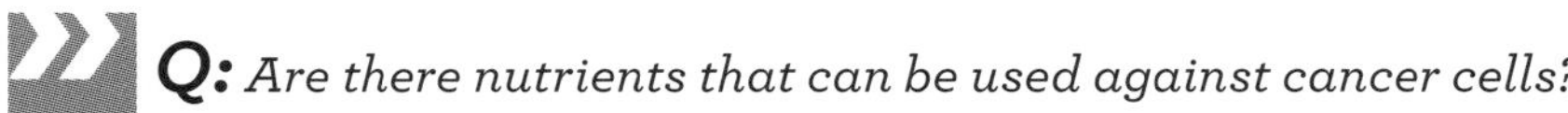

Q: *Are there nutrients that can be used against cancer cells?*

A: Scientists have determined that all cells produce certain proteins that are absolutely necessary for survival. Cancer cells are no exception. There are nutrients that can interfere with their production of essential proteins; these can stop or slow down tumor growth.

Over the last several decades, molecular biology has been gradually unraveling the way the body's cells work. "Signal transduction" refers to how cellular proteins undergo small and usually reversible changes in structure to induce alterations in cell behavior. The genetic material of cancer cells is typically altered in ways that over-activate intracellular signal transduction mechanisms; specifically, the ones related to cancer's malignant behavior. Some mechanisms prevent the process of apoptosis (programmed cell death) as well as support cellular multiplication, tissue invasion, and metastasis (the spread of cancer to distant organs), and resistance to being killed by chemo or radiation. Cell signal transduction therapy seeks to regulate the signaling pathways in cancer cells to make them easier to control or kill.

One most effective way to trip up cancer is to use nutrients, phytochemicals (natural plant-derived chemicals), and drugs to suppress overactive signal transduction pathways, or boost under-active pathways, in cancer cells. This inhibits their capacity to grow, spread to distant organs, and grow the new blood vessels necessary to feed tumors.

Let me share about the nutrients, phytochemicals, and safe drugs (drugs that cause no harmful or negative side effects) I use as part of cell signal transduction therapy. It includes familiar supplements—omega-3 fatty acids (fish oil), milk thistle extract (silibinin), and green tea extract—and less familiar substances, also, like boswellic acids, salsalate, diclofenac, and disulfiram.

Some Signaling Pathways Overactivated in Cancer Cells

In many cancers, one chronically overactive signaling pathway is known as "NF-kappaB"—short for "nuclear factor of kappa-light-chain-enhancer of activated B Cells." (Thank goodness for abbreviations!) This protein complex regulates the synthesis of a number of other proteins by binding to DNA in the cellular nucleus.

In a high proportion of advanced cancers, NF-kappaB is either continuously activated or rapidly activated in response to chemo.[1–5] One of its integral roles is boosting the production of proteins that act to prevent apoptosis,[6] the "cell suicide" process that cytotoxic ("toxic to cells") anticancer drugs are supposed to trigger. Moreover, it increases production of a "multi-drug resistance" membrane protein that functions to "pump" various cytotoxic chemicals, including many anticancer drugs, out of cells.[7] For these reasons, NF-kappaB activation, either as a natural condition of cancer cells or triggered by chemo, tends to protect cancer cells during chemotherapy. Conversely, many studies show that inhibitors of NF-kappaB activity can make resistant cancer cells much more sensitive to chemo and/or radiation.[8–11]

Chronic NF-kappaB activation also makes cancers act more aggressively, which results in increased production of angiogenic factors that promote development of new blood vessels required for cancer growth. In addition, it causes increased production of proteolytic enzymes (which break down proteins) that enable cancer cells to penetrate and migrate through tissues, and causes increased production of certain factors that promote rapid cellular multiplication.[12]

The bottom line: Cancers with high NF-kappaB activity tend to spread more rapidly and aggressively, and they're harder to kill. As if NF-kappaB weren't already pernicious enough, this factor is now known to be a key mediator of the muscle protein loss associated with cancer cachexia.[13] So effective inhibition of NF-kappaB likely has potential to help cancer patients preserve their muscle mass.

Another over-activated factor in many cancers is the enzyme cyclo-oxygenase-2 ("Cox-2"). This continuously active enzyme generates a group of hormone-like compounds known as prostanoids, many of which have inflammatory and pain-promoting activity. That's why Cox-2 inhibitors are frequently used to treat inflammatory conditions. However, some prostanoids produced by Cox-2 in cancer cells have growth-factor activity for these cancers[14] that promotes increased cancer proliferation, boosts angiogenesis, *and* can make cancers harder to kill.[15-19] Further, some prostanoids have local immunosuppressive activity that blunts the effectiveness of immune cells that attack the tumor.[20]

Both NF-kappaB and Cox-2 play a direct angiogenic role. Activation of these factors occurs in endothelial cells—the cells that give rise to new blood vessels during angiogenesis. This process is required for efficient production of new blood vessels;[21-23] inhibiting these proteins has the potential to directly suppress it by targeting endothelial cell function.

Still another enzyme expressed by many cancer cells that promotes cancer growth and survival is 5-lipoxygenase ("5-LPO"), which induces production of pro-inflammatory compounds known as leukotrienes. Just like the prostanoids Cox-2 produces, leukotrienes can promote growth and survival of certain cancers—including many with 5-LPO activity.[24-26] Inhibiting 5-LPO typically retards growth of cancer cell lines dependent on it and often increases the rate at which these cells die by apoptosis. Human cancer cell lines derived from prostatic, pancreatic, breast, esophageal, colorectal, bladder, gastric, and renal cancers, as well as mesotheliomas and leukemias, have shown 5-LPO dependency.[27-34]

Another overactive signaling pathway in many cancer cells is triggered by over-expression of the epidermal growth factor receptor (EGFR). Cancers that express EGFR also will usually make hormones that can activate this receptor or have enzymatic activities that can activate it from within the cell, bypassing the need for hormonal activation. Activated EGFR, like other growth factor receptors, promotes proliferation and spread of cancer cells while suppressing the apoptotic cell-death mechanism that enables chemo drugs to kill those cells.

A key growth factor many cancers produce is vascular endothelial growth factor (VEGF). Although VEGF has growth factor activity for some cancers, its bigger role in cancer spread is to promote angiogenesis by aiding multiplication and survival of the endothelial cells that form the new blood vessels. Our combined modality therapy (CMT) regimens seek to interfere with this by either suppressing tumor production of VEGF or blocking the receptors in endothelial cells that enable them to respond to VEGF. One way NF-kappaB and EGFR promote cancer spread is by boosting tumor production of VEGF and other angiogenic growth factors.

Now let's look at some of the agents—nutrients, phytochemicals, and safe drugs—that our regimens employ to inhibit the overactive signaling pathways that promote cancer survival and spread.

Fish Oil

Fish oil is a unique and rich source of the long-chain omega-3 fatty acids EPA (eicosapentaenoic acid) and DHA (docosahexaenoic acid). A small structural difference distinguishes these from the omega-6 fatty acids found in plant-derived oils.

EPA and DHA can play a valuable treatment role. A number of studies show that a diet rich in fish oil tends to slow tumor growth.[35-38] We can attribute at least part of this effect to a suppressive effect on angiogenesis—again, the process by which new blood vessels develop to enable tumor growth and spread.[39-40] EPA decreases the expression of a key receptor in endothelial cells that makes them responsive to VEGF.[41]

Cox-2, another key angiogenic factor, produces, in endothelial cells, prostanoids required for vascular tube formation.[42] A high intake of fish oil has potential to antagonize its role by decreasing this production *and* may blunt production of growth-promoting prostanoids in cancer cells.

Fish oil has the ability to fend off cachexia (severe muscle-mass loss that often complicates late-stage cancer).[43-46] Though usually it entails a loss of appetite that can contribute to weight loss by decreasing caloric intake, the commonly seen life-threatening selective muscle loss reflects a specific inflammatory process in muscle fibers not seen in healthy dieters. EPA interferes with the related inflammatory mechanisms.

Silibinin

Milk thistle extract has long been used in treating liver disorders. Approximately 80% of this extract consists of silymarin, a mixture of compounds known as flavonolignans. Silibinin, the most prominent, accounts for about 60% of silymarin's weight and is believed to cause most of the liver-protective activity. Within the last decade we've realized silibinin has considerable potential for preventing and treating cancer.

In concentrations that may be achievable with high-dose clinical regimens, silibinin has growth-inhibitory effects on a wide range of human cancer cell lines, including those arising from the prostate, breast, colon, lung, liver, bladder, and cervix.[47–54] It can suppress the proliferation of these cells while at the same time increasing the rate at which they die by apoptosis. In addition, it can sensitize cancer cell lines to the killing effects of certain cytotoxic chemotherapeutic drugs.[55] Thus, silibinin may have potential both for retarding the growth and spread of cancer and for boosting the response of cancers to chemotherapy.

The mechanisms that cause these effects have been studied most intensively in human prostate cancer cells.[56] Concentrations of silibinin, which retard the growth of these prostate cancers, do not influence the growth of healthy prostate cells. In other words, say these studies, silibinin's effects on cell proliferation appear to be specific to cancer cells.

Silibinin's anti-proliferative effects on prostate cancer cells have been traced to decreased function of the epidermal growth factor receptor (EGFR), a key mediator of growth signals in prostate and many other cancers.[57] Silibinin binds to this receptor and prevents it from interacting with hormones that activate it—some of which prostate cancers produce. Further, silibinin induces these cells to make more of a compound, IGFBP-3, that binds to and inhibits activity of insulin-like growth factor-1 (IGF-1), a key growth factor for many cancers (some cancers can even make their own IGF-1).[58]

As if these benefits weren't enough, silibinin also has been shown to suppress the NF-kappaB signaling pathway, an effect that helps to explain its ability to increase the sensitivity of cancers to certain chemo drugs. Its effects on EGFR also contribute in this regard.

The impact of orally administered silibinin on the growth of human tumors in immunodeficient mice has been studied with three different types of tumors: prostate, lung, and ovarian.[59] In each case, silibinin had a substantial and dose-dependent suppressive effect on tumor growth in doses that had no apparent toxicity to the treated animals.

Exams of the silibinin-treated tumors showed they had a much less developed vasculature than control tumors; there were fewer blood vessels to provide tumor nourishment and oxygen.[60] Follow-up studies found that in some cancers silibinin could suppress secretion of the pro-angiogenic factor VEGF. And, other studies show that clinically feasible silibinin concentration has a direct effect on endothelial cells; it can suppress their proliferation and reduce their ability to migrate, invade tissues, and roll themselves into tubes, which is how new blood vessels are formed.[61-62] These findings suggest that silibinin's growth-slowing impact on tumors reflects the interaction of at least three phenomena:

1. a direct anti-proliferative effect on cancer cells;
2. a suppression of VEGF production by these cells; and
3. a direct inhibitory effect on endothelial cells' capacity to build new blood vessels.

Silibinin deserves a gold medal!

Green Tea Extract

The Oasis of Hope strategy is to attack angiogenesis from as many angles as feasible for, hopefully, a cumulative effect that is a clinically worthwhile retardation of tumor growth.[63-66] The highly potent green tea extract we use comprises 98% polyphenols—plant substances, many of which have superb antioxidant activity. In green tea, the most prominent is the compound epigallocatechin-gallate (EGCG). Some of the first studies evaluating strategies for suppressing angiogenesis showed that oral administration of green tea could slow the process in mice. More recently, research shows that clinically achievable concentrations of EGCG can achieve partial inhibition of the receptor, in endothelial cells, that responds to VEGF. (Several costly new drugs that target VEGF's bioactivity also target this receptor, or the VEGF that activates it.)

Boswellic Acids

Boswellic acids are a group of closely related compounds found in salai guggul, a resinous extract from the tree Boswellia carteri. This is a substance traditionally used in Ayurveda (a traditional Indian medicine) as an anti-inflammatory agent.[67] In the early 1990s researchers discovered the mechanism of salai guggul's anti-inflammatory efficacy: boswellic acids are potent inhibitors of the enzyme 5-LPO and hence can suppress production of leukotrienes that act as cancer growth factors.

The impact of 5-LPO on the sensitivity of cancers to chemotherapy or radiotherapy has received little attention to the present. However, one fascinating recent report indicates that concurrent expression of 5-LPO is associated with substantial protection from the cytotoxicity of chemo drugs.[68] Conversely, suppression of 5-LPO in these cancers greatly enhances their sensitivity to these drugs, which implies that 5-LPO inhibitors, administered prior to and during chemo, should enhance the responsiveness of a high proportion of human cancers.

While a drug called Zileuton can inhibit 5-LPO and has shown cancer-retardant activity in hamsters with pancreatic cancer,[69] we've chosen instead to use boswellic acid-rich extracts in our regimens, for they're considerably less expensive and can be presumed safe based on centuries of use in traditional medicine. Moreover, cell culture studies indicate that these (most notably acetyl-11-keto-beta-boswellic acid) can slow proliferation and boost the death rate of various human cancer cell lines.[70-74] The only published clinical experience with boswellic acids in cancer treatment dealt with usage in children with progressing brain cancers.[75-76] Some experienced improved neurological function during this treatment, but that might have reflected an anti-inflammatory effect of leukotriene suppression rather than tumor regression. Even so, the observed benefit was worthwhile. In lab rats transplanted with gliomas, boswellic-acids treatment could more than double survival time.[77] We include a potent dose in both our CMT protocol and at-home regimen.

Salsalate

Fortunately, several drugs can suppress the signaling pathways activated by either NF-kappaB or Cox-2. One is salicylic acid, a natural compound found in white willow bark that's long been used to treat inflammatory disorders like rheumatoid arthritis. Chemists in the late nineteenth century first synthesized aspirin (acetylsalicylic acid) by adding an acetyl group to salicylic acid, which, like aspirin, can inhibit Cox enzymes. But its activity in this regard is weak and reversible—this explains why salicylic acid doesn't produce the side effects sometimes seen with chronic use of aspirin or related drugs (e.g., bleeding stomach ulcers, kidney damage).[78-80] Salicylic acid binds to and inhibits an enzyme usually required for NF-kappaB activation,[81-82] so its high-dose anti-inflammatory effects more likely reflect inhibition of that activation.

Pharmaceutical companies are working feverishly at expensive new inhibitors of NF-kappaB, yet few medical scientists have considered the possibility of using natural, inexpensive salicylate in cancer therapy.[83] Recent research establishes that it does have cancer-retardant and anti-angiogenic activity. We believe salicylic acid has considerable therapeutic potential (1) to potentiate the efficacy of chemotherapy in certain cancers, (2) to slow cancer's growth and spread during at-home therapy, and (3) to slow or prevent the progression of cachexic muscle degeneration.[84-85]

Several pharmaceutical forms are available. We've chosen Salsalate, a non-steroidal complex broken down in the intestinal tract to release free salicylic acid that's then absorbed.[86] Less likely to induce gastric irritation than other forms of salicylic acid, Salsalate was developed about fifty years ago for treating inflammatory disorders.

Salsalate won't produce dangerous toxicity when used as directed. Relatively high doses are needed for effective inhibition of NF-kappaB. In optimally effective anti-inflammatory doses, it can produce reversible ear dysfunction—tinnitus ("ringing in the ears") and mild hearing loss.[87] These issues resolve when the drug is discontinued, with no permanent damage. For the occasional patient in whom these side effects are highly troubling, a dosage reduction might solve the matter.

Diclofenac

Many drugs, commonly referred to as NSAIDs (non-steroidal anti-inflammatory drugs), can inhibit the Cox-2 enzyme. Some are relatively selective to Cox-2, including Vioxx—which ultimately was pulled off the market because it caused increased risk of heart disease—and Celebrex, a target of numerous lawsuits. Apart from their side effects, these drugs had little impact on the other form of cyclooxygenase (Cox-1). Prolonged effective inhibition of Cox-1 can lead to serious complications (e.g., bleeding stomach ulcerations, kidney damage), and so pharmaceutical companies have developed (and have highly marketed) Cox-2-specific inhibitors for treating inflammatory disorders.

Instead of these, we use a much older, much less expensive drug. Diclofenac has an activity spectrum nearly identical to that of Celebrex, producing effective Cox-2 inhibition in concentrations that only modestly impact Cox-1.[88] When administered in standard clinical doses, diclofenac is effective,[89] and while recently it has been shown to increase heart-attack risk (as do other Cox-2-specific inhibitors),[90] we always use it in conjunction with low-dose aspirin, likely to largely offset that risk.

Disulfiram

Another drug with potential for inhibiting NF-kappaB is disulfiram. More commonly known as "Antabuse," it was developed to help alcoholics abstain from alcohol. If they drink while using it, they become ill, owing to increased blood levels of the alcohol metabolite acetaldehyde. More recently it's been found that disulfiram can inhibit cellular components called proteasomes,[91–92] which degrade cellular proteins that have been specifically targeted for degradation. These play a crucial role in activation of NF-kappaB by degrading a protein that inhibits activation; thus, inhibition of proteasome function usually decreases NF-kappaB activity.[93]

Recent studies show that disulfiram and related sulfur-containing compounds can inhibit proteasomes and thereby suppress NF-kappaB activity in cancer cells. This renders them less aggressive and more susceptible to eradication. Disulfiram is reasonably well-tolerated in usual clinical doses as long as the patient drinks no alcohol.

Conclusion

Most people facing cancer want to know what causes it. Oncologists often don't discuss cell signal transduction with patients. But the health of the cell and its ability to generate a healthy replacement cell is the key to explain how cancer forms *and* how to reverse the process.

Pollution, chemicals, poor diet, lack of exercise, and other facets of life stress our bodies even at the cellular level. Stressed cells can undergo small and irreversible structural changes that alter their behaviors. If changes go uncontested, the cell can become unhealthy and mutate into a cancer cell that will begin to multiply, form a tumor, and spread.

Fortunately, research is uncovering information on how to re-regulate unhealthy cells' behaviors. Though this chapter was on the technical side, it's vital that you know the agents I've outlined are scientifically supported and can help regulate cellular behavior. If you were my loved one, I would not let you omit cell signal transduction from your treatment.

ACTION STEPS

1. Get a doctor on your team who can provide cell signal transduction.
2. Commit to doing therapies that build you up, not only treatments that tear down cancer.
3. Be open to ideas about which your oncologist may not be aware.

CANCER VICTOR TIPS

Marialuisa Pulido de Ruiz, México
Lung Cancer
Victor Since 2000

1. Care for your spiritual life. Put yourself in God's hands.
2. Take care of yourself. I recommend Oasis of Hope because its treatments are effective.
3. Follow the Oasis of Hope diet strictly.
4. Take your medication at the precise time prescribed.
5. Accept help from your family and friends.[94]

Cell Signal Transduction Therapy
https://vimeo.com/61060452

Chapter 5

Oxygen Therapies

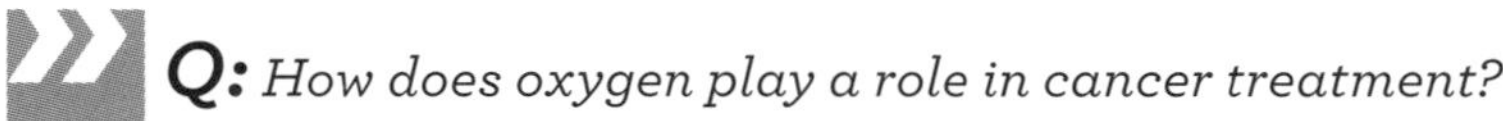

Q: *How does oxygen play a role in cancer treatment?*

A: Oxidation (increased oxygen concentration) is the most effective way to kill a cancer cell, so tumors have developed means to keep themselves hypoxic (low in oxygen). Successful oxidation can occur through natural therapies (high dose I.V. vitamin), chemical treatments (chemo), or physical interventions (radiation).

The book of Genesis tells how God created man, taking earth and giving the human body form but not life. *Then* God breathed life into Adam, and he lived. To this day we cannot live without air; our bodies depend 100% on the oxygen that comes from the breath of life.

Do you recall when your science teacher explained why we can't light a match in a vacuum—for instance, in outer space—because oxygen is required for combustion? Here's another oxygen fact: chemotherapy and radiation cannot destroy tumors without oxygen—they're oxidative therapies. To be effective, to create unbearable oxidative stress, they need sufficient oxygen levels within the tumors. This is a huge treatment problem, for tumors are hypoxic; oxygen levels inside them are low to nil. In this chapter I'll explain the obstacle and how to overcome it.

Ozone Autohemotherapy

Tumor hypoxia has been the stone in the oncologist's shoe since chemo and radiation were put into use. In 1992 the National Cancer Institute (NCI) sponsored a conference that emphasized the importance of developing methods to overcome it. More than a decade was needed for an answer to surface, but researchers did develop an effective technique, and in 2004 Bernardino Clavo and his colleagues reported that ozone therapy increases oxygenation in the most poorly oxygenated tumor tissues. Clinical studies demonstrate that it inhibits the growth of cancer cells of the lung, breast, uterus, prostate, and liver.[1]

Dr. Clavo recruited eighteen patients and used special needle probes to measure the oxygen content of their tumors before and after three sessions of ozone autohemotherapy (O_3-AHT), in which 200 milliliters of drawn blood is ozonated and then re-infused into the patient. He established that there were fewer hypoxic tumor regions following O_3-AHT because it makes blood less viscous, with red blood cells more flexible and prone to surrender oxygen.[2] He also found that O_3-AHT promotes vasodilation, widening of the blood vessels caused by release of nitric oxide from the endothelial lining of small arteries. The net therapeutic effect is a significant increase in delivery of oxygen to the tumor site.[3]

The conclusion from one study of seventy patients diagnosed with prostatic adenocarcinoma was that ozone therapy can continuously increase oxygen levels in micro-circulation, inhibiting cancer cell growth and metastasis.[4] It also increases the cellular antioxidant enzymes that can protect healthy cells against chemo and radiation damage. Further, it induces apoptosis and modulates the immune system, helping it recover its anti-tumor function.

• • • • • • • • • • • • •

O_3-AHT is one method we use at Oasis of Hope to oxygenate tumors as a preparatory step for intravenous vitamin C therapy, chemo, and radiation. In addition to oxygenating tumors, O_3-AHT presents a wide range of immune-stimulating effects that greatly benefit overall health. A study conducted on ozone use in patients with primary cancer of the liver showed that the therapy protects the liver, improves its function, and improves quality of life.[5]

This procedure is typically repeated several times weekly. We employ an O_3-AHT protocol that's been widely used in Europe with an excellent safety record. While ozone is unstable, none is directly infused into the body; we make sure it's completely dissipated in the ozone-treated blood before re-infusing, and so the body is exposed to the oxidation's positive byproducts rather than the ozone itself. The exposure of blood to ozone in clinically appropriate amounts does not damage the membranes of red blood cells or compromise growth and development of white blood cells. In fact, no evident side effects are noted in patients receiving O_3-AHT.

In some patients with stubborn, resilient tumors that present an imminent threat to life, we recommend chemotherapy, and now we can dramatically multiply its oxidizing effect by coupling it with intravenous vitamin C, vitamin K_3, and O_3-AHT. Our design is to leverage the therapies' complementary interactions so that destruction of cancer cells is maximized without an increase in toxic risk to healthy tissues.

HBO

Before Home Box Office there was hyperbaric oxygen, also known as HBO. Another treatment that can increase oxygen levels in tumors, HBO can be used safely in concert with radiation and chemo.[6] Critics of its use in cancer therapy have said it induces cancer cell growth, even though studies have proven otherwise;[7] oncologists who hold that it does simply have not reviewed the published results in peer-reviewed medical journals.

Some other oncologists believe HBO is a contraindication (scenario in which a treatment shouldn't be given) for use with certain chemo-types, including Cisplatin, on the grounds that it could contribute to renal failure. The findings reveal that one HBO treatment may reduce Cisplatin-induced nephrotoxicity, protecting kidney function.[8] Because the same study also found that two HBO treatments could increase nephrotoxicity, HBO frequency and duration must be controlled to avoid renal failure when used in conjunction with Cisplatin. The benefits outweigh the risks, which can be mitigated by proper use.

Conclusion

I'm a firm believer in ozone (or hyperbaric oxygen) therapy as an integral part of comprehensive cancer treatment. Decades of usage have demonstrated that in most cases this oxidizing strategy is efficient and effective. My patients frequently experience tumor reduction, increased longevity, and improved quality of life.

ACTION STEPS

1. Find a doctor who can administer O_3-AHT or provide hyperbaric oxygen sessions.
2. Protect your healthy cells, and potentiate any cytotoxic therapy with oxygen therapies.
3. Pray to God and give Him thanks for the breath of life. Use this breath to help you heal.

CANCER VICTOR TIPS

Bradley Palmer, Arkansas
Stage III Colorectal Cancer
Victor Since 2010

1. Nothing that comes our way has taken God by surprise. Surrender to Him; with this diagnosis will come the grace and strength you need.
2. There are many treatment options. Don't limit yourself to the first thing you hear.
3. What you eat and drink will have huge impact on your cancer journey.
4. Don't dwell on statistics. Every case is unique. Stay positive.
5. Learn a lifestyle that makes your body a cancer-fighting machine.[9]

Oxygen Therapies
https://vimeo.com/61062211

Chapter 6

Psycho-Oncology

Q: *How can counseling or support groups help me?*

A: Cancer strives pervasively to steal personal identity. As in, from her perspective, Jane Smith has become A Breast Cancer Patient. A counselor or group can help reframe her emotional status to regain her identity as a person—not patient—and overpower cancer.

I have selective memory, and nowhere more so than with movies. My mind remembers so many wonderful parts, so many fantastic messages, and for the most part it edits out the forgettable and the distasteful. And so I've learned the hard way that sometimes I need to re-view a "great movie" before asking others to watch with me. For example, I screened *Patch Adams*[1] for our patients. It's phenomenal; it's uplifting; yet in the opening scenes there's content inappropriate for children. I noticed this too late as some parents shot withering looks my way while escorting their kids from our dining commons.

I still like to show movies to my patients, though, because film can speak directly to a soul in a way lectures cannot. At the top of my must-see file is *The Bucket List*,[2] about Edward (Jack Nicholson) and Carter (Morgan Freeman), two complete strangers who become friends for life as they share the journey of cancer. Relatively few movies have the potential to make us laugh *and* cry so passionately. Its central message: a person shouldn't waste time waiting to die; instead, embrace each day of life and truly live it. The two make a list of the things they wish to do before they "kick the bucket," hence the term "Bucket List."

In one of my favorite scenes, Edward brings up the five stages of grief: denial, anger, bargaining, depression, and acceptance. When he's done sharing his wisdom on the subject, Carter asks, "What stage are you in?" Edward replies, "Denial."

• • • • • • • • • • • • •

Few words carry a punch like "You have cancer." Most who receive them go straight into denial. Among the expressions people use when sharing how they felt at diagnosis are "I was hit by a Mack truck," "I felt blindsided," and "It was a knockout punch—I was down for the count."

In most treatment centers, oncology is focused 100% on tumor eradication. Little if any attention is on helping patients cope with "cancer, the life-changing event." But sit in on a support group and you'll find that most conversations center on dealing with the stress, fear, and anxiety associated with the disease and its treatment's side effects.

Great minds like Plato, Aristotle, and Aquinas recognized the import of the soul-body connection and explained it through metaphysics and philosophical psychology.[3] I have explained it from a practitioner's point of view, leveraging scientific findings in the field of psychoendocrinology. Here's one point on which metaphysics, philosophy, psychology, and endocrinology agree: what happens in the soul affects the body.

Psycho-oncology considers the social and psychological aspects of cancer, it's goals being to alleviate emotional distress through various assessments, teachings, and therapies.[4] In treatment centers, most psycho-oncology is performed by nurses and social workers; they do look to identify emotional needs, empower patients, and provide coping strategies, but their approach is designed to be systematic—they work to help the patients communicate more effectively with the physicians.[5]

Counselors may have similar goals, but they're focused entirely on the patient—they have no need of trying to interface with the medical institution. The rest of this chapter is designed to help you see cancer through a counselor's lens of psycho-oncology. I hope that its information can help you to adjust and cope with your health challenge.

Psychological Challenges

Emotionally, cancer can be devastating. The main concerns that promote distress are the fear of death, anxiety about treatment, and issues of loss.

About 50% of patients experience emotional disturbances because of cancer, including adjustment disorder, depressive disorder, and post-traumatic stress disorder (PTSD).[6]

Let's take a closer look at these. If you've been experiencing intense feelings and thoughts, you are not alone.

Anxiety

It's normal for people to be nervous about cancer and its treatments. Anxiety levels have been found to increase in people feeling pain, nausea, and fatigue.[7] These symptoms can trigger negative emotions stimulated by the perception that the body is under attack or in danger.

Depression

The word *depression* often is mistakenly used to mean "sadness." Technically, to be diagnosed with depression, a person has to suffer from a number of symptoms that can include oversleeping or sleeplessness, weight gain or weight loss, apathy, continuous crying or numbness, and even suicidal ideation. It's easy to understand how cancer patients are under-diagnosed and under-treated for depression—these symptoms are very similar to the negative side effects of chemotherapy and radiation.

In one study that interviewed 330 cancer patients, more than 17% met the criteria to be diagnosed with clinical depression,[8] and close to 40% exhibited anxiety symptoms. In some, emotional stress builds up beyond the point of being able to cope. Many comment that the side effects of treatment are worse than the disease. Also, pain significantly increases the percentage of those who suffer depressive symptoms.[9]

Post-Traumatic Stress Disorder (PTSD)

The prevalence of PTSD in cancer patients is less than 3% as strictly defined in psychologists' diagnostic manual. But in some groups PTSD symptoms are reported in as many as 20% of post-treatment patients.[10]

Grief

It can exhibit similar symptoms, yet grief differs completely from depression. Most people think of grief in terms of dealing with a loved one's death, which is one situation that yields grief. Any loss sustained—even an anticipated loss—can put a person into a grieving process.

It's crucial to work through the grief of being diagnosed and treated for cancer, because patients grieving their situation have an increased tendency to want to die.[11] You must seek out counselors and support groups to help you grieve. This is a big generalization, but, overall, oncologists don't even think about these issues; if you find one who helps you cope with your grief, you are blessed!

I often work with young mothers, for whom it's common to grieve the possibility that they will no longer be alive to help their children grow up. People grieve about the dreams they've had that they never will get to fulfill. Yet there is no pill to cure grief; as Kay Cogswell, a great mentor of mine, once said, "You don't get over grief—you get through it."

Psychological Handles

In rumination, the cognitive process of repeatedly pondering issues that provoke stress, negative thoughts can race continuously through the mind. With cancer, it can be difficult to take your focus off the disease and place it on life. Let me recommend a couple handles to grab on to—grips to help you control what you can—for going through grief, or for when you find the time has come to battle fear, anxiety, or depression.

Ongoing Education

One of the motives for writing this book is that most hospital budgets do not afford providing counselors and social workers for their patients. I hope to share as much info as possible to help you better cope with what you're facing as a patient or caregiver. Do you know who else likely wants to do the same? Your nurse.

Nurses are just about my favorite people in treatment centers. Whereas doctors seem to excel in "drive-by" medicine, nurses administer the actual treatment and often will engage in conversation. They share some of the best facts and suggestions for stress management.

Make friends with your nurses! Go to them for input and feedback like you'd go to a well for water. One primary object of oncology nurses, social workers, and counselors is to inform you about diagnosis, treatment, symptoms, side effects, and coping strategies.[12] Knowledge is power, so whenever you can, take advantage of education opportunities.

Cognitive Restructuring

There are ways to substitute negative thoughts with positive, truth-based ones. Cognitive restructuring can be effective in dealing with rumination and alleviating PTSD symptoms by taking the focus off cancer's negative aspects.[13]

Cognitive restructuring is the process of identifying the negative thoughts that trigger emotional distress and generating positive thoughts to replace them.[14] One technique is called reframing, which is looking at the same situation from another perspective. For example, have you ever noticed how a painting can look much different or even completely dissimilar depending on the frame that's used? Scenarios and circumstances you face can likewise look very different when reframed.

In chapter 3, I explained how relieving emotional stress translates into an improved immune response against cancer. The end results of reframing can include better adaptation to stressful situations, improved coping, and development of more effective problem solving skills. Counselors often use such methods as logical disputation and Socratic questioning to help identify irrational thoughts; to effectively reframe a negative thought, a person first must identify it.

An effective way to identify your negative thoughts is through the ABC method, which psychologist Albert Ellis developed to help identify irrational beliefs.[15] Breaking it down into a process helps us begin to understand that stress doesn't just happen without any opportunities to manage it. In Ellis's model:

A = the perceived threat;
B = the irrational belief associated with the threat; and
C = the emotional, behavioral, or cognitive reaction to the threat.

The brilliance of ABC is in helping a person to see that there is more than a threat and a reaction; there's also a thought that determines the reaction to the perceived threat.

I use ABC with my patients as the first step in cognitive restructuring. I often say I've renamed it "Stop, drop and roll," a reference back to the nationwide training of how an elementary-aged child should respond if he or she smells smoke and suspects a fire.

My patients helped me develop the explanation this way:

Stop = When you perceive a threat, stop to find another (positive and tenable) way to look at the situation;
Drop = Get on your knees to pray for help during the difficult situation; and
Roll = Go on your way with the new thought and a plan for how to cope with or overcome the perceived threat.

I suggest that patients keep a "thought journal," where anytime they feel anxious they stop and identify the negative thought related to the anxious situation. They write that down and then come up with a replacement thought.

Here's one example:

Situation: I'm about to take a cycle of chemotherapy.
Negative thought: "Chemo makes me feel horribly sick."
Result: I feel anxious, and side effects may be exacerbated by the **anxiety.**

And, a substitute scenario:

Situation: I'm about to take a cycle of chemotherapy.
Negative thought: "Chemo makes me feel horribly sick."
Reframed thought: "The chemo is going to kill cancer cells, which I need. I'm grateful to have access to this treatment."

Result: Ability to manage the stress of treatment by placing focus onto its benefits instead of its side effects.

Want to give this a try right now? Think of a situation that makes you nervous. Why do you think it makes you nervous? Can you identify a negative thought that runs through your head when you face this?

Write down that thought. Try to look at the situation from another perspective. What statement can you make to yourself about a potential benefit or outcome you could experience in the difficult scenario? Write down that new perspective in one sentence. Then, next time you face this circumstance, repeat to yourself the new, positive thought.

Conclusion

Self-talk is powerful; what you tell yourself becomes the reality you experience. The soul (psyche) is the battlefield where a person either becomes a cancer victor or cancer victim, and yet it's estimated that only 10% of cancer patients ever seek out any form of counseling.[16] If you ever speak to some of our patients, they'll tell you the emotional and spiritual support we provide makes a huge difference in how they and their families are able to maintain hope and cope with cancer.

That you're reading this book makes me confident you're seeking answers and have set your feet on the path to victory. Though no one can determine how many days, months, and years he or she will continue to walk this earth, you decide how you will live each day. Being a cancer victor is having the conviction that you take on the disease on your terms; you refuse to let it define who you are.

ACTION STEPS

1. Start a thought journal. In one column, write down the situations that cause anxiety or stress. In a second, write down the negative thought(s) you associate with that event. In a third, write down a new thought to replace each negative thought. Whenever you face that scenario, stop a moment and repeat the positive thought until you feel more relaxed.
2. Seek out a counselor, social worker, support group, and/or nurse who can teach you effective coping skills.
3. Focus on getting through today; face tomorrow when it arrives. Each day, make a positive memory. Daily, make a journal entry, blog entry, or scrapbook page that shows you are actually living.

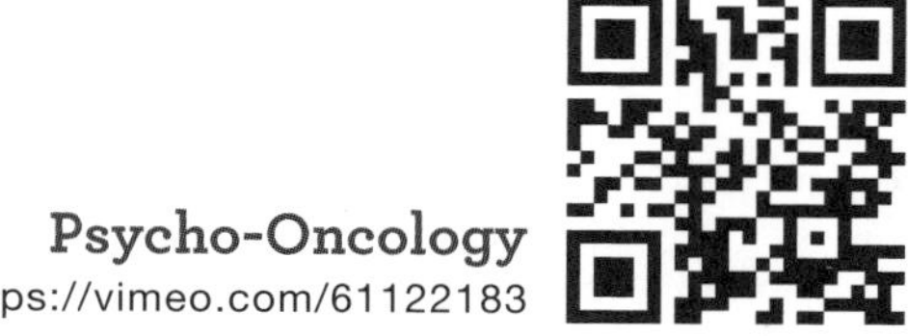

CANCER VICTOR TIPS

Rick Hill, California
High Grade Embryonal Cell Carcinoma
Victor Since 1974

1. *Be all in.* Keeping one foot in "Israel," one foot in "Egypt" won't work. You must commit 100% to the diet and detox for five solid years, then to a Mediterranean type diet thereafter: mostly organic vegetables, fruit, and small amounts of meat.
2. *Restart your life!* If you're in a career or a friendship that's draining you of your energy and enthusiasm, change it up. This is the time to set new goals and build a real support system.
3. *Recruit supportive friends.* If your friends say things like, "Now that you're back from La-La Land, let's go see a *real* doctor," or "We're going for pizza and beer tonight, and don't say no," ask them to stop. If they don't, get new friends.
4. *Learn to cook properly.* At cancersupportshow.com, you can check out Oasis of Hope cooking classes. Learn to shop organic, and gluten free, and to prepare foods below 186 degrees so you don't cook the life out of it. Make your diet 80% raw and organic at least for the first five years. For this to work, the buck stops with you.
5. *Be vocal, help others!* Be willing to speak at churches or civic groups about what Oasis of Hope is doing for cancer patients. When you learn about someone who has cancer, see what you can do for them.

Chapter 7

High-Dose Vitamin C Therapy

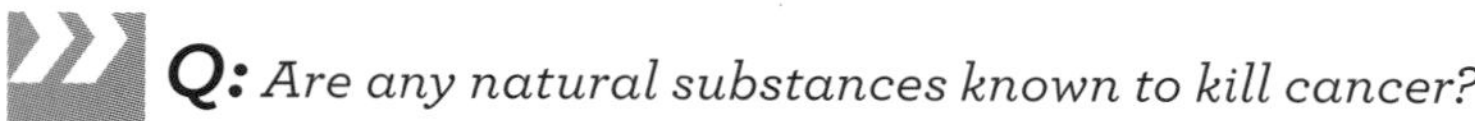

Q: *Are any natural substances known to kill cancer?*

A: It's a scientific fact: the antioxidant vitamin C will promote oxidation when it circulates in very high concentrations in highly oxygenated blood. Healthy cells tolerate high dosages because of catalase, an enzyme that neutralizes oxidation immediately. Catalase is abundant in our blood and normal tissues but generally scant in malignant tumors—this lack in cancerous tissues allows vitamin C's oxidative capacity to selectively kill malignant cells.

After President George W. Bush declared war on Iraq in 2003, the American public learned some terms and phrases. The first was "shock and awe," which civilians on the ground in Baghdad sure experienced in a different manner than those out of harm's way watching on TV. The second, "collateral damage," was used to label innocent lives lost who weren't an intended target. In all conflict, probable collateral damage ought to be estimated as part of deciding whether or not to initiate.

It's uncanny how fitting war analogies can be in explaining the fight against cancer. Conventional therapy produces significant collateral damage, by which I mean that while chemotherapy, radiation, and surgery are very effective at killing cancer cells, they don't discriminate—they also kill healthy cells, equally.

Some of the main cells that suffer are those of the immune system. Oncologists have to carefully estimate what the damage will be to healthy cells to avoid killing the patient with the very treatment intended to save him. That's why chemo and radiation must have breaks in their cycles.

I'm happy to share that there are natural therapies that produce no collateral damage. In some cases these work as effectively as chemo while not harming the patient. I want to introduce you to one of the oncology world's greatest secrets: high-dose intravenous vitamin C.

A Natural Anti-tumor Agent

Researchers have found that a highly concentrated vitamin C dose is "selectively" toxic to cancer cells, meaning the dose harms cancer cells but not healthy tissue. Yet when this treatment was coupled with the addition of catalase (an enzyme), the cancer-killing effect was reduced significantly. This led researchers to believe that the high-dose vitamin C infusion resulted in production of large quantities of hydrogen peroxide, which initially caused a cancer-killing effect that was then neutralized by the catalase. This suggested that cancer cells do not produce sufficient catalase to neutralize high levels of hydrogen peroxide on their own.

We now know that many cancer cells produce small amounts of catalase to sustain low concentrations of hydrogen peroxide.[1-3] This creates the cancer-friendly environment of mild oxidative stress that encourages rapid growth of and further aggression by malignant cells.[4-7] Fortunately, because a high proportion of cancers are only able to produce small amounts of catalase, they're vulnerable to the cancer-killing effect exhibited by high levels of hydrogen peroxide.

Dr. Mark Levine's National Institute of Health (NIH) team, analyzing vitamin C's cancer-killing effect, found that after a high dose and rapid IV infusion, large concentrations could be reached in the extracellular space. There, vitamin C reacts spontaneously with molecular oxygen within tumors, generating large amounts of hydrogen peroxide, lethal to tumor cells that produce only small amounts of catalase.[8-9]

The irony here is astounding. For many years vitamin C has been recognized as one of the most powerful known anti-oxidants. How can a substance with anti-oxidant properties produce levels of oxidative stress sufficient to kill cancer? Turns out, the answer is simple: the vitamin's effect within the body is dose dependent. Many substances render very different effects depending upon size of dose; the same substance can be a poison or a medicine depending on its quantity and concentration.

In the 1970s, double-Nobel-winner Linus Pauling, who believed antioxidant therapy was how to kill cancer cells, collaborated with Ewan Cameron to promote IV and oral administration of high-dose vitamin C for terminal cancer patients. They administered a ten-gram "megadose" intravenously, followed by ten more grams orally, and in two published clinical trials they reported that patients markedly prolonged their lives and enjoyed an improved quality of life.[10] Some peers claimed this dosing was irresponsible, and later, after controlled clinical studies at the Mayo Clinic, C. G. Moertel concluded that he couldn't replicate their results.[11]

Thereafter, many thought the case for high-dose vitamin C closed. But thirty years later, NIH researchers found it necessary to reopen the matter in view of recent discoveries. This is when Levine's team found that Moertel's studies failed because he only administered orally.

The NIH research has proven that to consistently achieve the vitamin-C concentration sufficient to provoke oxidation, a patient must receive dozens of grams intravenously; oral administration is useless in this regard.[12] A number of published case reports, which show that repeated high-dose IV treatments yield objective tumor regression,[13-15] are so compelling that NIH clinical trials are formally evaluating intravenous vitamin C therapy. Currently, we continue to look at dosing and treatment intervals as studies suggest that multiple, staged, and intermittent treatments may produce better anti-tumor effects than long high-dose single treatments.[16] This will also protect the kidneys from becoming saturated. At Oasis of Hope we're utilizing protocols with multiple treatments and pauses between doses to maintain the level of vitamin C within an optimal therapeutic window.

In theory, high-dose vitamin C should not cause toxic damage to healthy tissue because the body produces sufficient amounts of catalase to efficiently neutralize the hydrogen peroxide produced. My experience supports the theory. We've treated hundreds of patients in this manner with no side effects, and our current protocol ensures vitamin-C blood and tissue levels that are safe and effective to kill cancer cells.

• • • • • • • • • • • • •

Yet a burning question remains. *Why doesn't this therapy work for everyone?* Three variables can undermine its effectiveness.

First, some tumors produce larger amounts of catalase, which neutralizes the oxidizing effect of hydrogen peroxide.

Second, sometimes there are insufficient catalysts to promote the necessary transfer of electrons.

Third, sometimes in the extracellular space there is insufficient oxygen, which is needed for vitamin C to produce hydrogen peroxide.

For now, scientists have not found a way to selectively block production of catalase within tumors. However, we can definitively increase this therapy's effectiveness by providing two supporting agents: electron transfer catalysts and tumor oxygenating agents.

Specific Benefits: Vitamins C and K_3

Vitamin C's ability to generate hydrogen peroxide in tumors hinges on the presence of catalysts that can transfer electrons from the vitamin to oxygen molecules, generating an unstable compound superoxide, which rapidly converts to the hydrogen peroxide that has cancer-killing properties. One such well-known catalyst is menadione, also known as vitamin K_3.[17] Substantial research in both rodent and human studies demonstrates that supplementing intravenous vitamin C with injectable vitamin K_3 increases the therapy's effectiveness on cancer cells.

Catholic University of Louvain (Belgium) researchers have played a pioneering role in demonstrating the potential of the C/K_3 combination in cancer treatment. In particular, they've shown that the combined administration of these agents can retard cancer growth and metastasis in tumor-bearing rodents.[18-19] They also report that this therapy is well tolerated, without any evident damage to healthy tissues.

Further, they demonstrate that the C/K_3 combo can interact synergistically with certain cytotoxic chemo drugs in killing cancer cells. This is logical since, as mentioned before, some chemo drugs work by increasing the levels of oxidative stress within those cells. Indeed, there are reports that vitamin K_3 alone can increase the cytotoxicity of certain chemo agents, presumably because, in sufficiently high concentrations, K_3 helps generate oxidative stress by transferring electrons from intracellular molecules to oxygen.[20-21]

At the Oasis of Hope we inject vitamin K_3 just prior to the vitamin C infusions, with the hope and expectation that C/K_3 combination will markedly increase the production of hydrogen peroxide within tumors, enabling a more substantial cell kill in those cancers that produce sufficiently small amounts of catalase. While vitamin K_3 is an excellent electron transfer catalyst, the effectiveness of intravenous vitamin C therapy can still be crippled if oxygen levels within the tumor are poor. (Remember: Many common tumors create a hypoxic environment, so it's necessary to introduce agents that can efficiently oxygenate them.)

Increasing cellular oxygenation is so important that I dedicated chapter 5 to it. Please take a look there for further helpful information.

Conclusion

On July 20, 1969, in humankind's hugest-yet achievement in aerospace science, Neil Armstrong became the first human to set foot on the moon.[22] A billion people watched the lunar landing live. "Armstrong" became a household name.

In the same year, another major scientific discovery was published, in the field of medicine. Do you recognize the names "Benade," "Howard," or "Burke"? Probably not. But in 1969 they published their findings that vitamin C kills cancer cells.[23]

Why has vitamin C been overlooked? True, a natural vitamin treatment isn't rocket science. But while it may not be stellar news, it still may get you stellar results. I continue to use vitamin C in cancer treatment and am optimistic because the research community is seriously looking again at its action as a pro-drug to deliver malignant-cell-killing hydrogen peroxide to tissues.

High-Dose Vitamin C Therapy
https://vimeo.com/61133623

ACTION STEPS

1. Try to speak with others who've had high-dose vitamin C therapy; ask if it helped. Consider social networking to achieve this.
2. Look online for NIH studies on the use of vitamin C to treat cancer.
3. Find an integrative physician who administers high-dose vitamin C and consider whether the treatment is viable for you.

CANCER VICTOR TIPS

Julianna Jackson, Texas
Stage IV Ovarian Cancer
Victor Since 2008

1. Get anointed, as the Bible says in James 5:14.
2. Stop all sugar, no canned food; eat only what God made, but no meat.
3. Keep an open mind; search out alternative medicine.
4. Find a hospital that works on mind, body, spirit; all three work together to heal the body.
5. When you find one, get anointed again; sit back and enjoy the journey.

Chapter 8

Alkaline and Acid Balance:

The Foundation of Life

Q: *Are there ways we can influence the acid/alkaline balance in our body?*

A: While blood pH is almost impossible to influence through diet, it is possible to influence a tumor's pH environment through dietary, supplemental, and medical means. Tumor pH manipulation can directly kill or at least debilitate cancer cells, allowing anti-tumor therapies to be more effective.

Many alternative and holistic doctors recommend self-testing urine or saliva pH, to determine the overall body pH, so that through dietary adjustment (consuming alkaline or acid foods) an acceptable pH level is reached. Conversely, conventional doctors are skeptical of the idea, for our "body's" pH (usually meaning blood pH) won't be influenced by diet.

Both are right, and . . . both are wrong. Do not despair; I hope that after reading you'll have a grasp of this complex and challenging concept to where you can apply this knowledge practically and beneficially.

Most doctors really don't understand the intricacies of alkaline/acid balance. We have a good idea, but few are competent in this very basic yet complicated system that's so fundamental to life. While certainly there are experts in the field, most who claim to actually have little clue of the subject's profundity. Most of us don't appreciate the evolution of the technology relevant to pH and blood gas (oxygen and carbon dioxide) measurements, a scientific feat that's taken three centuries of research and more than three decades to develop instruments to make it practical for clinical application. I believe we're just scratching the surface of this incredible function of our bodies.

Understanding pH Balance

Søren Peder Lauritz Sørensen, a chemist, was the first to establish a scientific measure for acidity and alkalinity, introducing the concept of pH in 1909.[1] The "p" is for power or potential (or concentration), and "H" for hydrogen; "pH" stands for the power/concentration of hydrogen. To oversimplify, depending on hydrogen and hydroxide concentrations, a substance's chemical property will be acid, neutral, or alkaline on a scale of 0 to 14. A pH of 7 is neutral; < 7 is acidic; > 7 is alkaline (or "basic").

Pure water is neutral because its hydrogen ions and hydroxide ions exist in equilibrium; thus a pH of 7. *Both* H^+ (hydrogen) and OH^- (hydroxide) ions are present in any solution. A solution is acidic if the H^+ ions are in excess and basic (alakaline) if the OH^- ions are in excess.

All life systems function inside a very narrow pH range. Our pH system's balancing act is a thing of beauty and precision; our bodies have astounding capacity to neutralize acidity or alkalinity through an intricate chemical process called *buffering*. For instance, without enough acidity, buffers can increase acidity back to normal pH. Breathing out carbon dioxide gets rid of excess acidity, and some acidity is excreted (through urine, etc.). But even minute changes can cause havoc. Blood pH is neutral at 7.4; higher than 7.8 or lower than 7.0 leads to death.

There are lots of proteins in the body whose shape and chemical state depend on this narrow working range. For example, if your blood is much too acidic, hemoglobin structure changes so that oxygen uptake is compromised and your body's oxygen transport is reduced or disabled; circulating inoffensive microbes can change shape, mutate, and become pathogenic. Normal enzymes may become destructive; the assimilation of minerals can be compromised and affect function of the liver, kidneys, heart, et al. The body is so finicky about acid/alkaline equilibrium that it requires blood pH to be nearly perfect to keep us alive.

How to Affect the Body's pH

Back to the initial question: can we influence the pH balance in our body through diet or any other means? The first consideration is that there are many microsystems with their own particular acid/alkaline environments. The most sophisticated, and crucial to health, is the blood. So, restating the question, can we influence this balance in our *blood*? The answer is no, and thank God—otherwise the death rate would soar and humans would be virtually atop the endangered species list.

It takes ten gallons of water to neutralize the pH—2.5—of one 12-ounce can of Coca-Cola, so why don't we die after drinking a Coke if we don't follow it with ten gallons of water? Also, each day our stomach produces about half a gallon of gastric juice that's more acidic than Coke, and our blood's pH is unfazed. But does this mean that strongly acidic foods are healthy for us? Well, there are some very healthy acid foods, like citrus fruits; however, all processed foods are acid-forming and *un*healthy. That unhealthy acid foods do not influence blood pH doesn't mean there aren't consequences. Nutritionally savvy doctors are right in recommending pH-health-promoting foods instead of junk foods.

The reason we needn't take soft drinks with ten gallons of water is the aforementioned buffering system that keeps blood pH stable whether we eat acidic or basic foods. Buffers are like shock absorbers—if you cruise through a pothole in an expensive SUV, you may not feel much, but the SUV certainly does. Our lifestyle should be about protecting our protecting mechanisms instead of abusing them to the brink of a failure that translates into disease and shortened life expectancy.

• • • • • • • • • • • •

Three primary buffering systems maintain a constant and healthy pH in blood and other fluids to prevent acidosis or alkalosis.

First, the body fluids' chemical acid/base systems instantly combine with acid or base to prevent excessive change in hydrogen concentration. Most effective is the sodium bicarbonate-carbonic acid system; the phosphate system and the protein system also help regulate balance.

Second, the respiratory center regulates the removal of carbon dioxide (CO_2) and carbonic acid (H_2CO_3) from the extracellular fluid.

Third, during acidosis or alkalosis, the kidneys can excrete acidic or basic urine and thus readjust the extracellular fluid's hydrogen concentration toward normal.

Indirectly, that last factor means we can measure the stress our lifestyle is putting on our body (specifically, its buffering systems). For instance, if my urine's pH is too acidic, probably I'm ingesting too much acid-generating food. Referring back to the chapter's beginning, that's why measuring the pH of urine and saliva can be helpful. It's my opinion that we can avoid the need for this testing by reducing to the minimum possible our ingestion of processed foods (whose highly acidic pH ranges from 2.8 to 5.5). While our bodies are designed to buffer natural acidic and alkaline foods, because so much processed food is out there I do recommend we increase our intake of more natural alkaline foods.

Many resources in print or online show the pH value of foods and their potential to acidify or alkalinize our bodies. ("Potential" because a food's pH value does not necessarily translate in a direct impact.) Lemons, for example, are very acidic, but their byproducts after digestion and assimilation are very alkaline, so in the body lemons are alkaline-forming. On the flip side, the pH of meat is alkaline, but after digestion in our gut it leaves acidic byproducts (as do nearly all animal products).

As a general rule, a healthy diet should consist of 60% alkaline-forming and 40% acid-forming foods. If the aim is to restore health, make it 80% and 20%. A few examples:

Alkaline-forming: most fruits, green vegetables, peas, beans, lentils, spices, herbs, seasonings, seeds, nuts.

Acid-forming: meat, fish, poultry, eggs, refined grains, sugar, processed foods.

Again, within our bodies are independent micro-pH environments, including the stomach (very acidic, to promote food degradation) and the bladder (mildly acidic, to prevent infectious diseases). Let us look now into the abnormal low-pH environment of cancer. The reason tumors develop an acidic environment has to do with their aberrant structure and abnormal metabolism.

The Behavior of Cancer Cells

Mutated cancerous cells do not have an organized growth pattern, and they proliferate too fast for the supporting tissues to function in the way normal cells do (metabolically speaking), especially in terms of blood supply. Tumor vasculature is irregular and twisted, with areas of dilated and bulged vessels followed by constricted ones, or sharply bent and many times compressed by the tumor's uncontrolled growth. Hence a tumor's irrigation is sluggish and insufficient of various nutrients and oxygen to its cells. These conditions of hypoxia and undernourishment provoke a genetic adaptation for survival and make the tumor more effective at beating the odds—that is, more aggressive.

Normal cells generate energy (ATP, adenosine triphosphate) cost-effectively, leaving easily disposable waste materials like water and carbon dioxide; the malignant cell's genetic adaptations, in its hypoxic environs, lead cancer to generate energy via different pathways. Its cells obtain energy less effectively, through glycolysis, which generates lactic and carbonic acids, resulting in acidification of the tumor's environment.

We've long been addressing these microenvironmental differences because they provide certain advantages for tumors to thrive. In fact, tumor acidity is the driving force behind cancer's ability to invade other tissues and spread to other organs (metastases). A number of studies have shown that the extracellular pH in cancers is typically lower than that in normal tissue and that an acidic pH promotes invasive tumor growth in primary and metastatic cancers.[2] And it isn't easy to interfere with this abnormal environment—no matter how much alkaline and alkaline-generating food a person consumes, tumor acidity will not be affected; that must happen through specific chemical and metabolic pathways that directly affect the pH of malignant tumors.

About two decades ago Dr. Tullio Simoncini first proposed the use of sodium bicarbonate ($NaHCO_3$) as an anti-tumor therapy.[3] Though I do not agree with his whole theory that cancer is a fungal infection, there is sufficient scientific data to support sodium bicarbonate indeed selectively affecting the acidic environment of malignant tumors, reducing their ability to grow, invade surrounding tissues, or metastasize. *That* seems reason enough to include sodium bicarbonate in our oncological arsenal.

Drs. Ariosto S. Silva and Robert J. Gillie published a paper proving that intake of sodium bicarbonate, at dosages used in published clinical trials, reduces intratumoral and peritumoral acidosis and, as a result, significantly reduced tumor growth and invasion without altering the pH of blood or normal tissues.[4] Dr. Ian F. Robey also found that oral intake of sodium bicarbonate selectively alkalinized tumor pH and reduced the formation of spontaneous metastases in mouse models of metastatic breast cancer as well as reduced the rate of lymph node involvement and significantly reduced the formation of hepatic metastases.[5]

Together with this inexpensive pH buffer, at Oasis of Hope we also administer a well-known Proton Pump Inhibitor omeprazole (Prilosec). These types of drugs (PPIs) markedly inhibit gastric acid secretion; they also have been proven to work in cancer cells, reducing extracellular tumor acidity while lowering the intracellular pH of cancer cells, which slows proliferation and promotes apoptosis in various cancer cell lines. Well-tolerated doses have significantly hindered tumor growth and prolonged survival in mice implanted with a human melanoma.[6]

Tumor Acidity and Chemo Resistance

Knowing that tumor acidity likewise is a major factor in chemo resistance, one research group was able to prove that tumor pH manipulation makes resistant cancer cells sensitive to chemotherapies that usually do not work. Andrej Udelnow and his group decided to investigate pancreatic cancers (highly resistant to chemotherapy) using omeprazole as a modulator of tumor-chemo-resistance, measuring its pharmacodynamic, morphological, and biochemical effects on the cell lines. They found that it inhibits pancreatic cancer cell proliferation and enhances the cancer cell-killing effects of gemcitabine and 5-FU, two common chemo drugs that usually have no effect in pancreas cancer.[7]

More treatment avenues that leverage cancer's pH microenvironment are being investigated. The low pH can markedly affect tumors' response to treatments like chemo because some agents are mildly acidic and some mildly alkaline. Acidic pH increases the cellular uptake of weakly acidic drugs (e.g., Cyclophosphamide, Cisplatin), *increasing* their effect, whereas the same pH retards the uptake of weakly basic drugs (e.g., Doxorubicin, Vinblastine), *reducing* their effect.

For tumors sensitive to such chemo, one should not alkalinize them; in fact, administration of glucose has been proven to acidify tumors. If the chemo is a mild alkaline substance, then one should administer sodium bicarbonate. Dr. Leo E. Gerweck altered the extracellular pH of tumors and compared the effect of the resultant pH gradient change on the efficacy of a weak acid versus a weak base chemotherapy and demonstrated through this manipulation a 2.3-fold increase in efficacy.[8]

Conclusion

Tumor acidity not only influences chemotherapy but radiotherapy and hyperthermia as well. The radiation-induced apoptosis is suppressed by an acidic environment, whereas the hyperthermia-induced cell death is potentiated by an acidic environment. Better understanding of the control mechanisms of pH in tumors may lead us to devise more effective ways to determine when to alkalinize or when to acidify human tumors.

Now that you know more about the intricacies of our bodies' most important biochemical mechanisms, I encourage you to do the following.

ACTION STEPS

1. To protect your buffering systems, increase your consumption of natural alkaline foods.
2. Sodium bicarbonate (baking soda) is an effective tumor pH alkalinizing agent; add it to your supplement arsenal.
3. Seek an oncologist who's aware of the intricacies of tumor pH and can exploit it to your advantage.

CANCER VICTOR TIPS

Alicia Harrison, California
Breast Cancer
Victor Since 2007

1. Don't despair; there is hope. Trust in God, in whom all things are possible.
2. Find a practice that addresses spiritual, emotional, *and* physical wellness and includes both conventional and alternative treatments.
3. Don't talk about your sickness constantly with family and friends. Focusing on negative outcomes will not give you the hope you need.

4. Declare and believe that you'll be well. Quote the healing Scriptures that will cause faith to grow and keep your thoughts focused on life.
5. Never say, "This is too hard," or "I could never change my diet because I'd have to give up my favorite foods." Commit yourself to do whatever is necessary, and follow through to the end.

Alkaline and Acid Balance: The Foundation of Life
https://vimeo.com/61145515

Chapter 9

Emotional Roots of Cancer

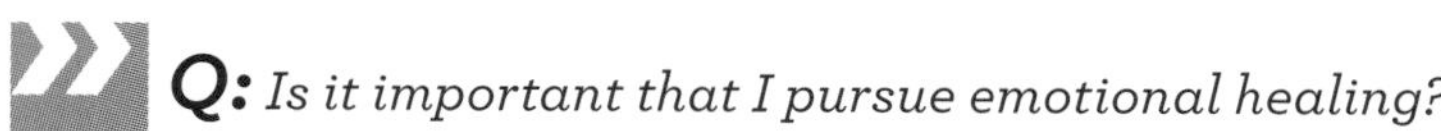

Q: *Is it important that I pursue emotional healing?*

A: Many studies confirm that a confluence of various strong emotional events will lead to immune deficiencies and the initiation of cancer. Resolving those issues or enabling a patient to effectively turn the page will invariably help restore proper immune function, which is absolutely necessary to beat cancer.

A sweet elderly patient approached after a group session where I'd had been teaching on the power of negative emotions to depress the immune system, focusing on the soul poison of guilt. In his beautiful German accent, the gentleman shared with me the tale of the two wolves, a Cherokee teaching of a grandfather and a grandson, passed down through generations in the storytelling tradition.

"A fight is going on inside me," he said to the boy. "It's a terrible fight, and it's between two wolves. One is evil—he is anger, envy, sorrow, regret, greed, arrogance, self-pity, guilt, resentment, inferiority, lies, false pride, superiority, and ego. The other is good—he is joy, peace, love, hope, serenity, humility, kindness, benevolence, empathy, generosity, truth, compassion, and faith. The same fight is going on inside you—and inside every other person, too."

The grandson thought a minute, then asked, "Which wolf will win?"

The grandfather replied, "The one you feed."[1]

Negative emotions leave the wreckage of emotional wounds in their wake. People who operate in them hurt others and themselves. When it comes to cancer, we cannot avoid this subject. Part of the reason tumors manifest is that the emotional and spiritual conflict in a person's life has been repressed or suppressed. If you have cancer, you can no longer put off dealing with the emotional pain inside.

• • • • • • • • • • • • •

Many years ago, my spiritually aware sister called and shared the details of a dream. She'd seen a person being attacked by demons whose claws were large hooks, trying to penetrate the skin. Wherever it was whole, the hook could not pierce, but at any open wound the hook would lodge itself and the demon would not let go. The openings were rooted in emotional wounds festering below the surface. She explained that God sent His son, Jesus Christ, to heal our emotional and spiritual wounds to protect us from attacks that would inflict further harm.

Clinical studies have identified the correlation between disease and negative emotions, repressed hurt, and suppressed grief.[2] My sister's dream was much more than a metaphor. One study conducted with forty-four men with cancer and forty-four without found that the former group had twice as many high-intensity emotional events as the latter.[3]

Emotional Correlates

Ryke Geerd Hamer's work on the emotional roots of disease began to get worldwide attention and scrutiny in the 1970s. Dr. Hamer amassed data from CT scans for more than 15,000 patients, then documented small marks on specific parts of the brain that indicate what type of emotional conflict had occurred in the patient and what organ was affected. He claimed that once the emotional conflict was resolved, the disease would simply go away. He noted on follow-up scans that the original marks blurred away, confirming the healing.

Recently I read a published article in which he explained the emotional cause for a number of skin conditions:[4]

SKIN CONDITION	EMOTIONAL CAUSE
Neurodermatitis: ulcer in skin.	Conflict shock of separation between child and parent or significant other.
Vitiligo: white patches on skin.	Brutal separation between two people; often a bloody (disfiguring) accident.
Alopecia: temporary hair loss.	Loss of someone dear who would pat the person on the head. When conflict is resolved, hair will grow back.
Neurofibromatosis: knot under skin.	A person does not want to be touched.

Hamer's work is more than controversial. In 1986 he was convicted of fraud and malpractice because many of his patients stopped all cancer treatment to do emotional healing only with him. He served time in Germany and later was also convicted and jailed in France. To say the least, scientists have questioned his methods. But his work is intriguing, and it may quite possibly be fifty to a hundred years ahead of its time.

Fantasy

There are psycho-oncologists, such as Sharone Bergner, who do not fully support the idea that cancer has emotional roots. She proposes that most patients have a theory, which she calls a fantasy, of why they have cancer. In "Seductive Symbolism, Psychoanalysis in the Context of Oncology,"[5] she shares a number of case studies where patients talked about how cancer was the consequence of negative behaviors from their past. A man with recurrent testicular cancer believed he deserved to get it because he was a sex addict. A woman with eczema outbreaks on one hand supposed it was due to suppressed aggression and violent tendencies. A mid-twenty-something man who had Hodgkin's lymphoma explained that his unhappiness resulted from anger at his parents; he was convinced that they preferred his older brother over him and believed that their inadequate way of loving him caused his cancer.

As you'll gather from chapter 47 (on beliefs and perception), I'm a firm supporter that a patient's belief will influence the treatment outcome almost as much as the medical therapy. Dr. Hamer may be overstating the significance of emotional root causes; Dr. Bergner may be dismissing its plausibility. For now, I believe psychoendoneuroimmunology supports emotional stress and distress having an effect on the immune system that's counterproductive to beating cancer. Let's take a look at a number of deep-rooted emotional issues I see frequently in patients.

Grief

Grief is about the loss of anything important to a person. Loss of a job or a home will cause grief. A student who doesn't get into the college of her dreams will grieve. Many people grieve that they never had a father, or that the father they had didn't meet their emotional needs.

Dr. Elizabeth Kübler-Ross described five stages of grief in people who are diagnosed with cancer and believe they're dying:[6] denial, anger, bargaining, depression, and acceptance. Most of my patients confirm passing through these stages, but through countless counseling sessions I've found that most have unresolved grief about issues that happened long before a cancer diagnosis. There's insufficient data supporting the idea that unresolved or complicated grief was responsible for the cancer.

Yet there *is* evidence that intense grieving results in a depressed immune system. A recent study, conducted with more than 1,500 soldiers who'd lost someone while deployed in Afghanistan or Iraq, found that 20% had difficulties coping and experienced poor health, increased medical services use, and impaired work performance due to illness.[7] Grieving takes its physical toll. When counseling in a bereavement center I noticed my clients commonly having colds, bronchitis, and sinusitis. Many also had eating problems and trouble sleeping. The combination of lack of rest, poor nutrition, and an increase in anxiety or depressive symptoms contribute to an immune system breakdown. To beat cancer, we need to boost that system. Therefore, it's important to identify the things you need to grieve. Most people have stuffed-down issues; if you're like most, it's time to identify your losses, grieve them, and move on.

I frequently use a timeline to help people document losses. I ask them to write down each issue and the age they were at the time of loss. It can be losing a first teddy bear, or the unwanted loss of virginity. It could be a death or a disillusionment the caused the sense of loss.

May I suggest you take a paper out now and copy the loss timeline diagram presented here. Above the line, write out the loss. Below, write the age you were when the loss occurred.

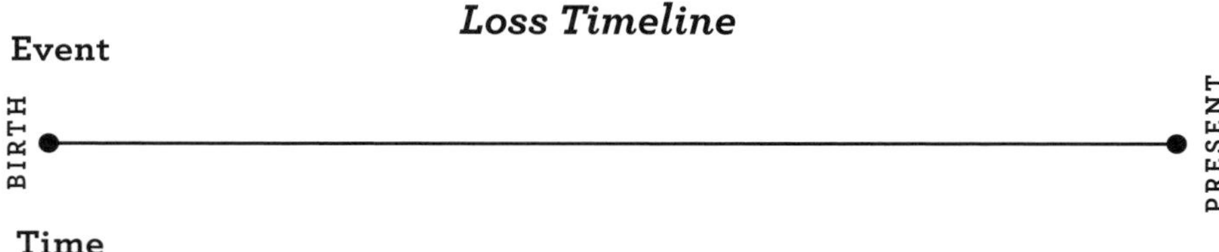

You may be surprised by the number of significant losses you've sustained over the years. If you can, try to find a counselor or a support group you can share your timeline with. Take time to consider each loss. You may need to cry about the loss and then surrender it.

One of my favorite stories about grief contains the Bible's shortest verse: "Jesus wept."[8] He had received the news that his friend Lazarus was gravely ill, but when he arrived in Bethany, Lazarus had died. The man's grieving sisters, Martha and Mary, approached Jesus, and when He saw Mary's deep sorrow, He was moved in spirit and wept with her. I always tell people that I believe our God shares every moment with us. You can trust Him; you can give Him your sorrows. Surrender your losses.

Anger, Guilt, and Love

It's generally accepted that smoking causes cancer. What's little known is that smoking alone may not be sufficient to produce it. A study in the 1960s concluded that smokers who suppressed emotion had five times the probability of developing cancer.[9] In fact, the more the person suppressed emotions, the less smoking was needed before cancer occurred. Another study confirmed that the incidence of cancer was forty times higher in smokers who had repressed anger issues than smokers who did not.[10] This actually suggests that smoking alone does not cause cancer—anger plus cigarettes does.

Sergio De La Mora, founding pastor of Cornerstone Church of San Diego, once preached, "Anger is the result of a person's need not being met."[11] One basic human need is to be loved. A small study with leukemia or lymphoma found that 85% of the patients reported feeling a loss through separation from a parent.[12] Another study with students found that 95% of the youth who rated their parents low on the caring and love scale suffered from some type of illness including heart disease, cancer, and asthma at midlife. Of the young adults who rated their parents high on caring and love, only 29% had any type of midlife illness.[13]

The hope is that if toxic emotions can be detected and remedied in children or adolescents, disease can be prevented.[14] Love and caring conquers all; even disease. If we consider that God is love, we must conclude that all healing come from God. In the same way a timeline can help identify feelings of loss, it can be used to identify events that triggered anger. Once the anger is identified, work toward releasing it.

Anger Timeline

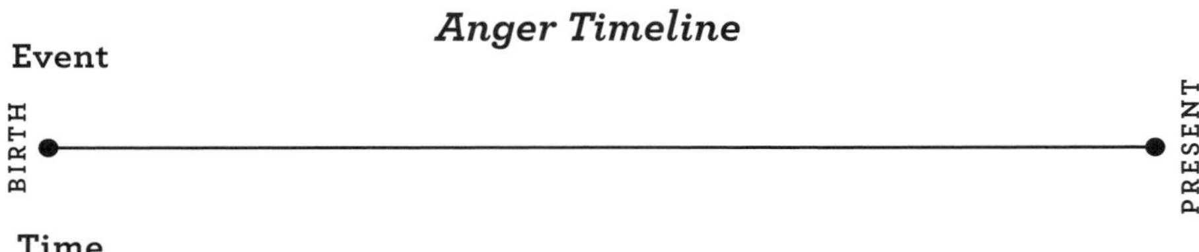

Another emotional issue many patients face is guilt. There may be things in their past eating them up on the inside, and many also feel a sense of responsibility for getting cancer.[15] Kay Cogswell, one of my greatest mentors, once said, "You can't live with guilt. You can live with regret." She invited grieving clients to shift their feelings of guilt to regret.

I encourage my patients to identify the things they feel guilty about on a guilt timeline and then reframe the way they look at the issue from self-blame to regret. Instead of saying, "It's my fault I crashed the car," he would say, "I regret being careless and crashing. I've learned from the accident and will be more attentive in the future." Take a moment to map out the things you feel guilty about and then shift your guilt about the issues to regret.

Guilt Timeline

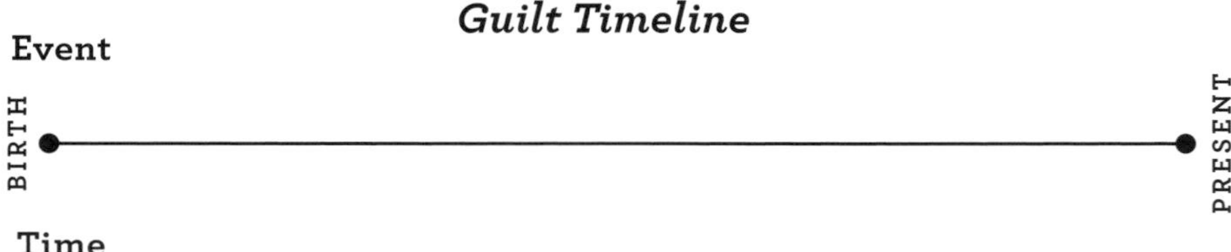

Forgiveness

We've come to the most important part of this chapter—forgiveness. In *Forgive for Good*, Dr. Fred Luskin states that forgiveness and self-forgiveness provide an opportunity for healing.[16] The topic was so important to Jesus that He included it in what we now call "The Lord's Prayer,"[17] asking God to forgive us as we forgive others. Clearly, we need forgiveness for offenses we've committed, and we need to forgive those who've hurt us. All emotional wounds and negative emotions can be healed through forgiveness. Take a moment and fill out a pain timeline, identifying the events where someone hurt you or vice versa.

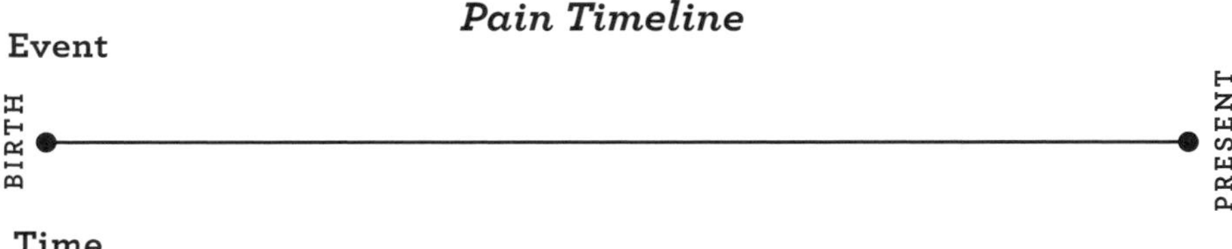

If you're able to ask forgiveness of the one you hurt, do. If you can make amends, do. Others may not ask forgiveness for hurting you, but you don't need them to ask. Simply forgive and move on with your life.

• • • • • • • • • • • •

Many people find it easy to forgive others but are unable to forgive themselves. But self-forgiveness is absolutely necessary. Consider what George Jacinto and Beverly Edwards wrote: "The act of forgiveness is the result of an individual giving up resentment and desire for retribution, the choice to cease rumination about being angry and resentful, and choosing to pardon the offending person or persons."[18]

Jacinto and Young Joon Hong developed these steps toward being able to forgive.[19] They suggest choosing the person to forgive, another or yourself, then visualizing the event that caused anger and expressing it with artwork. The drawing may express what words cannot as a positive way of externalizing the pain. Then, you can write down the experiences you've had with this person, good and bad. Reflect on these, then write a letter to him or her, expressing your pain and anger. You won't send it; you don't need to. You'll read the letter aloud, imagining that the one you need to forgive is listening. The final step is to let go and move on.

Try to apply this to yourself. Stop being angry. Give up self-hatred and criticism. Accept God's forgiveness and grace. Set yourself free.

Conclusion

Virginia Satir said, "We need 4 hugs a day for survival. We need 8 hugs a day for maintenance. We need 12 hugs a day for growth."[20] Once, when I ended a group session suggesting that everyone hug each other—I almost always end that way,[21] but that day was special—a woman stayed after. She had tears streaming down her face. When I asked what was going on, she said she lived alone and hadn't had a hug in ten years.

Be in contact with others daily. Hug, love, and live life to the fullest!

> The Holy Spirit produces this kind of fruit in our lives: love, joy, peace, patience, kindness, goodness, faithfulness, gentleness, and self-control. There is no law against these things![22]

Counselors recognize love, joy, peace, and hope as signs of spiritual health in a person.[23] Anger, resentment, bitterness, fear, hatred, envy, and anxiety are harmful to your soul; harmful to your body. Be filled instead with the fruit of the Spirit. Engage others with trust, honesty, compassion, and service. Health will ensue.

Let your spirit soar, and let your immune system rise with it.

ACTION STEPS

1. Use the timelines to identify and externalize negative emotions.
2. Write a letter about your pain. Read it aloud, make a statement of forgiveness, and dispose of it.
3. Give, and receive, healing hugs every day.

CANCER VICTOR TIPS

F. D., London, England
Stage IV Lung Cancer
Victor Since 1986

1. Seek a second opinion. Don't accept it when a doctor says, "There's nothing we can do for you."
2. Make amends with loved ones. Forgive others; ask for forgiveness.
3. Choose a doctor who knows how to integrate alternative and conventional treatments.
4. Get educated on the subject. What you know could save you.
5. After you're free of cancer, get regular check-ups and take natural preventative treatments periodically.

Emotional Roots of Cancer
https://vimeo.com/61545431

Chapter 10

Cancer Hand-Me-Downs

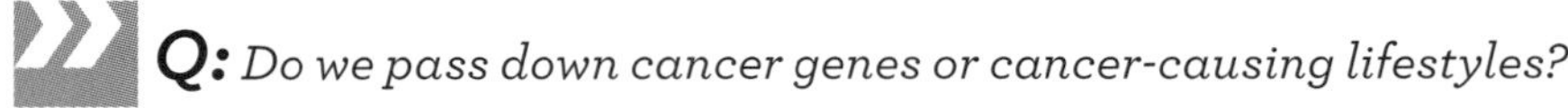

Q: *Do we pass down cancer genes or cancer-causing lifestyles?*

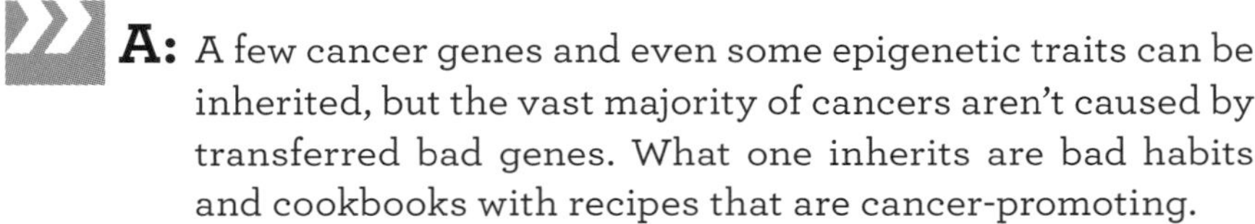

A: A few cancer genes and even some epigenetic traits can be inherited, but the vast majority of cancers aren't caused by transferred bad genes. What one inherits are bad habits and cookbooks with recipes that are cancer-promoting.

It's true, we are what we eat. And now we're learning that we also are what our parents ate. Researchers are uncovering the impact that our parent's diet, especially our mother's during pregnancy, has on modifying the behavior of specific genes that are essential for health maintenance. The better they ate, the better our genes will work for us.

Many genetic ailments and deficiencies are passed on due to what mothers eat, or don't eat, around the time they conceive. Under-nutrition can program their children's genes for trouble. Dr. Kevin Sinclair restricted mature female sheep's ingestion of folate, vitamin B_{12}, and the essential amino acid methionine during their mating period and found that their offspring developed into obese and significantly immune-challenged sheep in comparison to the ones from mothers fed the B vitamins and amino acids. It's clear that a diet deficient in methyl donor nutrients even for a short time around the time of conception can change DNA methylation of offspring and challenge their health for life.[1]

A research group led by Dr. Joanne Kotsopoulos proved that a low-folate diet for animals from post-weaning to puberty caused significant epigenetic changes that made them more susceptible to diseases in adulthood.[2]

In 2008 Dr. Karen Lillycrop investigated the effect in their juvenile and adult offspring of feeding pregnant rats a protein- and folic acid- restricted diet and reported that poor prenatal nutrition induces differential changes to methylation of individual genes in juveniles that persist in adults. This study was the first to demonstrate the epigenetic impact of diet on future generations.[3]

In another study, researchers found that parents' dietary patterns affect at least two future generations. Josep Jimenez-Chillaron and colleagues underfed and undernourished (low nutrition) pregnant mice, which then gave birth to low-weight offspring. The pups were skinny not only for lack of calories but also for a lack of methyl donor nutrients that caused epigenetic modification found to be associated with increased risk of obesity, diabetes, and cardiovascular disease during adulthood. Worse, they report, such risks may pass on to future generations.[4]

Epigenomes

Several research groups have used yellow agouti mice because of their peculiar agouti gene. These have a bright yellow coat, are obese, and are prone to cancer and diabetes. They have a sibling with the exact same genome but are called pseudoagouti because they look so different; these have a dark brown coat, are lean and healthy (very low propensity to cancer), and live longer. They're identical twins, so how do they look completely different and have such dissimilar health futures? While their genome is identical, their epigenome is not—it all has to do with methylation of their agouti gene. The obese yellow ones have it unmethylated; the lean brown ones have it methylated.

This gene, which we humans also carry, is easy to investigate. For instance, Dr. Robert Waterland tested two groups of yellow, fat, cancer-prone, pregnant agouti mice, giving one a diet rich in folic acid and vitamin B_{12} (well-known methyl donors), the other a B-vitamin-deficient diet. The yellow offspring of the latter developed into obese, health-challenged adults; the brown-coated pups of the fat yellow mothers developed into lean, mean (and healthy) machines! The oncologists got unhealthy agouti mothers to produce healthy brown pups of normal weight and not prone to diabetes or cancer, proving that the methyl donor nutrients (B vitamins) methylated (attached methyl groups to) the agouti gene.[5] Dr. Dana C. Dolinoy, another member of this team, was able to show similar results with the methyl donor genistein from soy.[6]

• • • • • • • • • • • • •

Obviously food *quality* is the primary concern, but, as Dr. Jimenez-Chillaron demonstrated, *quantity* also matters. Mothers, to give your children the best genetic platform, be careful what and how much you eat. And there's more: our fathers' diet is by no means irrelevant. Dr. Lars Bygren conducted an epidemiological study on the longevity of an agricultural community in Överkalix, in northern Sweden, during the nineteenth century and noticed a clear pattern of association between longevity and food availability. Weighing longevity of the descendants of well-fed boys during times of abundance vs. the descendants of famished boys during times of drought, he reported that the sons and grandsons of the former lived shorter lives than those of the latter. The differential was significant: The reward for boys who suffered the famine was grandchildren who outlived the grandsons of the overfed fortunate by at least six years. Further, when Bygren's team crunched the numbers, taking into account specific socioeconomic variations, difference in longevity jumped by an astonishing thirty-two years.[7–8]

The Dietary Need: Fewer Calories, More Nutrition

These studies correlate perfectly with one of the most effective ways to increase longevity: through a calorie-restricted but nutritionally rich diet, a case I made in *The Hope of Living Long and Well*.[9] Now we know that quality food in true moderation will reprogram our genes. We need no complicated data to see the obvious: We're witnessing a consequential explosion of obesity, diabetes, and cancer from environmental stressors on our epigenome: feasting on the wrong foods, exercising little, smoking, consuming too much alcohol, and abusing licit and illicit drugs.

Conclusion

The above studies clearly show that we cannot put all the blame on inherited genetic baggage—there *is* something we can do about it. What's exciting about genomics is that we can responsibly change the genetic abnormalities caused by environmental factors to modify the expression of critical genes linked to enhancing normal physiological events and to preventing and reversing pathologic processes, including obesity, aging, and cancer. A healthy lifestyle will eventually wipe away negative epigenetic marks, restoring your DNA code to its original programming. You can restore your health and foster the health of your dreams.

ACTION STEPS

1. Know that your genes do not determine your destiny.
2. Consume foods that will help reprogram your genes.
3. Rid yourself of dietary and lifestyle behaviors that stress your epigenome.

CANCER VICTOR TRIPS

Tine Hagedorn-Olsen, Denmark
Stage IV Breast Cancer and Ovarian Cancer
Victor Since 2001

1. Take charge, and seek knowledge. Demand answers from your inner soul; ask "What's the best treatment for me?"
2. Cleanse body and soul: Go on a vegan diet. Drink freshly made juice three times a day, and find a competent psychotherapist.
3. Pray and give thanks to God for the healing taking place in you, and visualize that every cell in your body is healed.
4. Accept your fear and use it to fuel your actions. Do all you can, and leave the rest to God.
5. Seek doctors who give you hope: Go to Oasis of Hope!

Cancer Hand-Me-Downs
https://vimeo.com/61292910

Chapter 11

The Cancer Genome

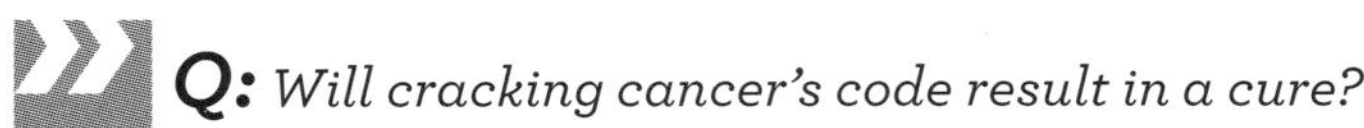

Q: *Will cracking cancer's code result in a cure?*

A: Cracking the human genome was difficult and expensive. Cracking cancer's genome is virtually impossible, for there are many cancer types, and each is singular to each patient. Efforts are now made to identify gene characteristics for each tumor, to establish sensitivity or susceptibility to specific drugs, with the goal of designing individualized therapies. But for some advances against breast cancer, researchers are far from making a dent in cancer on the whole.

One of history's most famous code-cracking devices was named for having been found in the Nile Delta town of Rashid (which means "Rosetta") by Pierre-François Bouchard in 1799 during a French expedition to Egypt. After the British won victory there two years later, the Rosetta Stone was transported to London; since 1802 it's been on public display as the most-visited object at the British Museum.

This artifact, a fragment of a much larger marker (*stele*), is the first ancient Egyptian object recovered in modern times engraved with trilingual text. In 196 BC King Ptolemy V moved to publish a decree, issued in Memphis, that he wished understood by all peoples, so he ordered it written in the era's three most common languages. The upper text is Egyptian hieroglyphs; the middle, Demotic script; the lower, Ancient Greek. The translational epiphanies made possible by the stone were elemental in deciphering the hieroglyph code that for so long had gone uncracked and ultimately revealing incalculable details about and insight into ancient Egyptian language and civilization.

• • • • • • • • • • • • •

All alphabets are codes that help us comprehend and explain the world around us through symbols. Since many words have the same letters, meaning is primarily determined by their sequence. For instance, two different sequences of our letters e, o, n and t have multiple and completely different meanings when combined as *note* and *tone*. Life's "alphabet" consists of just four—A, T, C and G—and their myriad sequences determine the code of our DNA, which is found in our genes. A gene is a portion, or a length, of DNA "letters," and its sequence contains the code (instructions) to make the specific chemicals, mainly proteins, that our body needs to survive. Proteins are our body's workforce: they control growth, generate defense mechanisms, break down food to release energy, and perform thousands of other vital tasks.

The Human Genome Project

Decode our DNA to help us understand our bodies—that was the purpose of the Human Genome Project, an incredible feat achieved by a code-cracking effort that mapped the blueprint for what makes us who we are. Begun in 1990 and completed in 2003, this gargantuan endeavor sequenced and identified all approximately 3.3 *billion* chemical units (known as base pairs) in the human genetic instruction set.

While this international undertaking was mostly sponsored by the US government through the Department of Energy and the National Institutes of Health (NIH), it also was aided considerably by funds and research from the UK, Japan, France, Germany, and Spain. In 2007, Craig Venter, founder of the parallel, private project Celera Genomics, led the group of scientists that published for the first time a complete DNA sequence of the six-billion-nucleotide genome of a single individual.[1]

Research continues. As of 2013, thousands of individual genomes have been completely sequenced, identifying the pairing of each chromosome within the DNA; many more have been mapped and are in the process of being sequenced. This info is used in multiple branches of science like biomedicine, anthropology, and forensics. The hope is that genomic studies will lead to advances in the prevention, diagnosis, and treatment of all diseases and to new insights in medicine and biology.

Cancer Is a Genetic Disease

At its root, cancer is a disease of genes. One in three people in the Western world will develop cancer, one in five will die of cancer; cancer is the most common genetic disease. All cancers develop due to DNA sequence errors (mutations) while replicating during routine cell regeneration; the result is the formation of aberrant, destructive tissue known as a malignant tumor. Such tumors, with their new genetic structures, establish a new set of rules through their mutated DNA sequences. In other words, they create their own genetic code.

This rogue genetic instructional manual enables cancer to thrive at the expense of other tissues, causing all kinds of havoc and destruction. The following are cancer's main lethal capabilities for overrunning normal tissue and spreading their terror throughout the body:

Proliferation. Malignant cells grow rapidly as their aberrant genes over-express growth factors and hormones to fuel multiplication.

Uncontrolled growth. Cancer cells become deaf to the antigrowth signals of normal tissues to establish their order and functionality.

"Immortality." For our protection, all normal cells have a planned-death ("expiration") date to be replaced by new ones; this is the process of apoptosis. Also, there's an intrinsic limit on the number of times a normal cell can divide; we call this a "cell line." Once every established replication has happened, this line—this family, so to say—is extinguished, and a new cell line appears, precisely to stop or delete any and all mutations from the former family.

1. Malignant cells disable the vital mechanism of apoptosis, which contributes even further to unopposed growth.
2. Cancer cell lines never extinguish and so continue to mutate and increase in aggression.

Angiogenesis (generation of blood vessels). Because tumors grow so rapidly, they need sustained blood vessel growth. To achieve this they over-express genes that produce the vasculo-endothelial growth factor (VEGF), a hormone-like protein that promotes new vessels' development to deliver the high-maintenance supplies.

Invasiveness. Cells of organs never invade other organs, no matter how close the contact is. For instance, a heart cell will never invade a lung or even a coronary vessel. Cancer cells defy multiple signals and forces that hold a cell in place and prevent it from traveling to (and thriving in) other tissues, a process called metastasis.

All these powers are enabled by abnormalities in cancer's DNA sequence, now called "the cancer genome." To improve diagnosis, treatment, and prevention through better understanding of the disease's molecular basis, scientists are striving to map out its genetic code using the knowledge, experience, and technology gathered by the Genome Project. To crack the code, they must identify all sequence variants and mutations that are critical in the development of human cancers.

Toward this goal, three ambitious projects got underway: The Cancer Genome Project (based at England's Wellcome Trust Sanger Institute), The Cancer Genome Atlas (funded by the National Cancer Institute [NCI] and the National Human Genome Research Institute), and The International Cancer Genome Consortium, a voluntary scientific organization that provides a forum for collaboration among the world's leading cancer and genomic researchers. All results are amalgamated and stored in the Catalogue of Somatic Mutations in Cancer (COSMIC) database. This approach has identified about 350 cancer-related genes and yielded many significant insights into this diabolical disease. It's estimated that through the project some two thousand genes for each of perhaps fifteen hundred tumor samples will be sequenced. To date hundreds of papers have been published on cancer genes, and tremendous progress is expected due to advances in computer sciences.

Even so, the more we learn about cancer's code the more we're stunned by its complexity. This is compounded by many cells also accumulating mutations that won't necessarily transform them into malignant cells. Further, it's necessary to identify and characterize all these changes to discover which mutations are unique to each cancer. Plus, there are both major ("driver") and minor ("passenger") mutations—drivers increase the growth rate and lead to more rapid tumor evolution and metastasis, while passengers (which are silent, or not important in the transformation process) are randomly distributed throughout the genome. Researchers estimate that the average tumor carries around eighty genetic mutations of which fewer than fifteen can be tagged as drivers. Thus one major sequencing goal is to identify driver mutations.

Environmental Factors

Believe it or not, this gets even more complicated. Mutations are not absolutely necessary for a cancerous transformation; environmental factors can influence perfect DNA to act malignantly without affecting its actual structure. This occurs in a process called epigenetics, which is the study of heritable changes in gene expression without changes in the DNA sequence. (The Greek *epi-* means "over," "above," or "outer"; thus the term basically means "on top of genetics" or "on top of the genes.") In essence, non-genetic factors cause the genes to behave (or, "express" themselves) differently, doing a lot more or a lot less of what they normally produce due to environmental mechanisms.

An "over-expressed" gene makes normal proteins but in dangerous or unhealthy amounts; when "under-expressed," it provides insufficient necessary proteins to maintain normalcy. These changes may remain through cell divisions for the remainder of the cell's life and even for multiple generations. So scientists are now also developing the *epi*genome, or the "epigenetic code," to describe the set of epigenetic features that create different phenotypes in different un-mutated cells.

Dr. Roger McLendon, using data from The Cancer Genome Atlas, found identifying characteristics in 206 glioblastomas (the most common type of adult brain cancer) and believes these findings establish the feasibility and power of The Atlas to "rapidly expand knowledge of the molecular basis of cancer."[2] Dr. Lijin Li is optimistic because of the revolution happening with new dramatic advances in DNA-sequencing platforms. His research group predicts that these technologies will make it possible within the next few years for a cancer patient to do a personal cancer genome test at an affordable cost of $1,000. They likewise maintain that tests like these will help "real-time decision-making with the potential to affect diagnosis, prognosis, and treatment, and have opened the door towards personalized medicine."[3]

Still in Development

As we'll soon observe (see chapter 12, under "Genetic Inheritance"), at present, personal-genomics analysis requires further research and development to become a practical application. Translating sequence information into a clinical treatment plan is highly complicated, requires experts of many different fields, and is not guaranteed to lead to effective treatment. Dr. Laura D. Wood conducted a large-scale screen for somatic mutations in breast and colorectal tumors and reported that many low-frequency mutations contribute to cancer development and growth; if cancer's survival depends on multiple mutations of small effect, she concludes that it's unlikely genome sequencing will uncover a single "Achilles' heel" target for anti-cancer drugs.[4]

As in so many other aspects of research, in this project, at least for now, there's been much effort with far too little gain. Up to 2010 the National Cancer Institute had invested $375 million; the International Cancer Genome Consortium, which aims to sequence 25,000 tumor samples, is expected to spend more than $1 billion.[5] Robert Allan Weinberg has said that this project is "money poured down a hole. Sequencing endless more cancer genomes isn't going to tell us more than we already know."[6]

Conclusion

Whether or not this is true today, I hope that in the future all the knowledge accumulated by these efforts and expenditures will translate into improved diagnosis, treatment, and prevention strategies. Even though I believe we're decades away for this technology to come full force to the trenches of cancer's battleground, there are some practical applications that we'll discuss in the upcoming chapters.

The Cancer Genome
https://vimeo.com/61302080

ACTION STEPS

1. Be careful about genetic testing, no matter how sophisticated. Many of the results are at best relative—again, currently we are far from decoding cancer.
2. Most tests on the market are done from blood samples. These are good for normal genome sequencing, but for a cancer genome the sample is best obtained from the tumor.
3. If you have a test done, be sure to consult an experienced oncologist who will put the results in the context of your condition.

CANCER VICTOR TRIPS

Al Harrison, Canada
Prostate Cancer
Victor Since 2007

1. When you're diagnosed, don't jump to any conclusions.
2. No matter what the doctors say, there is always hope. Trust in God.
3. In my opinion, don't take chemotherapy—it's poison that will kill off your body as well as some of the cancer.
4. Trust in the Lord. He said He won't give us more than we can handle.
5. In my opinion, always use alternative ways instead of Western ways to treat your cancer.
6. No doctor or treatment can help the person with cancer if he believes the cancer is going to kill him. Have faith. Your mind can rally the healing forces in your body to defeat the cancer.
7. Diet is a must to change, and you must stick to the diet or you're wasting your time. Stay away from animal protein; if you don't, the cancer will come back with a vengeance.

Chapter 12

Cancer Predictors

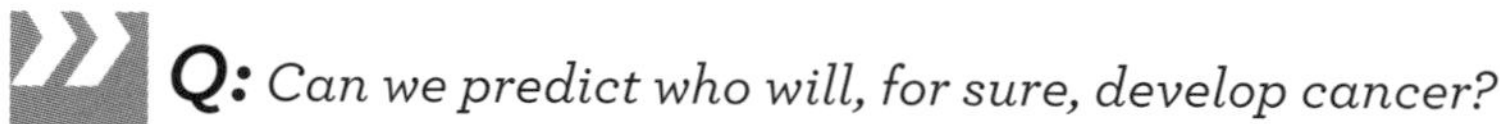

Q: *Can we predict who will, for sure, develop cancer?*

A: No. Some gene alterations may indicate an increased risk. Even without predictors, lifetime risk is 1 in 2 for men, 1 in 3 for women.[1] Regardless, you can greatly reduce risk by changing your lifestyle. You don't have to get cancer.

Predictions are one of humankind's most practiced pastimes, and we're getting better at them. Mathematical odds have proven accurate; the art of prognosticating more and more is fine-tuned by algorithmic models. The local news meteorologist probably is no longer such a target of regional scorn, and even polls on politicians are remarkably precise.

Regarding medicine, it's vital that we understand the implications of diseases and be able to estimate incidence, morbidity, and mortality in our populations as well as prognoses to establish proper individual treatments. For instance, acute bacterial infections, like "strep throat," need immediate treatment, whereas viral infections, such as the common cold, tend to be self-limited to three days. A well-trained pediatrician will only treat the symptoms of fever and pain if they persist after seventy-two hours. If they do, then most likely the infection is bacterial rather than viral, and now (but only now) should antibiotics be started.

For these and many other reasons, statisticians and clinicians for centuries have taken into account risk factors to determine the odds of persons and populations developing certain diseases. This data is analyzed and compiled in the hope that practitioners and the general populace take advantage of the info to reduce the possibility of falling prey.

Risk Factors: Two Types

Generally, risks are either modifiable (avoidable) or un-modifiable (unavoidable). Too often we choose to put our health at risk through irresponsible choices like smoking, drinking, consuming junk foods, not exercising, and so on. These factors we certainly can do something about. Simultaneously, just being a man puts him at risk of developing prostate cancer, relieves him of any ovarian cancer risk, and minimizes his risk of breast cancer; one un-modifiable risk is gender. Another could be age, in that some cancers are common in children and others after sixty. Another is genetic baggage, for diseases that run in the family.

As certain mutated-cancer-causing genes are discovered, many people are hoping that eventually we'll be able not only to predict each individual's risk for a given cancer but also to determine precise therapy with drugs that exclusively kill a diagnosed patient's particular tumor. Imagine knowing that our blueprints show no cancer on the horizon.

At the same time, our world is imperfect. One intrinsic downside of this technology is that a person who tested negative likely would sense a false security in regard to modifiable risk factors. A second is that a person found to have some rogue genes would be as likely (or more so) to feel, in terms of cancer, that it's not a matter of if but of when. As we'll see (here and in chapter 14), the truth is that a healthy and responsible lifestyle pays high dividends regardless of genetic heritage. Even for the exceptions or rarities—e.g., those who abuse their bodies immensely while never developing cancer, or the lifelong health fanatics who develop cancer in their thirties—genes are not necessarily the culprit.

Family ties often are blamed for tumors, especially those of breast cancer. It's said that if a couple close relatives (say, mother and aunt) have been diagnosed, then your risk increases exponentially—in other words, is genetically inherited. This hypothesis was validated, somewhat, by the discovery in the Ashkenazi (Eastern European) Jewish population of mutations called Breast Cancer Genes 1 and 2 (BRCA1, BRCA2). UC Berkeley in 1990 was first to describe BRCA1; in 1994 other scientists first cloned it; one year later still others cloned BRCA2.

Both mutated genes produce proteins that block DNA repair, thus promoting malignant cell growth. Different research groups report different incidence statistics, but the latest (2012) estimates that women with an abnormal BRCA1 or BRCA2 have up to a 60% risk of developing breast cancer by age 90 (vs. 13% minus the genetic alterations) and, for ovarian cancer, about 55% and about 25% for women with BRCA1 and BRCA2 mutations, respectively (vs. 1.6% for non-carriers).[2]

According to the above mentioned study, these mutations affect at most 5% of all women with breast cancer. Let me put this in perspective. First, of all who develop breast cancer, the vast majority—*95%*—does not have breast cancer genes. One study found that less than 1% of breast cancer patients actually had the mutated genes.[3] But, even though just 5% of women suffering breast cancer have hereditary BRCA 1 or 2 abnormalities, most researchers and clinicians *still* consider family history the strongest contributing risk factor. *Why?*

Knowledge Is Not Equivalent to Wisdom

Due to the established doctrine that genes determine fate, women have been lured into preemptively removing their breasts (bilateral prophylactic mastectomy) and/or ovaries when considered high-risk because of family history (defined as two or more first-degree diagnosed relatives). I'll repeat this: *Some women are choosing the surgical removal of both healthy breasts to prevent a cancer that may never appear.*

This practice increased when BRCA 1 and 2 first came into the picture. For instance, led by Lynn C. Hartmann, Mayo Clinic surgeons retrospectively reviewed the results of 639 women who'd undergone this procedure between 1960 and 1993 with a family history of breast cancer. Their finding? "Prophylactic mastectomy was associated with a reduction in the incidence of breast cancer of at least 90%."[4] Their basis? Among the 639, twenty breast-cancer-related deaths were expected during the observation period, and only two occurred, "equal to" 90% efficacy. They *assumed* that eighteen women had been saved by the procedure.

However, consider the way they reached their conclusions. First, we're discussing outcomes from a retrospective (backward-looking) analysis, which in the research world is suboptimal at best. Second, they expressed results in relative terms—"two deaths instead of twenty means '90% effective.'" By the absolute numbers, 621 women who likely would've survived without prophylactic mastectomy paid a price that, were it not for prediction-induced fear, most would have rejected if they'd known their true odds of dying from breast cancer. Even if the relative number is correct, for every death avoided, thirty-five women underwent a disfiguring, psychologically damaging operation.[5]

Dr. Deborah Schrag evaluated the absolute results of prophylactic bilateral mastectomy and crafted a computer model to predict the average life expectancy among women with BRCA mutations. In the aptly titled "*BRCA* Genes—Bookmaking, Fortunetelling, and Medical Care," the late Dr. Healy Bernadine, first woman ever to be NIH director, said of Schrag's model,

> Adding one statistical prophecy to another, they estimate that prophylactic mastectomy leads to about 3 to 5 years of additional life expectancy and prophylactic oophorectomy [ovarian removal] 4 to 20 months, depending on the levels of risk used.[6]

Is it really worth having your body mutilated for such meager gains, especially when the odds are on your side of never even developing breast cancer? Healy concluded, "Information about the value of a preemptive strike against cancer in carriers of *BRCA* mutations is at best primitive, and better data will take years to obtain from controlled clinical trials."[7]

She was right. In 2008, Dr. Sarah Fuller did a mathematical analysis (qualitative review) of the publications on primary prevention strategies against BRCA mutations. Crunching the numbers from ten of these to evaluate the efficacy of prophylactic bilateral mastectomy, prophylactic bilateral oophorectomy (removal of both ovaries), and tamoxifen prevention, she found that three of the ten, including the Mayo study mentioned above, reported a reduction of more than 95% of the incidence of breast cancer in women who had the surgical procedure. Nonetheless, she concluded, "These trials are of insufficient methodological quality."[8] In other words, the results aren't reliable.

Fuller also stated, "The data on the effectiveness of prophylactic bilateral mastectomy on mortality is not available." Six other studies had better methodology to evaluate the efficacy of prophylactic bilateral salpingo-oophorectomy (removal of both ovaries and Fallopian tubes) and reported a reduction of approximately 50% in the incidence of breast cancer; only one trial reveals a mortality reduction after bilateral salpingo-oophorectomy. The other study Fuller and her team reviewed was of chemoprevention with tamoxifen, which did not yield significant improvement in incidence or mortality.

Fuller recommended in 2008 exactly what Healy stated in 1997: that more studies, especially controlled and prospective (vs. retrospective), should be done in order to accurately evaluate the efficacy of these procedures. The obvious message to surgical oncologists is that we need to know more before we recommend these mastectomies to women with actual or supposed high-risk factors for breast cancer.

Hyper-Caution May Cause Unnecessary Suffering

There are clear precedents for the precautionary position I've been describing. One example: for decades doctors recommended hormone replacement therapy to menopausal woman to prevent heart disease, even though we knew it increased the risk of breast cancer, because more women would die from heart disease than from cancer. These recommendations were based on observational and retrospective studies without data from controlled studies. Finally, a prospective study, known as the Women's Health Initiative, was designed to evaluate efficacy, but it had to be stopped early because the risks outweighed the benefits.

In fact, the most dramatic decrease in breast cancer incidence ever registered by the American Cancer Society's "Cancer Facts & Figures" has been attributed to reductions in the use of menopausal hormone therapy, previously known as hormone replacement therapy, following publication of results from the Women's Health Initiative.[9] This study found that use of combined estrogen plus progestin was associated with an increased risk of coronary heart disease *and* of breast cancer!

Geneticists and clinicians have established inherited cancers as a category. I disagree that this should be a category. I'll explain this later (see chapter 14); for the moment, let us not forget that inherited forms of cancer are rare (only about 5% of all adult-onset cancers), even as we must be aware that inherited-cancer-promoting genes are aggressive.

Another gene causing terror is CDH1 (discovered in 1998), which is responsible for aggressive cancers like hereditary diffuse gastric cancer, hereditary nonpolyposis colorectal cancer, and familial adenomatous polyposis. As with breast cancer, persons with strong family ties to these diseases have been treated with prophylactic surgeries. To the gastric cancer, the response has been total gastrectomy (stomach removal); to the other two colon conditions, total colectomy (colon removal). These surgery types are far more complication-prone and more damaging to quality of life than mastectomies, just as these cancers are highly lethal in comparison to breast cancer.

Dr. H. J. Järvinen conducted a fifteen-year, controlled, prospective study to evaluate alternative methods to prophylactic surgery with persons at high risk to hereditary colorectal cancers. His hypothesis was simple: when in doubt, err on the side of caution. Because we don't know who will develop cancer due to genetic mutations, or when, and because we now have superb screening technology, close surveillance is a viable and safe option to prophylactic surgery. The study included 252 high-risk CDH1 gene carriers of twenty-two different families. About half were screened with colonoscopies; the other half, the control group, went without. The screened group had 66% fewer colorectal cancers than the control group and, because of early detection, suffered no deaths from cancer, whereas there were nine in the control group.[10]

Predictor Models

Mathematical and computer models have helped political scientists and meteorologists improve their prognostic accuracy; the cancer-gene-sequencing field hasn't gotten the same results. Concern is mounting for the lack of practical applications; some researchers say current risk-prediction algorithms underperform by not allowing for potential synergistic effects. After billions of research dollars, skepticism that personalized genomics will be of clinical benefit is growing.

Recently, Harvard School of Public Health scientists examined in detail the relationship between the genetic variants of breast cancer and environmental risk factors. It's the first study to evaluate the claims, or hopes, that genetics can improve disease-risk prediction enough to aid in prevention and treatment. Lead researcher Hugues Aschard incorporated the most advanced algorithms and analytical models (including potential synergistic effects) for the evaluation of three common diseases including cancer of the breast. He considered fifteen common genetic variations associated with breast cancer risk (not just BRCAs) as well as environmental factors like age of first menstruation, age at first time giving birth, and number of close relatives who developed breast cancer.

The models generated a variety of statistical combinations of genetic and environmental factors, but none produced marked improvement in predicting disease risk over lifestyle factors alone. So, old school (inexpensively) still rules. While optimistic about the future of genomics, Dr. Aschard said we're far from understanding the complexity of genetic testing to correctly interpreting their results; furthermore, that "[t]he road to efficient genetic risk prediction, if it exists, is likely to be long."[11]

Conclusion

What then can we do to assure frightened women with heavy genetic baggage? One of this book's main purposes is to provide information to inspire confidence that even if your genes seem stacked against you, you have means at your disposal to come out on top. I believe we can use the dramatic advances in genetics to apply better means against rogue genes. Taking into account that prophylactic surgery leaves women disfigured and distraught, that its results are suspect, and that preventive gastrectomies and colectomies have high morbidity and mortality rates, the possibility of effective, nonsurgical, humane prophylaxis for those with cancer-prone genetic material is invigorating.

I've made the argument that up to now genetic testing is not mature enough for us to make preemptive therapeutic decisions because we still lack the tools to fully understand or correctly interpret the test results. Until then, let us provide without bias ample info about all implications and limitations tied to genetic testing. With time, experience, and better protocols, genetic evaluations will be a tremendous tool for better preventing, diagnosing, and treating disease. The discovery and identification of cancer-susceptibility genes (especially the BRCAs) has opened the door to an intense gene-hunting effort for more predicting traits, an important step toward a better understanding of cancer's biology. It also set the stage for the pursuit of mapping all our genes (known as The Human Genome Project—see chapter 11).

Cancer Predictors
https://vimeo.com/61362038

ACTION STEPS

1. No genes cause cancer. There are mutations that can make a person more prone to it, but no available test tags a label of cancer to a person. Your lifestyle decisions are more powerful than genes.
2. Some genetic tests are available. If you opt to do them, take the results and recommendations as suggestions to consider; seek the opinions of experienced oncologists.
3. Read on. You'll find information to counter any genetic baggage.

CANCER VICTOR TRIPS

SueAnne Bassett, Georgia
Stage IV Cervical Cancer
Victor Since 2004

1. Submit yourself wholly to the Lord Jesus Christ. *Then*, be determined, and single-minded, to fight the cancer battle and *believe* you will be healed. Read God's Word, and claim His promises for healing.
2. Change to a vegan diet immediately. Eat as many organic whole foods as you can without frying, grilling, or adding a lot of ingredients.
3. Begin drinking fresh (preferably organic) vegetable juices (esp. green and carrot). Try starting off with two quarts daily, and try to drink them when they're fresh.
4. If you're physically able to exercise, start walking daily in the fresh air; go for two to five miles, briskly, if you can. While walking, begin praising the Lord with each step. Quote Scriptures that encourage you and strengthen you; know that it is God who is our Healer!
5. If you have surgery to remove as much cancer as possible, get whole-body alternative/holistic treatment to build your body's good cells to fight and win the tough battle *before* submitting to conventional therapy (chemo/radiation). I suggest Oasis of Hope, and I suggest you listen and do everything the doctors say to do while you're there. *Do your own research* so that you're equipped to battle as naturally and effectively as possible; statistics show that chemo and radiation alone don't have a good track record for healing.

Chapter **13**

Targeted Cancer Therapy

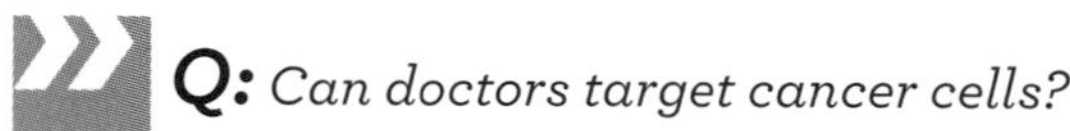

Q: *Can doctors target cancer cells?*

A: Yes. Researchers are investing vast resources in search of genes for this purpose. We can also target effectively and much less expensively with therapies like high-dose vitamin C and signaling transduction.

The aim of the genome projects is to develop personalized therapies based on genetic profiling; however, the complexity of cancer continues to challenge our efforts, intelligence, and patience. If genes so far have been ineffective in *predicting* cancer, what other practical applications can we glean from the wealth of accruing information?

Marksmanship vs. the Shotgun Approach

In the late seventies, based on the incontrovertible fact that only a small percentage of patients respond to strict orthodox protocols designed for specific malignancies, we began to design more flexible protocols to treat our patients (instead of their cancers), taking into account their singular interaction with their tumors. In other words, we began profiling our patients to tailor therapies to individual needs.

At an oncological meet in 1977 I was criticized for this approach. I responded that the reason for much of the failure in results was the notion that a patient must fit into a protocol rather than fitting the protocol to the patient. Typical orthodox therapies are akin to shoe stores that would offer nothing but size eights—to all clients. I'm so thankful that now we actually want to offer shoes of all sizes by genetically profiling them; the oncological community is finally seeking to leave behind the shotgun approach to treating cancer.

Though the Cancer Genome Project carries many objectives, its main goal is to find the genetic roots of disease, develop effective treatments and, ultimately, identify both the genetic variants that increase their risk and possible means to prevent them. Interpretation of genome data is still in its initial stages, but we're already using our deeper understanding to explore potential therapeutic approaches. DNA sequencing provides priceless data at the molecular level, for it helps to determine the fundamental pathways of cellular processes that may facilitate curative means that heretofore were unavailable.

This approach is particularly needed in cancer therapy, where oft-used agents are ineffective in many patients and where side effects are common, given the nonspecific action mechanism of most chemo drugs. For instance, Dr. Bernard F. Cole did a meta-analysis (mathematical and statistical examination) of all major chemo trials for breast cancer and found that most still-menstruating women with early stage breast cancer are given adjuvant chemo.[1] They receive this extremely toxic and often cancer-*causing* treatment after surgery because it's shown to reduce the possibility of the tumor coming back; however, its absolute survival benefit is only 3% at five years and 5% at ten years. In other words, 95% to 97% of the patients are being over-treated. In fact, Donald J. Brennan estimates that 70% to 80% of these inherently low-risk patients would also have survived without adjuvant therapy and thereby avoided potentially toxic side effects.[2]

• • • • • • • • • • • •

For patients with all cancers and in all stages, unfortunately, much chemotherapy is administered as a shot in the dark. Why? Because to date there's no reliable method to establish whether a patient needs chemo, and, if so, to which chemo the malignancy will be sensitive. Many researchers believe the light at tunnel's end is pharmacogenomics, a new discipline wherein drugs are developed based on the genetic structure of pathological entities (e.g., tumors). Some believe it could be the ultimate in patient-treatment individualization as the genomics-based approach would (theoretically) accurately predict his/her response to medications. While efforts to date have not yielded practical applications, researchers are inching ever closer, and perhaps soon we may have the methodology to tap into this extraordinarily complex genetic mesh and couple the right pharmaceutical or nutraceutical to its suitable cancerous cell.

As scientists race toward "chemosensitivity profiles" for thousands of chemical compounds, advanced DNA microarray technology allows them to simultaneously evaluate thousands of genes, gene sequencing, and gene expression to gather and process data. For instance, Jane E. Staunton and her Harvard group, who've developed an algorithm to ascertain malignant-cell chemosensitivity based on gene expression profiles alone,[3] were able to determine the expression levels of 6,817 genes from a panel of sixty human cancer-cell lines kept at the National Cancer Institute. They used these "expression signatures" to classify the sensitivity or resistance for 232 drugs. The accuracy of chemosensitivity prediction was considerably better than would be expected by chance, and they concluded that, at least for a subset of compounds, genomic approaches to chemosensitivity prediction are feasible.

Genetic Profiling

The long-term apex of this phenomenal technology is in its potential to reduce the number of patients who receive chemo ineffectively and to accurately establish a reliable prognosis. Still, the real question is, *will* genetic profiling prolong survival and decrease cancer's devastating death rate? More than forty studies profiling breast cancer genetically with this technology have been published, with over-optimistic results; the data was not uniformly established and cross-validation has been problematic, especially because most studies were retrospective. To resolve these shortcomings and seek practical implementation, in 2004 the European Organization for Research and Treatment of Cancer (EORTC) and the Breast International Group (BIG) established TRANSBIG—a "sister network of excellence"—dedicated to multinational translational research. BIG headquarters manages and oversees the collaboration between twenty-eight institutions in eleven nations.

The main goal of MINDACT (Microarray In Node-negative Disease . . . may Avoid ChemoTherapy), the first TRANSBIG mega-study aimed at "translating" molecular knowledge into improved treatment tailoring for early breast cancer management, is to genetically profile patients and identify those unlikely to benefit from adjuvant chemo. Hypothetically, the number of women exposed could be reduced by as much as 25% without increasing the risk of local (primary-tumor) or distant (metastatic) recurrence. Recruitment was completed with 6,700 patients enrolled from 119 participating institutions in nine European countries. Anticipated date of completion is January 2017.

Some preliminary results are not encouraging. Following the analysis of 291 independent samples from six independent institutions, the MINDACT research trial had to be redesigned because, according to Dr. Rabiya S. Tuma, the number crunching showed increased risk for metastasis in early stage breast cancer in comparison with the original validation studies.[4] Lead researcher Dr. Martine Piccart also stated the obvious: proving statistically that one treatment option is better than the other is very difficult. The changes, she hopes, will not alter the goal of treating 25% fewer women with chemo.

So we must wait until 2017 or thereabouts to see if genetic profiling is helpful in establishing prognostic value and therapeutic impact for patients with early breast cancer. If you have any other kind of malignancy, the wait is much, much longer.

• • • • • • • • • • • •

There's no question genomic profiling research is provocative, that identifying patients who can avoid prolonged, toxic regimens is a major advance. Nevertheless, to date, predicting a tumor's sensitivity to a given chemotherapy is particularly challenging; further, genetic signature is only one of many factors that determine whether or not a drug will kill a cancer cell. In truth, the mechanisms by which a malignant cell resists or protects itself from the chemo attack are still poorly understood.

It's unquestionable that DNA microarray studies will help to develop individualized therapy, but its actual benefit in the clinical setting is debatable. I agree that avoiding toxicity and expense is a worthy goal; unfortunately, that in itself does not greatly increase the overall number of patients cured, and in that sense the absolute survival and death rates of cancer patients will be unaffected.

We must understand that this marvelous technology is only being used to determine if a tumor is sensitive or resistant to chemotherapy—drugs that have been proven highly ineffective in the war against cancer. *To improve cancer survival we must develop more effective and less toxic therapeutic agents.* The Cancer Genome Project no doubt will yield results, but we do not necessarily need to wait for scientists to intrude into the most intimate area of people and their malignancies to tailor-make the most effective therapies; we already have at our disposal sufficient means to tailor therapies for patient-specific needs.

Conclusion

For decades at Oasis of Hope we've been profiling our patients' malignancies in relation to their immune system's quality. Based on this, we've tailored their therapies to provide physical, emotional, and spiritual resources to fight their cancers. We're eager and willing to apply innovative technologies to improve individual and collective outcomes, but we're more interested in designing more effective therapies than in rehashing ineffective and toxic drugs in newer settings. For this reason we always are reviewing the medical literature for new findings and seeking better ways to make them practical to today's cancer challenges.

ACTION STEPS

1. Be always on the lookout for new technologies. Evaluate whether they're ready now or if they're a hope for a future generation of patients. Support research in any way you can.
2. Even if the full impact is not immediate, find out if any part of it is available for your benefit. For instance, right now there's sufficient genetic profiling that has practical treatment implications for some aggressive breast cancers called "triple negative."
3. Find doctors and institutions that keep up with nonstop worldwide cancer research so you know that all angles of your specific situation will be addressed.

CANCER VICTOR TIPS

Suzie T., Australia
Breast Cancer
Victor Since 2011

1. Find a hospital specializing in cancer treatment, that has published statistics on survival rates, and that encourages you to talk to past patients to determine if it's right for you.
2. Find a hospital whose philosophy is based on spiritual principles (love, faith, compassion, respect, etc.) and explains the facts in a balanced, truthful way so you feel safe and calm. Avoid any hospital that engages in fear marketing, which only serves to heighten anxiety and distress.
3. Ensure that it has an integrated approach to treatment, wherein the doctors, nurses, patient care staff, et al., discuss your case and, as a team, find the best solution using a holistic approach (i.e., taking into consideration not just the cancer but also your living situation, career, emotions, personality, spirituality, and future quality of life).
4. Make sure it has a comforting environment (nice décor and gardens, clean rooms without being sterile, pleasant smelling rather than of toxic fumes from cleaning agents) and a healthy, caring culture (compassionate staff, fresh organic food, happy staff and nurses who encourage fun, laughter, music, positivity, etc.).
5. Know that it provides a long-term follow-up program, with backup support, for when you leave and continue the healing process at home.

Targeted Cancer Therapy
https://vimeo.com/61378255

Chapter 14

Epigenetics

Q: *Can we do something about our genetic baggage?*

A: The real genetic baggage we're carrying is epigenetic. These genetic changes are in fact reversible in one generation through lifestyle changes.

The Epigenome

There are so many hopes that deciphering our genetic code will allow us to read our destiny, predicting if and which diseases are found within our blueprint and when they will or won't strike. Ideally, we'll design ways and means (therapies) that interfere with our imperfect genetic structure and change fate. However, after sequencing the three billion-plus nucleotides (for about a dollar each) of the twenty-some-thousand genes that make our DNA, the somber conclusion of the Human Genome Project, the most critical scientific enterprise ever undertaken, is that we've found our makeup to be so complex that we still must wait for benefits to be reaped. And, by wait, I mean *really* wait.

For now we're left with a sense that we must resign to our DNA destiny since, for the time being, it cannot be altered. How true is this? Well, there's a lot of evidence that the DNA we were born with does *not* completely determine our future. Mutations aren't even necessary for diseases or differences to occur. For instance, "identical" twins have exactly the same DNA, having come from a single fertilized egg cell (zygote); yet, though very similar, they're not identical at all.

In 2008, Robert Kucharski and his colleagues investigated the reason for the differentiation between worker bees and queen bees, which are genetically identical.[1] Why, if their DNA is exactly the same, do the queens develop fertility capabilities (like functional ovaries and a larger abdomen for egg-laying) while workers remain sterile? Why do queens develop behaviors such as killing rival queens, "piping" (communication sounds), and going on mating flights while the worker bees have no fun?

The difference, Dr. Kucharski reports, is the queen's diet. The larva that becomes a queen is the one that gobbles the largest quantities of royal jelly that, appropriately, is secreted from glands on worker bee heads. Royal jelly is exclusively the queen's diet for the rest of her life.

Bee larvae by default develop into the "worker" variety due to one specific gene. It's the complex, protein-rich royal honey, according to these scientists, that silences or turns off this key gene, triggering other normally silenced genes to jump into action (be turned on), converting the lucky larvae into queens. In other words, the royal jelly causes major larvae differentiation without structural changes of the bees' DNA.

This fascinating discovery offers an explanation for the "identical" twin differentiation, for example, how one can develop diabetes or cancer and the other doesn't. Environmental factors must cause the differences observed between the individuals that share the same genome; these factors can also be internal and not necessarily detrimental. All our cells have the same genetic code, yet some will become liver cells, others skin, kidney, et al, depending on which genes are turned on and which off.

Epigenetic Marks

As mentioned in chapter 11, epigenetics, the science that studies these non-structural DNA changes, literally means "on top of the genes." The way these environmental factors modify gene activity is by attaching a chemical to a normal nucleotide sequence (DNA code or "alphabet"), causing abnormal gene behavior. These chemicals are earmarks (called epigenetic marks) that scientifically are known as DNA methylation, histone modification, and chromatin remodeling.

Epigenetic marks are fascinating and complex, but basically it takes only the addition of a methyl group (DNA methylation) to change a gene's agenda. A gene's main function is to produce the proteins necessary to create cells and tissues and to sustain life. Genes must produce specific proteins in specific amounts at the specific time needed for the task at hand. Potentially, any glitches in the process can be lethal—health is predicated on good gene behavior. Scientifically, we say genes "express" themselves when they do their thing (e.g., produce proteins).

Epigenetic marks alter a gene's expression, turning it off or on, dampening it or making it louder. In other words, the proteins needed may not be produced at all, or produced in less than or in excess of desirable amounts, none of which is healthy. But some marks are absolutely necessary to maintain health, jump-starting good genes that extend life and silencing bad genes to prevent disease. If these marks don't work properly, mistakes in gene expression happen, and cancer development or cell death can be the consequence.

Until recently we believed our genome controlled the totality of gene expression. Epigenetics has changed that view. Now we know that a large percentage of (if not most) gene behavior depends on epigenetic marks. For this reason, and because epigenetics had become central in biology, in 2008 NIH director Elias Zerhouni announced a nationwide initiative to study the epigenetic processes with an initial grant of $190 million.

This is a drop in the genetic research bucket; again, consider that it took $3 billion to map the human genome (less than twenty-five thousand genes). Our *epigenome* consists of variables of patterns of epigenetic marks. According to Dr. Joseph R. Ecker, a leading authority on molecular biology and genetics, the number of variants is certainly in the millions. "A full epigenome map" he says, "will require major advances in computing power. When completed, the Human Epigenome Project (already underway in Europe) will make the Human Genome Project look like homework that 15th century kids did with an abacus."[2]

Epigenetic marks have been studied since at least the 1970s and always have been understood to be important for cell differentiation, but they long were obscured by the star, the earlier Genome Project. In my opinion, the genome will be the foundation for epigenomic progress because the former is akin to the hardware and the latter to the software. No matter how expensive and sophisticated your computer, it's only as powerful and effective as the software you install on it.

The scientific community is excited and chilled about epigenetics, perhaps the most important breakthrough since the genome, because it shifts the paradigm from nature to nurture. In other words, *we no longer can blame our genes; we must take responsibility for our behavior.* There's evidence that lifestyle choices like smoking and overeating can change the epigenetic marks to cause the genes for obesity to express themselves too strongly and the genes for longevity to express themselves too weakly. We all know you can truncate your own life if you smoke or overeat; what's *chilling* is that those same behaviors can also predispose your kids—before they're even conceived—to disease and early death.

What's *exciting* is that if you change your behavior, your genes change too! A bad habit by our parents or ourselves epigenetically programs our genes to work against us. By improving our habits we can epigenetically reprogram genes to work for us with the added advantage that we will bestow upon our next generation a better epigenome.

Conclusion

For years I've fought the concept that we're inheriting bad genes, especially for breast cancer-prone families. I maintained that what these women were inheriting was bad habits and family cookbooks. Though I accept that we inherit high-risk genetic traits, because of these findings I feel partially vindicated; what's passed on to us are un-mutated genes, epigenetically altered by our ancestors' habits. Normally we do adopt, implement, and pass these on—but we can change all that! Even if our destiny were written in our DNA, we can rewrite it by espousing diet, lifestyle, and environmental changes to switch on genes that promote health and switch off genes that lead to diseases.

ACTION STEPS

1. Adopt an anti-cancer (e.g., vegan) diet.
2. Walk briskly for thirty minutes, three to four times a week.
3. If you smoke, quit now.

CANCER VICTOR TIPS

Caleb Dominguez, California
Acute Lymphoblastic Leukemia (Cerebrospinal Fluid/Brain Metastasis)
Victor Since 1996

1. *Do not try to take on cancer alone.* Put aside pride; don't believe you are a burden. Include as many people as possible in your struggle, sharing as much detail as you feel comfortable with but enough so they can contribute to your recovery. Be straightforward with

needs; let them know how they can help. Many times friends and family are afraid to ask, not knowing what to do or wondering how to assist.

2. *Take an active role: Be in charge of your battle to take back your health.* You may feel all your control is lost with a diagnosis, but you can still greatly affect your outcome. Trusting your doctors to give the right medicines or supplements, take them faithfully and willingly. Also, be involved in any support groups or events that will encourage and can only benefit you. Being passive or defiant only harms you.
3. *Let your food be your medicine and your medicine be your food.* What you put in your body will give you life or take it away. Changing what you eat has a tremendous impact. Eat what your body needs to fight back and to live. With cancer or after cancer, food must take on a new meaning with a new purpose for the rest of your life.
4. *Be physically active from the start of diagnosis through the day cancer is no longer in your body.* Then, keep going. Exercising and being as fit as possible throughout your cancer journey will increase your chances of getting through treatment as planned and to completion. Be up and out of your bed when you can, for however long you can, and you'll find you have improved mood, less side effects, and decreased need for additional medications. Bottom line: reduce your chances of relapse.
5. *Pray.* This goes back to Tip 1. If you don't pray, or don't like to pray, find someone who does. Speaking as a survivor of three battles with cancer, you can count on this—there will be times when things go wrong, and all else fails, and you feel all you have is a prayer. Don't wait to get to that point. I know: prayer changes things. Believe in the God of the Bible and His words in it. Make it a part of you as often as you breathe. It will change how you think, speak, and act in your fight to overcome daily challenges on the way to defeating cancer.

Epigenetics
https://vimeo.com/67659031

Chapter **15**

Chemotherapy:
Today and in the Future

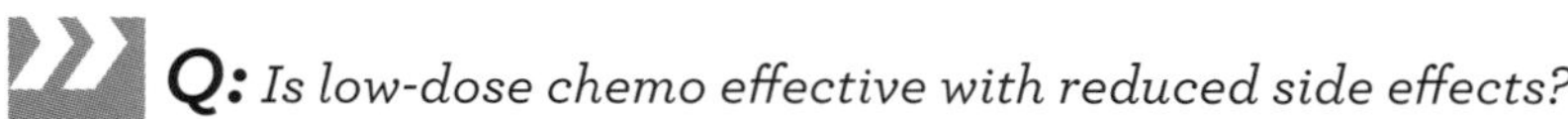

Q: *Is low-dose chemo effective with reduced side effects?*

A: Researchers are finding more and more ways to increase its cancer-killing effect while lessening side effects. At Oasis of Hope we precondition our patients thoroughly and often utilize low-dose, even minute-dose, metronomic chemo. Few experience excessive nausea, weakness, suppressed immunity, or hair loss.

In May 2009 Daniel Hauser, thirteen, refused chemotherapy when diagnosed with Hodgkin's lymphoma.[1] His mother, Colleen, honored his wishes, and they left home, apparently headed to Mexico for alternative therapy. When various networks invited me to speak about the family's decision,[2] I wasn't sure what they expected me to say, considering that my father is the icon for alternative medicine in Mexico. I shared what I would do: If Daniel Hauser were my own son, I'd go forward with chemo because it has a 95% cure rate for Hodgkin's lymphoma.

Eventually he went back and took chemo; he's in remission today. Though it was his best option, it isn't in every case. Only clinical experience teaches an oncologist when and how chemo can be of benefit.

I believe chemotherapy is no stand-alone solution. Some colleagues would agree; some would not. In this chapter I'll present an overview of when chemo is effective, when it isn't, and how it can be used innovatively for better results and diminished side effects.

Chemo Sometimes *Is* the Best Option

If we were to play word association with *chemotherapy*, most people would say, for example, "nausea," "hair loss," "ineffective," or "necessary evil." This is understandable, as chemo drugs are cytotoxic—that is, toxic to cells. Of the many types developed with the purpose of killing cancer cells, most have severe side effects: those mentioned above plus immune suppression, flu-like symptoms, dry mouth, loss of appetite, and other non-desirable physical effects. As people are always weighing the ratio between efficacy and negative side effects, we must realize that, for a few types of cancer, the scale is weighted completely to the side of efficacy:[3]

- choriocarcinoma, 90%
- Burkitt's lymphoma (Stage I), 90%
- testicular carcinoma (Stages II–IV), 95%
- childhood sarcomas (w/ radiation & surgery), 70–90%
- nodular mixed lymphoma, 75%
- childhood lymphomas, 75%
- diffuse histiocytic lymphoma, 70%
- acute lymphocytic leukemia, 60%
- Hodgkin's lymphoma (Stage I) 95%
- Hodgkin's disease (Stages III–IV), 60%

These success rates represent an impressive record! In fact, whenever I encounter a patient with one of these cancers, I quickly recommend the chemotherapy protocol that's yielded these results.

Conversely, in regard to cancer's most common forms (lung, breast, prostate, colon, stomach, pancreas, bladder, ovary, head, neck, etc.), which account for close to 90% of cancer deaths in the industrialized world, clinicians tend to agree that chemotherapy alone is of little help.

Dr. Ulrich Abel, a cancer biostatistician, spent over a decade evaluating the published results for thousands of patients treated with all kinds of chemo protocols. In 1990 he released his seminal *Chemotherapy of Advanced Epithelial Cancer*, which stated that for "most of today's common solid cancers, the ones that cause 90% of the cancer deaths each year, chemotherapy has never proven to do any good at all."[4]

Then another renowned scientist raised a red flag. Dr. Albert Braverman said no solid tumor that was incurable in 1976 became curable by

1991. In "Medical Oncology in the 1990s" he said, "The time has come to cut back on the clinical investigation of new chemotherapeutic regimens for cancer and to cast a critical eye on the way chemotherapeutic treatment is now being administered."[5] A few years earlier, Dr. John Bailar III had already expressed his concerns. After carefully evaluating the national cancer program, he said it was "in big trouble" and concluded that "some 35 years of intense effort focused on improving treatment must be judged as a qualified failure."[6]

Why am I quoting studies from the eighties and nineties? I'm simply trying to illustrate the sad reality that, in this regard, not much has changed since. Consider this overarching statement on chemotherapy in the new millennium: In 2007, the American Cancer Society said, in its prestigious annual "Cancer Facts & Figures," "Surgery, radiation therapy and chemotherapy . . . seldom produce a cure."[7]

Chemotherapy: Strengths and Weaknesses

Not all the related news is bad.

In 2006 the Centers for Disease Control and Prevention said the five-year survival rate for cancer patients had gone from 50% in 1971 up to 63% in 2003.[8] Chemotherapy may have played a role in this success, even though the data is insufficient to credit chemo alone for this boost, for, again, it's been shown to increase the longevity of patients with a number of cancers, such as those with ovarian cancer (for years), or those with high-grade non-Hodgkin's lymphoma or localized cancer of the small intestines (at least for months).

Many statisticians criticize the vast majority of studies that tout chemo's efficacy because the data in support of such claims is woefully lacking.[9] According to a report published in the *British Medical Journal* about the efficacy of two Bristol-Myers chemo drugs, only 11% of patients taking carboplatin and only 15% taking cisplatin had a total response to the drugs. In the cases studied, the patients experienced remission for an average of one year and survived an average of two.[10]

To the drugs' manufacturers, *effectiveness* is defined by the FDA, which deems an effective chemotherapeutic agent as achieving a 50% or more reduction in tumor size for twenty-eight days.[11] Again, does this definition assess whether the therapy can halt progression of the disease and significantly prolong life? No. To the oncologist, efficacy *also* is defined, regrettably, by the degree to which a therapy can be endorsed without fear of legal repercussion.

What *does* an oncologist mean, exactly, by the terms *response*, *remission*, and *cure*? Total "response" is when the tumor disappears completely; partial response is when the tumor is reduced by at least 50%; a failed response is when it's reduced by anything less than 50%. "Remission" refers to the time period a response lasts, and "cure" refers to a total response with a remission lasting five consecutive years; in some cancers, remission has to last ten years.

Cancer patients talking with an oncologist want to know what the chances are that a given chemotherapy will (1) halt the disease's progression, (2) prolong their life significantly, and (3) secure quality of life for them. But oncologists often frame their responses in a language that's unequivocally unforgiving because, "in the trenches," they live with the fact that chemo usually doesn't cure cancer, extend life significantly, or improve the quality of a patient's life.

I've written on this subject for years, and I still feel that chemo, if used as the solitary weapon in the fight against cancer, is wrong and generally bad for the patient. Here's a case in point: In 2004 a study took the data reported in the cancer registry data in Australia and from the Surveillance Epidemiology and End Result (SEER program) for new diagnoses of twenty-two major adult cancers treated with chemotherapy.[12] With disheartening results, the researchers concluded, "The overall contribution of curative and adjuvant cytotoxic chemotherapy to 5-year survival in adults was estimated to be 2.3% in Australia and 2.1% in the USA." Please understand, this does not mean that if you have cancer your survival probability is 2.1%. It does strongly suggest that oncologists cannot look at chemo as a stand-alone therapy.

Facts to Remember

Before we write off chemotherapy completely, let's take a look at some noteworthy facts.

First, chemo tears down tumors fast, much faster than any non-toxic therapy available. No one can argue with that.

Second, cancer cells mutate in ways that make them resistant to chemotherapy. Now, not all chemo drugs are created equal—there are many differences—but for the sake of this discussion I will group them by level of toxicity, from mild to extreme. Oncologists almost always initiate as effective a drug as they can that is the least aggressive chemotherapeutic agent to minimize negative side effects for the patient.

It's fair to say that most patients will "respond" to chemo drugs during the first round of treatment. Unfortunately, if the tumor comes back, which happens too frequently, the cells, through a number of adaptability mechanisms, regularly have developed a resistance to the previously used drug, rendering ineffective the once-effective treatment. Even more disturbing, the stress the therapy causes often compels the cancer cells to mutate so as to render them more aggressive and difficult-to-treat. For example, a drug may destroy 99% of a moderately aggressive cancer, but the 1% that survives can mutate into a highly aggressive cancer that no longer responds to drugs. This is why manufacturers have had to develop second and third lines of chemo drugs, with each presenting an increase in toxicity and dangerous side effects.

Third, chemo is toxic and does cause serious side effects. Patient tolerance varies. Some die from exposure to the least aggressive drugs; others experience virtually no adverse reactions to drugs so toxic that even those administering them wear rubber gloves. Besides nausea, vomiting, and hair loss, some cause muscle mass loss, blood disorders, or heart and lung damage; others, nerve or kidney damage, hearing loss, seizures, loss of motor function, bone marrow suppression, and blindness. Up to 60% of patients receiving chemo will experience anemia, which causes great fatigue and is a predictor of shorter survival rates.[13]

A most dreaded complication is mucositis, an inflammation of the mucus membranes in the mouth and stomach lining that can lead to life-threatening diarrhea and bleeding. Some chemo drugs can destroy bile ducts, cause bone tissue death or infertility, restrict growth, lower white and red cell counts, and lead to intestinal and lactose malabsorption.

Because chemotherapy is so effective initially at breaking down malignant cells, I've dedicated the last ten years of research to finding ways to leverage its cancer-killing potential, re-sensitize resistant tumors to mildly toxic chemo drugs, and protect healthy cells from the treatment's onslaught, thus reducing side effects to a minimum. Read on. This chapter will end on a positive note—I promise.

New Strategies: Maximal Efficiency, Minimal Side Effects

Earlier I indicated that chemotherapy offers very little hope to patients with breast cancer. I stand by that statement because it's true when chemo is used without any other intervention. I am encouraged that researchers are finally abandoning the idea of finding a single drug to cure illness. Instead, strategies are emerging to utilize combinations of therapy to create synergistic results.

I conducted a five-year clinical trial with stage IV (advanced) breast cancer including metastasis to lungs or liver. There were two groups: patients treated with conventional therapy before they became my patient, and patients who had no treatment before becoming my patient. Because cancers of the breast are chemo-sensitive, I administered chemo to all the patients but in combination with therapies that blocked estrogen receptors as well as natural treatments to increase intra-tumoral oxygen levels and provoke apoptosis.

The results were published in September 2011.[14] According to the NIH's SEER program, the average stage IV breast cancer five-year-survival rate is 20%. With this combo therapy, the rate increased to 45% for my patients already devastated by conventional therapy. For my patients who'd not undergone any treatment before seeing me, the rate skyrocketed to 75%. If all the patients received chemo, what made the difference between the results of 20%, 45% and 75%? It was all about new treatment combinations versus single-drug therapy.

Biomarkers and Targeted Therapies

The notion of one-size- (or one-drug-) fits-all is starting to fade. With the understanding that chemotherapy can be devastating, intensive effort has been made to find specific therapies that will target specific cancer types. Not all breast cancer is the same. With biomarkers, breakthroughs are being made in personalization development that could potentially predict a patient's therapeutic response to different treatments.[15]

Combination and Multitasking Drugs

Just a few years ago, when oncologists spoke of combination therapies they were referring to the mix of two or more chemotherapies. Many of us now combine non-cancer drugs to either inhibit cancer's ability to spread, provoke malignant cell death, or cut off the tumor's ability to form new blood vessels to feed itself and grow. For example, the new drug cabozantinib ("cabo") can block the c-MET cancer cell's receptors, which will inhibit the tumor's ability to spread and cut off its blood supply.[16] Using cabo could substantially weaken the tumor to where an oncologist may be able to use a less aggressive chemotherapy and get wonderful results without the negative side effects.

Another interesting therapy combo is bringing about survival benefits for the first time in thirty years for patients with multiple myeloma. Doctors are utilizing autologous stem cell transplants after chemo and combining bortezomib, thalidomide, and lenalidomide.[17] Outside-the-box thinking *is* providing new hope. (Researchers also do point out that some of the new protocols could produce toxicity issues and are better reserved for patients in good general health.[18])

Cell Signaling Transduction

Researchers in the US and abroad are reporting that, through cancer cell signaling transduction, a number of nutrients can effectively counter a cancer cell's resistance mechanisms. In practical terms, this means we can use first-line chemo drugs again and again because it's now possible to re-sensitize cancers to them with lower toxicity levels.

Not only that, but more and more research is showing that it's possible to protect normal tissues and internal organs from chemo's negative and destructive effects. How? With nutrients! Their medicinal power is a reality integrative oncologists have championed for decades.

Low-Dose Chemotherapy

The current treatment buzzword is low-dose chemo. Numerous studies in leading oncology journals report that in many cancers, low-dose results are superior to standard dosing. For instance, low-dose metronomic oral chemotherapy is proving effective against lymphoma.[19] I'm particularly encouraged by a study on the use of low-dose chemo for the chemo-resistant stage IV lung cancer, because currently the five-year survival rate is less than 2%.[20] I've been able to increase it to 9% using high-dose vitamin C and ozone, and I'm tracking the results with patients also receiving low-dose chemo. Many of the superior results can be attributed to our pre-conditioning, cell signaling transduction, minimized side effects, preservation of the immune system, prolonged treatment duration, and the potentiating agents we utilize (e.g., insulin).

Conclusion

Many patients come after chemo failed them and they were sent home to die. You could say they were running from chemotherapy. It takes some trust-building to where they'll allow me to educate them on new strategies for effectively using it. I explain how chemo often is used as 80% of the treatment; how the other 20% of what oncologists prescribe is only to help ease suffering from side effects. In my practice, chemo, low-dose chemo, and even high-dose vitamin C only represent 15% of the treatment because of the comprehensiveness of our protocols.

How do we use chemo at Oasis of Hope? Because "chemotherapy" is a very broad term, this question is somewhat loaded. Chemo is an anticancer therapy that uses cytotoxic drugs to kill cancer cells. There's an incredible array of cytotoxic drugs and an infinite number of ways to combine and administer them. The precise treatment administered will depend on a number of variables, including type of cancer, stage of development, patient's physical status, prior chemo treatments received, response to prior treatment, likelihood that side effects would eliminate the possibility of further treatment, and many other factors.

Suffice it to say, we employ oncologists who specialize in nouveau applications of non-aggressive chemotherapies and alternatives to chemo. We thoroughly evaluate each patient to tailor treatment in regard to drug choice, dosage, and duration. Two factors separate our protocols from those around the world: first, the preparation our patients undergo to enhance the therapy's cancer-killing effect; second, the umbrella of protection we create over them, designed to reduce side effects.

ACTION STEPS

1. Find an oncologist who offers immune-system-protecting therapies.
2. Work with a nutritionist who'll help you boost your immune system and keep your weight on.
3. If you're taking chemo and it isn't working, consider alternative cancer treatment or low-dose chemotherapy.

CANCER VICTOR TIPS

Marilyn Bennett, Australia
Stage IV Inoperable Ovarian Cancer
Victor Since 2008

1. Do *whatever* it takes to develop a positive, grateful, "I'm being healed" attitude.
2. Incorporating natural therapies makes your journey much easier.
3. Make plans for when you're healed—keep looking forward.
4. Identify the pre-cancer stresses in your life and *actively* reduce them.
5. Ensure you make plenty of time for yourself, for reflection and pampering; that is, *whatever* makes *you* feel good and/or relaxed.

Chemotherapy: Today and in the Future
https://vimeo.com/61548899

Chapter 16

Radiation:
A New Era of Precision

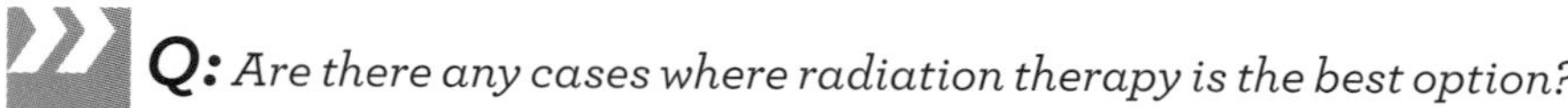

Q: *Are there any cases where radiation therapy is the best option?*

A: In the past, when radiation was so toxic that it devastated the patient, the answer was no. This is changing. Newer delivery systems are making radiation extremely precise, reducing the "burn" of normal tissue and thus making this therapy more effective and much less toxic.

A Cornerstone Treatment

Using high-energy radiation to shrink and kill cancerous tumors dates back to the early 1900s, when doctors in Vienna successfully treated a patient with pharyngeal carcinoma. Marie Curie is generally honored with having discovered radiation, but what she really found, in 1898, was the element *radium*, an accomplishment that ultimately would make her the first woman to receive a Nobel Prize.

Three years earlier, Wilhelm Röntgen had discovered X-rays, a phenomenon Curie associated with "radioactivity," the term she coined as associating with anything that emits these rays. This discovery, along with the search for its source by Henri Becquerel, was the basis for Curie's research that led her to radium.

There's a common misconception that the use of older cancer therapies like radiation is on the decline. It may seem that this more-than-a-century-old method has been somewhat obscured by numerous innovative advances, such as the advent of monoclonal antibodies (see chapters 31–32), signal transduction inhibitors (see chapters 4 and 13), and other targeted agents. Yet radiation oncology actually remains a treatment cornerstone; it's one of medicine's most sophisticated and quickly evolving areas. The annual percentage of recipients is on the rise—for example, an estimated one million patients in the US were treated with radiation in 2010, an increase of 15% from 2007.[1]

Today, radiation therapy is on the rise especially in certain specific cancers—for instance, within the span of one decade the number rose from 26% to 51% in prostate cancer patients and from 33% to 47% among breast cancer patients.[2] Some scientists are convinced that still not nearly enough patients are receiving it.[3] What's evident is that with the American Cancer Society expecting approximately 1,660,290 new cancer cases to be diagnosed in 2013,[4] tens of thousands of patients will be treated with some form of radiation therapy.

Improving Precision

Researchers have worked hard to hone in the radiation onto the tumors while shielding the normal cells. From computer-assisted techniques to the application of particle physics, innovations have improved efficacy and reduced collateral damage.

The word *radiation* itself commands awe and fear at the same time because of the hope it may represent but also the harm it can cause. Electromagnetic radiation consists of a stream of charged particles that, though invisible, damages the DNA of cells, impeding their reproduction. The delivery systems are, basically,

1. external beam machines, the most popular and practical option;
2. internal beam probes placed close to or within the tumors; and
3. systemic radiation where radiopharmaceuticals are injected intravenously to seek and destroy cancer cells.

Medical engineers have utilized the flood of new technologies to improve efficacy and reduce risk; in other words, to better destroy cancer cells and minimize damage to normal cells. The following is a very basic "tour" of some newer options.

Intensity-modulated radiation therapy (IMRT, aka 3D delivery system or tomotherapy) is a major external-radiation breakthrough. In the old days of the twentieth century we used two-dimensional (2D) radiotherapy, with a single beam from one to four directions. Beam setups were relatively simple; plans frequently consisted of opposed lateral fields, or four-field "boxes," which meant (1) there was much exposed normal tissue *and* (2) the amount of radiation to the tumor was limited. Today, computed tomography- (CT-) based planning takes into consideration our actual anatomy and complex tissue contours (e.g., the hourglass shape of the neck and shoulders). With more sophisticated software we can create detailed 3D maps to precisely plot location, size, and shapes of a tumor, of surrounding organs, and of sensitive tissue, then use these images to determine the exact dosage of radiation needed. IMRT reduces the radiation to normal tissue and increases it to the tumor by delivering thousands of thin beams that enter the body from hundreds of angles, intersecting the cancer with high precision.

At this stage we still have faced another complication. Most tumors "move with us" when we breathe, or with peristalsis (the natural movement of our bowels); though this shifting is subtle, high-dose radiation still burns the normal tissue that moves into the beam. So, human ingenuity soon will come to the rescue once again. Next-generation radiation oncology that accounts for this movement is being called four-dimensional conformal radiotherapy (4DCRT). Tumor tracking is now possible through a small wireless device, akin to a global positioning system (GPS), that doctors can implant in the tumor to track its position in real time. The intensity-modulated radiation stops whenever the tumor is out of the allowed area. This system is now being used in treating prostate cancer and is sure to soon be instituted in treating many other cancers.

4D will be complemented by another in-the-works development: megavoltage computed tomography. MVCT will allow for reconstruction of the actual daily-delivered dose based on the patient's anatomy in real time—the machine will detect and adjust to whatever changes the therapy causes to the tumor. This is called "adaptive radiotherapy," the modulation and delivery of the ideal daily (as opposed to planned) dose.

Gamma Knife, Brachytherapy, and MRT

Gamma Knife technology, another development, delivers a single high radiation dose (rather than multiple smaller doses). This system is used widely and effectively for brain and spine cancers, especially for patients with painful or function-interfering tumors in these areas. Technicians are now developing Gamma Knife applications for other tumors, such as lung cancer.

One limitation is that radiation therapy in general can only treat one tumor at a time, but with a new technology called Total Metastases Irradiation, it's now possible to simultaneously target tumors in multiple areas with high doses while still limiting damage to healthy tissue.

Computer technology has also advanced brachytherapy to enable delivery of concentrated radiation doses to a very limited area with short exposure time. This high-dose-rate (HDR) therapy is a tremendous benefit; with the old method patients were hospitalized several days in a shielded room, confined to bed and totally isolated because the implanted radiation source would affect anyone who came in contact. Now they come to an office, have a ten-to-twenty-minute session, then go home; if necessary, the patient has HRD therapy for several days. (External radiation therapy takes six to eight weeks.) Plus, HDR poses little risk of radiation injury to the rest of the body or to caretakers.

One advancement that significantly reduces radiation for breast cancer is MammoSite® radiation therapy (MRT), used after a lumpectomy (surgical removal of a breast tumor) to prevent a recurrence. A small balloon-shaped catheter, inserted into the cavity where the tissue was removed, is loaded with a radioactive pellet. MRT is far less invasive than external radiation and can help doctors preserve as much healthy breast tissue as possible.

Additionally, it's now possible to use highly targeted treatment methods by placing microscopic glass beads to deliver radiation inside a tumor with the help of advanced imaging. Once a tumor has been mapped and its main feeding artery found through computerized angiography, with the aid of a fluoroscope, we can place a catheter in that artery. For example, TheraSphere® treats liver metastasis with beads that contain the radioactive isotope Yttrium-90. Theoretically the beads are precisely sized to lodge in the blood vessels associated with the cancerous tissue but not in the blood vessels of the liver's healthy parts, thus the term "highly targeted." Time will reveal its effectiveness.

Proton Therapy

All of this notwithstanding, the hope and future of radiation therapy rests on the shoulders of protons. Most radiation today is delivered by X-rays or electrons (photons), which have a negative charge. *Protons* are positively charged elementary particles found in the nuclei of all atoms. When directed with magnetic fields, they emit a high radiation dose with very little spillage, enabling us to deliver an extremely aggressive yet precise dose to the tumor. Proton radiation's major advantage is that it gives up its energy only when hitting its intended target, the tumor; it does not then continue through the body and damage normal cells. There's no question that sufficiently high radiation can kill most if not all tumors; the unfortunate limitation is radiation's collateral damage. But proton therapy may prove to be an answer unlike one we've yet found.

Even though proton therapy has proven remarkably effective against many cancers, especially prostate, lung, and breast, the data is insufficient to demonstrate without a doubt that it's superior to photon (typical) radiation therapy. The main reason is its absurd cost, about $200 million per machine (with that money you can install about twenty of the most avant-garde radiation therapy machines, like the linear accelerators) making the cost unreachable for most cancer patients or insurance companies.

Limitations, to Date

Despite the improvements in 3D and 4D image-guided radiotherapy, brachytherapy, and proton therapy to target tumors more precisely, exposure and injury to surrounding tissues and organs with serious and often permanent side effects still limits the amount of radiation therapy that can be administered to a patient undergoing cancer treatment.

Furthermore, the state-of-the-art technology, developed to increase efficacy and reduce injury, is so complex that human and mechanical error still is inevitable due to software flaws, faulty programming, poor safety procedures, or inadequate staffing and training. The problem is compounded by how difficult radiation injuries are to identify. Complications due to organ damage and radiation-induced cancer are not apparent for many years, even decades; meanwhile, insufficient dosing is impossible to detect or interpreted as failure to respond to treatment.

According to the *New York Times,* accidents are chronically underreported. In June 2010 a Philadelphia hospital gave the wrong radiation dose to more than ninety patients with prostate cancer, and in 2005 a Florida hospital disclosed that seventy-seven brain cancer patients had received

50% more radiation than prescribed because one of the most powerful—and supposedly precise—linear accelerators had been programmed incorrectly for nearly a year. The article's author concluded, "Regulators and researchers can only guess how often radiotherapy accidents occur."[5]

And, again, because of the incredible advances in imaging and therapy, people today receive far more medical radiation than ever before. The California Society of Radiologic Technologists reports that the average lifetime diagnostic radiation dose has increased sevenfold since 1980, and more than half of all cancer patients receive radiation therapy.[6] Also, a study conducted in US emergency departments indicated that CT scans of pediatric patients have increased fivefold over a thirteen-year period ending in 2008.[7]

Health professionals may be the one remaining large group of highly exposed workers of any type, especially if we focus on exposures to the head. While radiologists may have been the most highly exposed medical workers before, today cardiologists have twice the average annual exposure rate, due to their high use of fluoroscopy,[8] an X-ray apparatus that gives real-time images during a procedure. A 1999 study found that brain cancer incidence had increased among physicians in general.[9]

Protection from Radiation

In short, though, these implements are here to stay, and radiation therapy innovations will continue. While the benefits seem to outweigh the risks, some of us are working to shield patients and doctors from actual and potential threats, particularly with radioprotector products.

To date, the only FDA-approved medication to prevent radiation damage is Ethyol® (amifostine), originally discovered through the U.S. Army Research and Development Command's Anti-radiation Drug Development program. That project was intended to search for ideal protective agents for a variety of exposure scenarios, such as nuclear war and industrial accidents. Ethyol, a prodrug, is converted in the body's tissues to an active metabolite that can scavenge reactive oxygen species (ROS) generated by exposure to either chemo or radiation therapy. Unfortunately, it has generated unfavorable side-effect ratios; nearly one third of patients endured Grade 3 or higher nausea/vomiting, and nearly two-thirds developed abnormally low blood pressure (hypotension). Obviously this has greatly limited Ethyol's product acceptance.

Aeolus Pharmaceuticals is developing a metalloporphyrin (compound) that scavenges ROS at the cellular level, mimicking the effect of the body's own natural superoxide dismutase (SOD; an antioxidant enzyme).[10] If these products are developed to mimic such natural agents, why not just use the natural agents? In the wake of industrial accidents (like with Japan's Fukushima nuclear reactors), at Oasis of Hope we've developed a natural compound to help protect people from the exposure to radiation with all-natural elements (described below.)

• • • • • • • • • • • • • •

Let me further explain *why* you need to protect yourself from radiation and *how* natural elements can help you do so. Ionizing radiation damages cellular molecules in both direct and indirect ways. It splits directly hit molecules into highly reactive fragments known as free radicals. These, in turn, can attack other molecules they encounter in a continuing and damaging chain reaction.

Fortunately, our cells contain molecules known as antioxidants that can readily donate electrons to molecules damaged by free radicals, thus stopping this train of events. One key damage target in irradiated cells is DNA, which acts as a crucial blueprint for cellular function. Severe damage to DNA can induce cell death, and this effect is an important mediator of lethal radiation toxicity. But more limited damage to DNA, if it isn't rapidly repaired by antioxidants or certain protective enzymes, can result in permanent changes—mutations—in the DNA base code, potentially leading to cancer induction in the future. Radiation can attack DNA directly, but more often DNA is damaged by hydroxyl radicals formed when radiation interacts with water molecules in the body.

Nutrients and phytochemicals (compounds in plants) can boost our cells' capacity to quickly repair damage to DNA and other vital cellular components. The following are the elements in the formula we developed.

Glutathione, a crucial antioxidant compound produced in our cells, can prevent or repair radiation-caused oxidative damage, and we can support efficient cellular synthesis of glutathione by two complementary mechanisms (on the second, see chapter 4).

First, N-acetylcysteine is a supplement that increases cellular levels of the amino acid cysteine, the rate-limiting precursor for glutathione synthesis.

Second, lipoic acid, green tea polyphenols, silymarin, and curcumin stimulate our cells to make increased levels of the key enzyme required for glutathione synthesis. These components also increase cellular expression of a wide range of antioxidant enzymes that, like glutathione, can help cells cope with radiation-induced oxidative stress. One of these, glutathione peroxidase, requires the essential mineral selenium. Also, biopterin can improve intestinal absorption of curcumin and silymarin. Taking these nutrients is a smart way to ensure that your cells' natural radioprotective mechanisms are operating at peak effectiveness.

Conclusion

Once again, radiation therapy commands awe and fear, and rightly so. If it's recommended for your case or that of your loved one, make sure you do it at an experienced center with the latest available technology. This chapter has given you the tools to ask the right questions and to take the steps to do all you can to protect your normal tissues with radiation-protective nutrients.

ACTION STEPS

1. Discuss with your oncologist the possibility of using non-invasive targeted radiation.
2. Protect yourself from radiation damage with nutrients like glutathione, lipoic acid, and green tea polyphenols.
3. Enhance radiation's efficacy with ozone autohemotherapy or hyperbaric oxygen (see chapter 5).

CANCER VICTOR TIPS

T. Hill, Maryland
Waldenström's Macroglobulinemia
Victor Since 2005

1. Keep God in the picture. If your relationship is weak, strengthen it. If it's strong, continue to nurture it. Turning to God can help keep you going.
2. Don't waste time asking, "Why me?" Ask, "What can I learn from this?"
3. Live! Take the time to do things big and small that you've been wanting to do.
4. On treatments, don't let anyone talk you out of doing what you think is best for you, and don't let yourself be forced into doing anything you don't feel is right for you. Do your research and trust your gut.
5. Don't let cancer be your only focus. Take time for your friends. If you're feeling down, help someone else.

Radiation: A New Era of Precision
https://vimeo.com/61552420

Chapter 17

Surgery:
Coming of Age

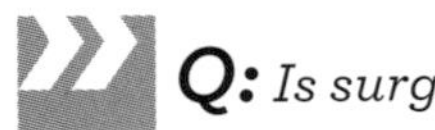

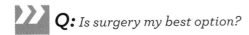

Q: *Is surgery my best option?*

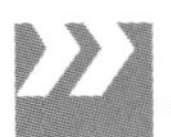

A: Surgery is the most effective treatment for early stage cancers, which is why early detection is so important. Because of its efficacy, oncologists tried for years to develop procedures for later-staged cancers, with results ranging from devastating to inhumane. Thank God almost all of those went into disuse. Most cancer surgeries now are conservative and aimed at improving quality of life.

Surgery is and will continue to be one of the most important weapons in the anti-cancer arsenal against tumors. Let me take you through a brief history of its development. I was blessed to do my surgical training in one of the world's most prominent surgical institutions, the University of Vienna Surgical Department, where historical giants walked the halls and many procedures were developed.

An Historical Overview

In the 1600s Ambroise Paré said we perform surgery "to eliminate that which is superfluous, restore that which has been dislocated, separate that which has been united, join that which has been divided and repair the defects of nature."[1] This continues to be true, even though at that time the "handy work," which is what *surgery* literally means (from the Greek *cheiro-urgia*, from *cheir* ["hand"] + *ergon* ["work"]), was eerily and brutally done by barbers and second-class medical personnel.

Artifacts and documents have shown that surgery was performed much earlier. Trepanation, drilling a hole in the skull, is one of the most documented ancient surgeries, from Egypt to China. Hippocrates mentioned the procedure four hundred years before Christ. At a French burial site, of 120 skulls found, forty had trepanation holes, and those human remains were calculated to be around eight thousand years old.

The Babylonians had an established, legislated surgical community two centuries before Christ; the Code of Hammurabi (a law book) dates to about 1772 BC. Some regulations are intriguing. For instance, code 215 says, "If a physician make a large incision with an operating knife and cure it, or if he open a tumor (over the eye) with an operating knife, and saves the eye, he shall receive ten shekels in money." Code 218 incentivized surgeons to stay honest: "If a physician make a large incision with the operating knife, and kill him, or open a tumor with the operating knife, and cut out the eye, his hands shall be cut off."[2]

Adina Sherer, a pediatric neurosurgeon in Israel, researched Hua Tuo, an Eastern Han-era Chinese surgeon, and found that he put his patients under a sort of anesthesia, sixteen centuries before Europe "invented" anesthesia.[3] The Spanish historian Manuel Lucena Salmoral wrote about the daily life of the Aztecs and other indigenous peoples of Mexico when the Spaniards came to the New World more than five centuries ago and describes their advanced medical practices. For example, not only did they resolve fractured bones, but "the broken bone had to be splinted, extended and adjusted, and if this was not sufficient an incision was made at the end of the bone, and a branch of fir was inserted into the cavity of the medulla"![4] Not until *1939* did the Europeans come up with implanting an intramedullary rod (nail) when Gerhard Küntscher first used this device to treat soldiers with fractures of the femur.[5]

In India, ancient surgeons pioneered plastic surgery and became proficient with nose jobs (rhinoplasty), for among Hindus and Buddhists anyone who stole a large animal or abetted a thief or an adulterer had his nose and ears cut off.[6]

Before Anesthesia

For us, the history of surgery before anesthesia is unimaginable—it was treacherous, bloody, and brutal. Barber-surgeons cut hair, pulled teeth, set bones, and amputated limbs. Today the barber's sign seems innocuous, but the white and red striped pole outside their workplace once represented blood and bandages, and those in need of their services teetered, thinking of them more as executioner than as savior. Sounds of thrashing and screaming filled their shops and larger operating rooms. To minimize shock and pain, speed was more important than precision; they had to be time-driven gladiators, fast and furious.

Supposedly the speediest of all was Robert Liston, a British surgeon who reputedly amputated limbs so rapidly that operating-theater gallery spectators would take out pocket watches to time him. One surgery took twenty-five *seconds* from incision to wound closure, a spectator said, "Liston operated so fast that he accidentally amputated an assistant's fingers along with a patient's leg." A couple days later, "The patient and the assistant both died of sepsis, and a spectator reportedly died of shock, resulting in the only known procedure with a 300% mortality."[7]

This story reminds me of a father who, wanting to show off his son's mathematical quickness, prompted friends to quiz him. So one asked the prodigy, "How much is 5 times 7?" The kid immediately barked, "25!" "What? That's not right!" the man exclaimed, perplexed. "Hey," said the dad, holding up his hands, "I said he's quick; I didn't say he's precise."

At any rate, the eighteenth-century surgeon William Hunter was right when he taught his medical students, "Anatomy is the Basis of Surgery, it informs the Head, guides the hand, and familiarizes the heart to a kind of necessary inhumanity."[8]

Surgery, then, has existed since humans first learned to make and handle tools, and while the sophistication of tools and techniques evolved through the centuries, the professionalization of the European barber-surgeons into hospital-surgeons is what brought surgery fully into the medical field. Further, the Industrial Revolution brought the means to overcome surgery's threefold roadblock: pain, bleeding, and infection.

Due to anesthesia, effective anti-bleeding techniques, blood transfusions, and antibiotics, in the last two centuries surgery has become one of the most respected medical fields. Most of us will need a surgery or two during our lifetimes—for a broken bone, a cataract, a tumor, a cesarean section, a joint replacement, a coronary bypass. . . . Surgeons have more than 2,500 procedures to offer—some the "old-fashioned" way, some with the aid of laparoscopy, some even robotically aided. And, more often than not, we will view them as saviors rather than executioners.

Present-Tense Extremes

However, though the barbaric era is long gone, the threat of misuse still lingers. Because of their relative safety and efficacy, we've seen an explosion in number and frequency of surgeries—at least fifty million annually in the US alone.[9] A high percentage are unnecessary. For example, a study was conducted on 34,000 women screened for ovarian cancer whose blood tests came back positive and underwent surgery. Out of every hundred women who tested positive and had the procedure, less than *2%* had cancer.[10]

In addition, due to advancements in techniques and tools, surgeons, especially cancer specialists, have developed some disturbing procedures. For example:

1. The *extended radical mastectomy*; removal of the entire breast, the pectoral muscles, and the armpit's and chest wall's lymphatic-bearing tissues, leaving only skin to cover the ribs; the woman is severely mutilated.
2. The *COMMANDO* (*COMbined MAndibulectomy and Neck Dissection Operation*), a complicated procedure for stage I malignancy of the tongue; removal of the tongue, half of the jaw, and all of the neck lymph nodes of the side of the original tumor (in tongue).
3. *Pelvic exenteration* (or *evisceration*); removal of all organs (urinary bladder, urethra, rectum, anus) from the pelvic cavity; leaves the person with a permanent colostomy and the ureters connected to the small intestine; vagina, cervix, uterus, Fallopian tubes, ovaries, and (in some cases) vulva are removed; prostate is removed [men].
4. *Hemicorporectomy* (or *translumbar amputation*, or *halfectomy*); the most radical surgery ever devised; amputation of the body below the waist (legs, genitalia [internal and external], urinary system, pelvic bones, anus, and rectum), transecting the lumbar spine; a severely mutilating procedure recommended only as a last resort.

Conclusion

As a surgical oncologist I opine that these surgeries do flirt with the barbaric. Thank God most surgeons worldwide frown upon most of them, for many if not most survivors will later die not of complications but of psychological deterioration. The peak of this type of surgical obscenity was in the 60s—since then the goal of oncological procedures has been more and more conservative, more intent on improving quality of life.

And, again, surgery continues to be the most effective anticancer therapy for cancers found in early stages. The stage I cure rate reaches percentages in the high 80s to 90s. When early detection has failed, the second goal is to improve quality of life by removing tumors that impede organ function or that cause untreatable pain.

ACTION STEPS

1. Find out whether you're a good candidate for surgery.
2. Ensure that the recommended surgery is for curative or palliative reasons; make an educated decision on the procedure's temporary and permanent consequences.
3. Seek as many different opinions as you need from oncologists who also understand alternative therapies.

CANCER VICTOR TIPS

Richard Shea, California
Stage IV Prostate Cancer
Victor Since 2010

1. Change your diet to the Hallelujah diet.
2. Power walk everyday for one hour.
3. No meat, dairy, white flower, caffeine, and most of all no sugar!
4. Drink carrot juice.
5. Buy organic food. It's worth the extra money.

Surgery: Coming of Age
https://vimeo.com/61554539

Chapter 18

Empowerment

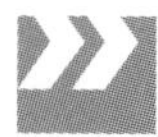 **Q:** *How can I help my doctor to help me?*

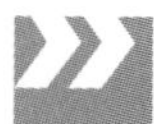 **A:** Be informed and proactive. You'll gain your physicians' respect and cooperation if your treatment team sees that in your therapy you're an active participant and a decision maker.

A few years back a friend of mine referred his uncle to us for cancer treatment. He called and explained one of his major concerns: his uncle had already given up, even though the cancer was at an early stage. On the day he was diagnosed, he stopped going to work, church, family events, or any other gathering, and now he sat alone in his dark house.

I found his uncle in our dining commons, eating lunch in silence. I introduced myself and asked if we could chat. After he invited me up to his third-floor room, the first thing I noticed was that he bypassed the elevator and took the stairs. I commented that he looked very strong, and he replied that he felt quite well.

This led me to ask why he'd cut all ties. He responded with five words: "I am going to die."

I asked how old he was when he first contemplated his mortality—when he realized that one day he would die. He said he'd faced that reality when he was seventeen.

I asked if he severed all ties with society at age seventeen. He looked at me questioningly and said he hadn't—he'd actually gone on to get an education, marry, have kids, and start a prosperous business.

I asked how he found the motivation to go on after age seventeen when he discovered that one day he would die. And suddenly, a peace came over his face. *Now* he instantly embraced that basic truth, that all of us one day will die. A diagnosis of cancer doesn't change this reality.

I said that the most important thing to do is live each day to the fullest and make a lifetime worth of memories; a collection of significant, meaningful moments. I suggested he spend as much time as possible with his grandchildren to pour into their lives his years of wisdom.

That was all it took. He checked out of the hospital, went back to work, and spent as much time as possible with his family. It was as if he needed to receive permission to still live after a diagnosis that looked like a death sentence.

This is what patient empowerment is all about: helping them to see they are not powerless over what they're going through.

Empowerment's Role and Goal

The aim of empowering a patient is to help train and motivate him to make informed decisions and take positive steps toward improving the quality of his life.[1] Helped to realize more about the illness and about treatments, self-awareness, and self-care activities, he can increase his coping skills and have positive input on how he's treated.

For example, a patient may discover that a round of chemotherapy makes her feel bad enough that subsequently she loses two days of work. Through this self-awareness and understanding of the side effects, she might use self-advocacy to request that treatments be done on Friday so she can have the weekend to recover and get back to work on Monday. By missing less work, she also feels she's maintaining some sort of normalcy, which increases her perception of her life's quality.

While reviewing medical and psychological peer-reviewed literature, I came across a study that defined disempowerment as, "Dependency on caregivers, from asymmetric power relations between professionals and patients, and from that one's life is planned around treatment calendars over which the patient has little or no control."[2] Comparing empowerment and disempowerment paints a broader picture and reveals further opportunities for people to improve their quality of life. It also helps me promote two goals for my patients:

- Do not allow cancer to determine your identity. Be you. Deal with cancer—do not become a cancer patient, and do not give your sense of self to the illness.

- Do not let cancer become a prison from which you have no freedom to decide how to spend your day. Do not let treatment schedules put you on lockdown, and do not let nurses and doctors tell you what you can and cannot do.

Interventions

The word "intervention" may bring to mind the image of a family and friends confronting a person about substance abuse. That's an example of one kind of intervention; social workers and counselors use this word to refer to any activity used with a client to produce a desired outcome. Most interventions are designed to educate patients, help them find their voice for self-advocacy, develop an awareness of limiting conditions, and bring about alternative actions, liberation, illumination, and mastery of life. It's not really about seizing control; it's about doing the possible and finding peace when dealing with the impossible.

In the chapters on psycho-oncology and noetic therapies, I explain interventions for coping and empowerment. I refer you to those (chapters 6 and 48) to begin or to continue your process of becoming empowered.

Conclusion

Bernie Siegel, one of our generation's most knowledgeable and articulate teachers of patient empowerment, helps strengthen people to find significance through being self-transparent and in touch with their intuition and feelings. In an interview about *101 Exercises for the Soul*,[3] he explains, "We are just getting to the most important breakthrough, and that is to understand that our internal environment selects the genetic blueprint that affects our physical health and bodies."[4]

Dr. Siegel says the soul is, "Who I really am, and the life I will live when I am being my true self and not the life others impose upon me."[5] This is the heart of empowerment. When facing cancer, you will enjoy a higher quality of life if you're true to yourself and do not succumb to the existence that the disease and treatments impose.

ACTION STEPS

1. Be your own advocate. There's no one better for the job.
2. Attend a self-help group, and pick up coping tips from other patients.
3. Don't forget who you are, and remember to do the things you love when you can.

CANCER VICTOR TIPS

Ivonne Arrache, México
Breast Cancer
Victor Since 1995

1. Eliminate stress.
2. Have a close relationship with God.
3. Do not harbor resentment.
4. Diligently watch what you eat. Especially avoid processed foods. Eat lots of raw fruits and vegetables. Don't drink milk or milk products. Don't eat red meat, fish, or chicken.
5. Keep a positive attitude, even in difficult circumstances.

Empowerment
https://vimeo.com/61282374

Chapter 19

Meaning

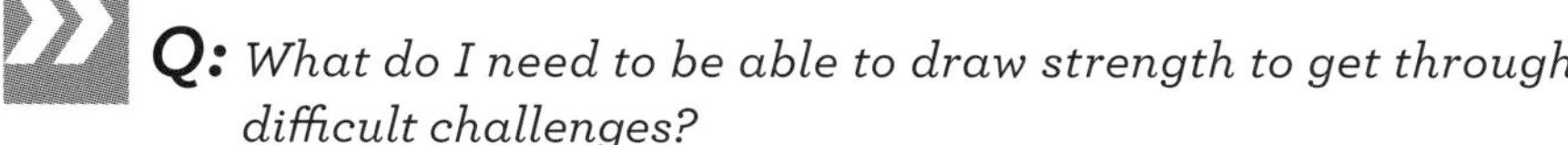

Q: *What do I need to be able to draw strength to get through difficult challenges?*

A: If you choose your attitude, you choose your destiny. Many things are beyond your control, but how you face them is always your choice. No matter how dire the situation, a positive attitude always works in your favor.

My father, Dr. Ernesto Contreras Sr., founded Oasis of Hope. At this writing we're celebrating fifty years of treating the whole patient, body, mind, and spirit; sharing the healing power of faith, hope, and love; and, one patient at a time, advancing medical science to put an end to cancer.

My father was the visionary. My mother, Rita, was the architect, engineer, administrator, coordinator, and more. She never achieved a college degree, yet she's raised six children, built Oasis of Hope Hospital and our laboratory, built numerous churches, financially supported hundreds of pastors, and put many, many orphans through school. My brother is a clinical oncologist; I'm a surgical oncologist. Her four daughters all became schoolteachers; all married pastors, and, arguably, all preach better than their husbands.

My mother's name is Rita. She has a daughter named Rita, a granddaughter named Rita, and a great-granddaughter named Rita. When her great-granddaughter married, my mother, herself an incredible visionary, offered to pay all the medical expenses if she and her husband had their first child within a year. They had a baby girl, and they named her . . . Agnes. (I'm kidding. They named her Rita.)

My mother is about to celebrate her ninety-third birthday. What's the secret to her longevity? Her life is meaningful. She has found purpose in all that she's done. She maintained our hospital for half a century to help tens of thousands of patients who came for care from more than sixty countries, and now she continues to pray her children, twenty grandchildren, forty-seven great-grandchildren (and counting), and great-great-grandchild (and counting) into God's kingdom. Her life's meaning has been to bring glory to God.

A Reason to Live

Perhaps no one has been a greater existential teacher than Viktor Frankl, who, in *Man's Search for Meaning,* tells of his holocaust experience.[1] Dr. Frankl was a graduate of my alma mater, the University of Vienna, where he specialized in psychiatry. As Adolf Hitler stockpiled power and initiated World War II, Frankl, a Jew, was no longer allowed to treat patients of Aryan decent. Then, one fateful day, his family was separated and shipped off to concentration camps. He never saw his wife again. Immersed in furious chaos, he tried to save his life's work, a manuscript, by sewing it into the lining of his overcoat. But his coat, and all his clothing, was taken from him and burned.

Frankl taught that while no one can control all the circumstances life delivers, he can control his reactions to circumstances. His reaction to the loss of his family and his life's work was to survive at any cost to retell the story and to rebuild his theory of psychology. He did both, and his landmark book contains both his memoirs of daily life in Auschwitz and an introduction to his theory.[2]

Logotherapy is considered the third school of psychiatry to come out of Vienna, after Sigmund Freud's Psychoanalysis[3] and Alfred Adler's Individual Psychology.[4] Its basic tenets assert that "(a) Human life has meaning, (b) human beings long to experience their own sense of personal life meaning, and (c) human beings have the potential to experience life meaning under all circumstances."[5] *Humans have the potential to experience life meaning under* all *circumstances, including cancer.* Friedrich Nietzsche stated it this way: "If we have our own why in life, we shall get along with almost any how."[6]

• • • • • • • • • • • • •

If you were progressing right along on your life plan and suddenly everything changed when the doctor said, "You have cancer," you're not alone.

If everything you thought you knew instantly became ambiguous and inconsequential, this is not to be unexpected.[7] Your world just got rocked. You may feel you've lost your way, your drive, your purpose. You may feel you're spiraling in an existential free-fall. You're in a crisis.

In Mandarin, the word "crisis" does not exist. Instead, two symbols are grouped to give the meaning: *wēi*(危), which means "danger," and *jī*(机), which means "crucial point." Cancer represents danger, and the moment of diagnosis is a crucial point to make decisions that will impact your life forever. *Crisis can be transformed into opportunity by the discovery of meaning.*

Meaning-Centered Strategies

Hong Kong's Haven of Hope Hospital found three conditions of existential distress: "Anticipation of a negative future, failure to engage in meaningful activities and relationships, and having regrets."[8] In the table below, I list the opposites of the conditions:

EXISTENTIAL-DISTRESS CONDITION	MEANING-CENTERED STRATEGY
Anticipation of a negative future	Take one day at a time, finding meaning throughout each day.
Failure to engage in meaningful activities and relationships	Converse with others, and make affirming statements to them.
Having regrets	Forgive others and forgive yourself. Forgiveness is the key to freedom.

Mindy Greenstein and William Breitbart, physicians at Memorial Sloan-Kettering Cancer Center, encourage patients to "focus on what has been and can still be meaningful in their lives given the circumstances, and to further develop their ability to reframe their experience from that of dying to that of living despite the threat of death."[9]

One of our goals is to help patients change the paradigm from "dying with cancer" to "living and dealing with cancer." Made successfully, this shift frees up emotional energy for focusing on quality of life. It helps diminish fear and grow faith. It can help a patient cope with a seemingly unbearable situation.

While there's clinical data that supports this, it's my personal experience that convinces me of its importance. Our cancer hospital has become a beacon of hope! I rejoice because I see smiles on the majority of my patients' faces and frequently hear laughter in the hallways. Just today I was overjoyed as I heard their voices spilling out of our prayer and healing room, singing, "Sing Hosanna, sing Hosanna, sing Hosanna to the King of Kings."[10] Their jubilance reassured me that my patients, though dealing with cancer, were really living. In fact, over the years many of them have taught me great lessons about the meaning of life.

Conclusion

I'll wrap up with the story of a former patient I'll call J.R. When he was diagnosed with advanced cancer, J.R. took some time to reflect on his life. He realized he hadn't truly lived before, had been caught up in pursuit of material gain. As a traveling salesman, he said, he'd been surviving mostly on candy bars.

But instead of looking at cancer as a death sentence and letting everything stay at a screeching halt, J.R. reframed it to be a new birth. He termed it a wakeup call. He determined he *would* begin to truly live.

When J.R. started looking for info on getting help, he found that resources were in abundance for aid with certain other cancers but that very little was available for the type he had. He found meaning through his mission to raise general awareness about that type with the objective of raising funds for new research. He was so successful that he was invited to carry the Olympic torch part of the way across the US to the 1996 Summer Games in Atlanta.

J.R. met the danger of cancer at the crucial point and made the rest of his life meaningful. He found purpose. He found a reason to live. He was so grateful for the opportunity cancer provided him to reevaluate his life that he wrote a list of the hundred benefits of being diagnosed. Three he included were: never missed a sunset again, took walks on the beach with his wife every day, and was kinder to his dog.

I included his list in *The Hope of Living Cancer Free.*[11] It might help inspire you to continue finding your own meaning.

ACTION STEPS

1. Write a list of ten things you're grateful for today.
2. Purpose yourself to do meaningful things each day.
3. Write a list of ten good things that have happened to you that may not have happened had you not been diagnosed with cancer.

CANCER VICTOR TIPS

Kathy Cooke, California
Adenocarcinoma with Liver and Bone Metastases
Victor Since 2011

1. God alone knows the number of your days. Don't let doctors tell you otherwise.
2. Stay optimistic! Live as if you're cured. Find reasons to be joyful now.
3. Help other people—you'll forget your trials for a while.
4. Surround yourself with Christian music, books, pictures of family events, holidays, and vacations.
5. Work closely with your doctor; be open-minded and informed.

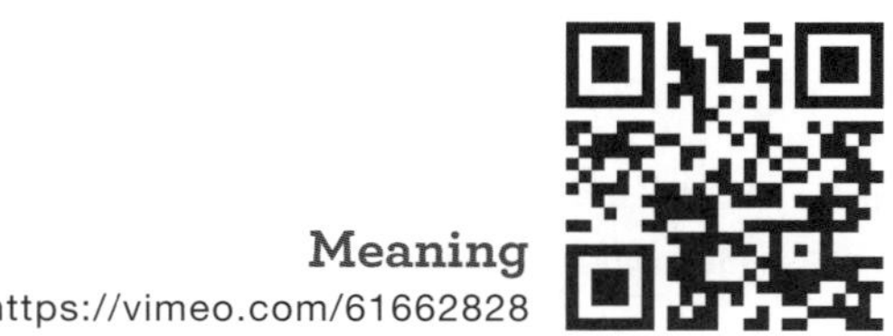

Chapter 20

Positive Resolve

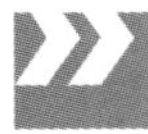 **Q:** *What's the most important component for helping me stare fear in the face?*

 **A:** Your attitude, which is absolutely dependent on your spiritual fortitude.

At the 1992 Summer Olympic Games in Barcelona, a most amazing testament to human courage and resolve unfolded during the men's 400-meter track and field semifinal. Derek Redmond of the UK was favored to win gold—he'd posted the top qualifying time and had won his quarterfinal heat—and, seconds after the starter's gun fired it appeared he'd have no real trouble here either.[1] Yet as he was nearing the 150-meter mark, anguish suddenly ripped across his face and showed through his body as he tore a hamstring and collapsed, writhing in agony. His dream had vanished in the blink of an eye, lost to debilitating injury. It was the USA's Quincy Watts who'd go on not only to win the gold but also to better the world record.

Redmond had lain on the track in excruciating pain. Most people naturally expected the stricken runner to be carried off. But then, to widespread surprise, he stood up and, haltingly, began hobbling toward the finish line. In an overwhelmingly emotional moment, his father, Jim, jumped up and shot onto the track. The son wrapped his arms around his dad, and the two of them completed the race together.

Redmond earned no medal, but his resolve to complete what he'd started continues to encourage and inspire more than two decades later.

Winning the Race for Life

Today, Derek Redmond often speaks at business and leadership conferences. He teaches how the slightest competitive edge can be the difference between losing and winning. In 1991, when he and his teammates ran the 400 relay at the World Championships, a simple and unexpected switching of their running order[2] provided just enough difference—four-hundredths of a second—for them to shock the favored Americans and go home with gold *and* finish with the second-best time ever run. For a person in a fight for his life, the smallest change may provide the competitive edge to beat cancer. Usually that change doesn't involve the medical treatment; it usually revolves around attitude, perseverance, and resolve.

I cannot overstate the power of positive resolve—it's a determining factor in whether a patient lives or dies. I find it a powerful experience when a patient looks me straight in the eye and says with conviction, "Doctor, I'm going to beat this thing." When I look through the window to the soul and see she really means what she says, I know she has given herself the highest probability she can have.

• • • • • • • • • • • • •

Maintaining a positive attitude is clinically proven to lower cancer-related distress and improve one's ability to cope.[3] Last chapter I shared about Viktor Frankl, who held that though you cannot control everything that happens to you, you can determine your attitude. No one else chooses it. It's your decision and yours alone.

Cancer patients with a hopeless mindset have a significantly lower probability of survival.[4] Now, many factors can affect one's ability to maintain positivity,[5] and patients don't like to be told they must be positive. What they really need is positivity in the people around them.

The diagnosis is shocking. Treatments may have side effects that can promote negative emotions. Pain is a real test of one's ability to keep perspective. But no matter your circumstances, you *can* find a way to be positive. My patients who keep positive always fare better.

"I Will"

I'll never forget receiving a patient with stage IV lung cancer that had spread to the liver and spine. The statistics said he had less than 2% probability of surviving five years; he was so weak he was brought in on a stretcher. His pain was unmanageable, and it was doubtful he could tolerate any treatment. Yet seeing the concern on my father's face, he reassured, "Don't worry, Dr. Contreras. I know I'm going to get well."

We gave him laetrile, which has a natural analgesic effect. The pain came under control, and he responded to treatment involving many therapies outlined in this book. He felt so well he started to walk again. In two *weeks* he'd checked himself out before the treatment was done.

My father asked why he was quitting treatment when he was doing so well. The man said he wasn't quitting—he had something crucial to take care of. He would do that, then come back later to continue.

After ten days he rechecked himself in. When my father went by and asked what he'd been doing, he said that years before he'd had a falling out with his adult children and they'd stopped all communication with him. He said he knew he needed to make things right with them—that's what he'd gone to do. They'd forgiven him; he was relieved and strengthened to continue his fight against cancer.

That was a quarter century ago. We still talk from time to time.

Perseverance starts with the words "I will." Our new friend showed us what this looked like. He was determined to get well; determined to make amends with his children; determined to go on living. He allowed no room for doubt or maybes to be a part of his battle plan. He had the will to overcome. And his resolve to beat cancer came down to two words.

• • • • • • • • • • • • • •

Psalm 118:17 gives one of the strongest "I will" statements: "*I will* not die but live, and *will* proclaim what the Lord has done."[6] Those who put their faith in God will never taste death. Jesus Christ laid down His life to give all who believe eternal life. Standing between us and eternity is only the mortal shell we occupy. Physical death is merely a transition from this life to the next—it's not final. Still, eternal life starts here. Choose to live today, in this world, and declare the glory of the Lord.

You Can Live Worry Free

In 1995, David Kennedy was diagnosed with renal cancer. When the doctor said, "David, you have cancer," he replied, "I understand," then smiled and thanked him. The doctor, thinking he hadn't grasped the situation's gravity, said, "I don't think you completely understand. You have a malignant tumor in your kidney. Left untreated, it could kill you." David replied, "I heard you, and I understand. But my whole life I've sought to honor God and be grateful. I can't wait for the day I get to see Jesus face to face."

Today, David Kennedy continues to live with his wife, cancer free. His spiritual fortitude gave him the attitude and the resolve to live worry free. His example is a testimony to how we can lay down our burdens and give our worries over to God.

That is surrender. That is freedom. That is victory over cancer.[7]

Conclusion

Few stories pack as much impact as that of Shadrach, Meshach, and Abednego,[8] who lived in Babylon under the reign of Nebuchadnezzar. The king, being full of himself, built a huge gold idol and ordered everyone in the kingdom to bow and worship it whenever they heard his musicians play. Word soon reached him that these three men refused to bow to his image and would worship only the One True God. Livid, he threatened them with death in a white-hot furnace.

Resolved to acknowledge no god but Yahweh, they answered,

> King Nebuchadnezzar, we do not need to defend ourselves before you in this matter. If we are thrown into the blazing furnace, the God we serve is able to deliver us from it, and he will deliver us from Your Majesty's hand. But even if he does not, we want you to know, Your Majesty, that we will not serve your gods or worship the image of gold you have set up.[9]

They were 100% committed to their course of action. They chose to fear God and not fear the fire. They trusted that He would deliver them either through a miraculous rescue or through into the next, better world. Their resolve gave them the courage to face imminent death.

And their resolve resulted in life. They *were* thrown into the furnace, heated to seven times its normal fury. They were not burned. Not even their clothing was singed.

When the king looked in, he saw them accompanied by a figure that looked like "a son of the gods."[10] He asked, "Weren't there three men? I see four!" In the midst of their trial by fire, *God was with them*.

You may feel like you're in the furnace and the heat is rising. You may see no way out. Resolve in your heart to trust in God. He will give you the courage to face difficulties with a positive attitude. He will deliver you. You can live worry free when you know He is sovereign and that He either will give you a miraculous healing or will pick you up and carry you into eternity, where there is no disease, no sorrow, and no pain.

ACTION STEPS

1. Resolve to beat cancer.
2. Choose to be positive.
3. Every day you wake up, say, "*I will* persevere."

CANCER VICTOR TIPS

David Kennedy, Indiana
Renal Cancer[11]
Victor Since 1995

1. Know that God knows and cares.
2. Learn what you can about your cancer.
3. Ask for prayer support from family and church.
4. Get other professional opinions.
5. Adjust your diet for optimal health.

Positive Resolve
https://vimeo.com/61760115

Chapter 21

The War on Cancer

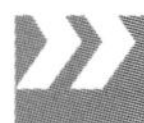 **Q:** *Are we winning the war on cancer?*

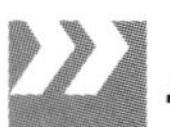 **A:** In my opinion, we are not, and the tide won't change until the established methodology, goals, principles, and philosophy to face cancer change. The medical and scientific communities must stop putting all efforts on destroying tumors and start putting more emphasis on aiding patients in restoring health.

On December 23, 1971, President Richard Nixon signed PUBLIC LAW 92-218, 92ND CONGRESS, S. 1828, known as the National Cancer Act of 1971, to form the National Cancer Institute, in which the program director would answer directly to the president's cancer panel, which reported directly to him.[1] Nixon urged the federal government to commit to finding the cure; the NCI's clinical-trial funding was increased tenfold in under ten years. The act promised the disease's cure would be found within a decade if adequate funds were allocated.

About thirty years after the act was signed, former NCI director Dr. Vincent DeVita Jr. stated, "The full promise of the original Cancer Act could not be reached despite the fact that over 40 billion dollars of public funds have been expended on cancer research."[2] In support of a new cancer act being promoted by Senator Dianne Feinstein in 2002, he said,

> Given the current favorable trends in national statistics and the power of the new discoveries, with a concerted effort to use and improve the structure provided by the original Cancer Act, cancer, still the most feared disease in the minds of the American public, will become a far less threatening killer within the next two decades.[3]

Today, approaching forty-five years after President Nixon's promise, the question remains: *Are* we winning? The answer depends on whom you talk with and how they utilize statistics to back their stance. Every few years, writers publish articles like "We're Winning The War Against Cancer,"[4] and "We Fought Cancer...And Cancer Won."[5] So while the jury's still deliberating, let me present support for both points of view.

We *Are* Winning the War on Cancer

If we relied on population-adjusted stats from the NCI and the Centers for Disease Control, we'd conclude that we're winning. According to a published CDC report, three million cancer survivors (1.5% of the population) were living in 1971; that number was 9.8 million (3.5%) in 2001 and 11.7 million (3.9%) in 2007.[6] By this interpretation,

> The population of cancer survivors continued to grow, both in number and as a percentage of the U.S. population, from 2001 to 2007. This growth can be attributed to multiple factors, including earlier detection, improved diagnostic methods, more effective treatment, improved clinical follow-up after treatment, and an aging U.S. population.[7]

The NCI began tracking cancer stats with its SEER program in 1975. According to its data, the overall (combined) cancer mortality rate declined by 11.4% from 1975 to 2009.[8] Also, the combined (all types) five-year survival rate increased from 36% in 1950 to 64.4% in 2008.[9]

The National Institutes of Health reported that from 1975 to 2000, 795,000 lung cancer deaths were prevented.[10] But the NIH-provided explanation had nothing to do with research or treatment. The saved lives resulted from the decrease in smoking in the US—the report itself went on to say that if Americans would have dropped the smoking habit in 1964, when Surgeon General Luther Terry published his report on smoking and health, 2.5 million deaths would have been prevented.[11]

Even so, overall the information published by government research departments supports the idea that we're winning the war on cancer.

We Are Not Winning the War on Cancer

If when looking at the statistics we focus on the absolute numbers—the figures not adjusted for population or other factors—we see that the results are sobering at best. Consider just the following:

1971[12]	2013[13]
Estimated cancer deaths: 335,000	Estimated cancer deaths: 580,350
New cancer cases: 635,000	New cancer cases: 1,660,290
Number of people in the US living with cancer: 3 million	Number of people in the US living with cancer: 13.7 million

Conclusion

I kept this chapter short and to the point, with little personal opinion, because the numbers are overwhelming. For you the most important point is not whether we're all winning the war but whether you are winning the battle. This book's main purpose is to help you get answers to crucial questions for support in developing and implementing your own action plan.

ACTION STEPS

1. Focus on actions you can take to beat cancer.
2. Do not let information overwhelm you or compromise your resolve.
3. Interpret data to your own advantage.

CANCER VICTOR TIPS

Angela Fenter, Massachusetts
Stage II Invasive Breast Cancer
Victor Since 2008

1. Believe in the power of God to heal you.
2. Be positive. "A cheerful heart is good medicine."
3. Eat healthy (80% fruits, vegetables, and whole grains).

4. Surround yourself with upbeat, positive people.
5. Treasure each day; not because you were diagnosed but because it's a gift from God.

The War on Cancer
https://vimeo.com/61676971

Chapter 22

Statistics

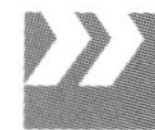 **Q:** *What do cancer statistics mean in my case?*

 **A:** Stats have very little to do with you. Think about it: Even with odds against them, people defy probability all the time, every day. And miracles do happen.

In 1924 Joseph Stalin succeeded Vladimir Ilyich Lenin as leader of the USSR and began a rule characterized by paranoia and tyranny, one responsible for killing tens of millions. The man's real surname was "Dzhugashvili," but he had changed it; "Stalin means "man of steel."[1] When questioned about mass deaths, his answer was as hard and cold as steel: *"A single death is a tragedy; a million deaths is a statistic."*[2]

Cancer statistics also send a chill down the spine. The American Cancer Society reported the following domestic (US) numbers for 2012:[3]

- Probability That a Person Will Develop or Die from Cancer Over the Course of a Lifetime: *men, 1 in 2; women, 1 in 3*
- People Alive Today Who've Ever Had Cancer: *13.7 million*
- New Cases Expected to Occur This Year: *1,660,290*
- People Expected to Die of Cancer This Year: *580,350*
- Percentage of People Who Survive Cancer: *The combined five-year survival rate for all cancer types is 67%.*

The question still remains: "What do these statistics mean in my case?" Part of the answer is, you determine what they mean for you.

• • • • • • • • • • • • •

Imagine a young boy who's intent on playing in the NFL. Consider that, even for high school players, the odds of doing so are 4,000 to 1—only 250 of every million will make it to the league for even a single play.[4]

What about a teen girl who dreams of becoming a *prima ballerina*? Only 2% of all women even have the physical attributes required. From there, competition is so fierce, and the bestowal of the honor so rare, that the probability of achieving such a goal is less than 1 in 1.6 billion.

Odds of becoming a rock star? Said to be around 10,000 to 1. But Kelly Clarkson, urged by friends and family, auditioned for *American Idol* and, out of many thousands, became its first winner. More than a decade later she continues to make hits (as of this writing *eighty-two* have reached *Billboard's* #1) and has sold close to twenty-five million albums.

Many people won't even try when the statistics say the odds make success very unlikely. Yet what the numbers say doesn't determine whether or not we succeed. I'll never forget being twelve and facing a huge sixteen-year-old pitcher whose fastball was topping 90mph. I was so intimidated by this MLB-bound slinger that I watched three pitches zoom right by me. I heard the ump yell, "Strike 1!" and "Strike 2!" and "Strike 3, you're out!" but never even started swinging the bat. I learned that day that the only way failure is 100% guaranteed is if I fail to try.

The Uncertainty of Certainty

If a doctor says your probability of surviving is less than 7%, or that you have six months to live, why simply believe it and wait to die? The reality is, *no one knows your treatment outcome with certainty*. Data is gathered and analyzed to generate statistics intended to help doctors make treatment decisions. Martin Brown, the NCI's chief of Health Services and Economics, said documenting a correlation between cancer control and outcomes is a key goal for surveillance, as difficult as it is.[5] The NCI utilizes many data-gathering techniques and technologies to generate stats that the American Cancer Society publishes: physician questionnaires, phone surveys with cancer survivors, reviews of clinical-trial publications, and reports from HMOs and private research organizations that participate in programs (for example). The numbers are projections, estimations, based on large sample groups. They definitely don't take into account every detail of your personal case. They look precise when put into print but are no more than approximations.

Lifetime Risk

When a person hears that half of all men will get cancer at some point, it sounds like every man is a 50/50. What the stats don't explain is that each person is different, or how much influence lifestyle choices and self-care can have on placing you in one 50% or the other. Did you know that eating five portions of vegetables and fruits,[6] exercising about five hours a week, and cutting your animal protein consumption to below 17% of your total diet can lower your personal risk of getting cancer by 50% to 60%?[7] *When looking at lifetime risk, be motivated to be proactive.*

Among the models used to predict lifetime risk are crude incidence rate, age-standardized incidence rate, cumulative rate, cumulative risk, current probability, and multiple-primaries adjusted method.[8] As you can see, researchers aren't satisfied with the validity of the projections and continue to search out methods and means to improve accuracy.

Calculating a Prognosis

If you've received a prognosis—a prediction of probable outcome—you may wonder how your doctor came up with the number. (I'm pretty sure there's no iPhone app for it.) Survival-rate statistics factor in incidence, mortality, and rates for each cancer, and much of the data is acquired through national surveys. For many cancers there are also microarray studies that consist of gene lists for estimating potential outcomes based on specific types and associated treatments.[9]

If your prognosis is recorded in your mind, I'd like to urge you to take the number away from the forefront of your thinking and move it to background noise. Stats have so many variables that by nature they're overgeneralized. When you hear about specific cancer-cell microassays, you may think, "It can't get more precise than an actual analysis of the same type of cancer cell I have and its response to the exact treatment I'm taking." But in reality most of these statistics are based on gene sets versus individual sets. In other words, the numbers are based on cells that may or may not even be similar to the cancer you're dealing with.

Five-Year Survival Rate

Stats for the five-year survival rate, which predicts the probability that a person will survive a specific type of cancer from the time of diagnosis, are calculated using data collected on hundreds of thousands of patients of all ages and races. As a patient, you'd look at the numbers and conclude that they're telling you your chances of being cured. I want to caution you to avoid this thinking. The experts are not in agreement on the validity of using these rates to predict cancer cure.

Frank Lichtenberg conducted a 2010 meta-analysis on numerous studies reporting on five-year survival rates. After review of the medical literature he concluded, "There is a highly significant correlation, in both the U.S. and Australia, between the change in 5-year survival for a specific tumor and the change in tumor-related mortality."[10]

Yet other studies discount these rates' value. One points out that not all cancers reveal their outcomes or tendencies within five years; each has a specific threshold. For example, the threshold to calculate statistical cure for pancreatic cancer is 2.6 years, whereas it's 25.2 years for cancer of the salivary gland.[11] This underscores my general point: *you cannot, so do not, base your hope or lack thereof on the numbers.*

We also must consider that the five-year rate changes over time from date of diagnosis.[12] The further a person is from the diagnosis, the more the rate increases in some cancers, while in others it decreases. This is what's meant by the term *conditional survival*. Each cancer differs in its conditional survival; the published numbers don't explain this.

Net Survival

Cancer survival rates represent the net survival; that is, the excess mortality due to cancer.[13] This is significant, because people who have cancer may die from another cause, the term for which is *comorbidity*. There's a saying about prostate cancer—not 100% accurate, but a great illustration of comorbidity: "All men will eventually get prostate cancer, but no one will die of it." More precisely, the survival rate for prostate cancer is so high that most men will die of old age or another cause.

"Personal cure" occurs when a person is successfully treated from cancer and later dies from another cause. It's vital that you consider this, too, because the survival rates do not reflect personal cure. Once again, there are too many variables when it comes to cancer for you to to look at a statistic and apply it to yourself.

The Proper Use of Statistics

A study published in 2012 found that few physicians comprehend cancer statistics.[14] One oft-misunderstood issue is the difference between survival rates and mortality. A phenomenon of over-diagnosis is on the rise, due to many new screening tests; cancers that would have never progressed if left untreated are now factoring into survival rates. This is resulting in physicians becoming more enthusiastic about survival when in countless cases the probable mortality does not justify the outlook. Another reality that makes it difficult to settle on the appropriate use of stats is that there are so many variables along the lines of race, age, smoking habits, diet, lifestyle, occupation, regional environmental factors, and more that make the numbers generalizations at most.[15]

I believe cancer statistics are about as useful to us as bumpers are to bowling. They ensure that the ball won't go into the gutter; they guarantee some degree of success without increasing the probability of a strike. Cancer stats will help an oncologist make decisions that are within an appropriate range. What will increase the accuracy of those decisions and improve the treatment outcome will be the actual clinical experience he or she has acquired while treating patients.

Conclusion

Once, lecturing in London, I pointed to some stats and asked, "What do these numbers mean to you?" One patient said, "They mean that cancer is a death sentence." When I asked if someone would reframe that outlook, another jumped up and exclaimed, *"I am not a statistic!"*

You can choose to be a cancer *victor*. My hope is that you will look at numbers, not live by numbers. Cancer statistics serve as a rough reference. They don't tell your story, and they don't predict your future.

ACTION STEPS

1. Make decisions based on useful information, not statistics.
2. Live by vision, not by numbers.
3. Decide that you'll be a cancer victor—no matter the odds.

CANCER VICTOR TIPS

Kate Pickford, Colorado
Stage 3c Ovarian Cancer
Victor Since 2009

1. Research all treatment options before committing. Understand the success rate of conventional treatment for your cancer before agreeing.
2. Adopt a diet that's anti-cancer.
3. Find a way to manage your stress level.
4. Prioritize your needs.
5. Rid yourself of toxic chemicals and toxic people.

Statistics
https://vimeo.com/61724635

Chapter 23

Defining Success

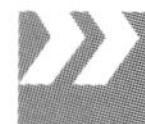 **Q:** *What should my treatment goals be?*

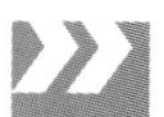 **A:** Most people believe success is getting rid of the cancer at whatever cost. With that measure of success, many suffer greatly or even die from aggressive treatments on the path to tumor eradication. A treatment that destroys the tumor but also destroys quality of life is what I call "a successful failure." To me, success is preserving and promoting an excellent quality of life at whatever cost. This is mostly achieved not by getting rid of a tumor but by taking away its threat on life. With this philosophy we have many patients alive and well with controlled cancers, in what I call "failed successes."

In the early 1980s, my father was invited to present his case studies at the World Congress on Cancer in Argentina. As part of the process, he was asked to present his best cases for peer review at Memorial Sloan-Kettering Cancer Center in New York. I was in medical school at the time.

Entering the boardroom, we were met by a few top oncologists and asked to present. My father put up a number of before-and-after X-rays and began to explain the success. Before he could finish with the first, though, another oncologist stood and said, "But there are still tumors present after treatment—that's not a success."

He told us to wait a moment, left, then returned with X-rays of his own. He showed a "before," with tumors, and an "after," tumor free. My father congratulated him and asked how the patient was doing. The oncologist replied that he'd passed away.

My father's case, considered by the review board a failure, was of a still-living man with lung cancer. Yes, there were still tumors, but the time difference between X-rays was ten years; the tumors didn't grow, and the patient didn't die. Nonetheless, his cases were stamped as failures and he was dropped from the World Congress.

It was quite redeeming in 1994 when he was invited to present his life's work at the World Congress in Australia. He received a standing ovation as he explained that tumor eradication should be secondary to preserving quality of life and adding years of quality living.

New-School Oncology

I am encouraged to see oncology evolving and tumor eradication no longer the gold standard. This is the new successful-treatment definition:

> When the mortality among a cancer patient group returns to the same level as in the general population, that is, the patients no longer experience excess mortality, the patients still alive are considered "statistically cured."[1]

Any oncologist can destroy tumors with conventional treatments. Once again, aggressive chemo is a highly effective tumor killer. High-dose radiation can wipe out tumors, and surgery can cut out any tumor. The problem is, a patient can die in the process or suffer so much that death becomes a welcomed result. *The art of cancer treatment is preserving the quality of life and adding years of quality living.*

Cancer Cure Vs. Cancer Control

As an integrative oncologist, my goal is not cancer cure but cancer control. Patients can learn to live many peaceful years *with* cancer. We regard it success if through effective treatment we're able to slow down or even reverse the disease's progression and the patient is able to go on living a fairly normal life, even if the markers indicate there's still some tumor activity. Remember, we're seeking for the patient to be able to live as long as a cancer-free person would live. I add to this the goal that not only will he or she live as long but also live as well and as productively. That's why our focus is not on cancer but on life.

Let me illustrate this with the testimony of a patient who came to Oasis of Hope in 1987. In her own words:

> In the summer, when my daughter had turned eleven, I'd just gone to the doctor and had my second pregnancy confirmed; of course I was very happy. At the same time, however, there was a suspicion of breast cancer, confirmed two days later. So the doctor basically told me that to save my own life I'd have to follow the therapeutic plan: (1) therapeutic abortion; (2) mastectomy; (3) radiation; and (4) chemotherapy. All this, one month after the diagnosis. I prayed to the Holy Spirit that night, and the next morning I knew I was going to keep the baby. We lived in Colorado then; we went to the University Hospital and told the doctor, "We're keeping the baby."
>
> The rest of my pregnancy was really happy. After we'd decided, I called Dr. Contreras, Sr. I'd heard his lecture at a 1984 health conference in Arizona and said to myself that if we ever needed anybody to help us in the field of cancer, his approach made sense, and he was a beautiful warm person. I said we're keeping the baby and asked what he suggested. He said everything we'd decided was okay and asked me to visit after the baby was a few months old. Now my baby is twenty-six! I think God is with me.
>
> The cancer did come back. I did well for a while; I also had some setbacks. In autumn 1991 we moved back to Europe (I was raised in Germany), but I've continued returning to the Oasis of Hope. All the spiritual and emotional support I've received is with me. . . . I still have cancer in my back and in my collarbone, but it has been stable since 2000. I am very grateful for that and for Oasis of Hope. If you or any of your loved ones have cancer, check it out. It's a holistic place, they just don't treat the body; they treat the person. Everyone there has the same great spirit. (Burga Theresia Ratti)

Medically speaking, our dear friend Burga still has cancer. But she is living well; living strong. She has many wonderful years ahead to enjoy her grandchildren. If you come to see us in the summer you'll probably get to meet her personally; she comes every year and spends a couple weeks volunteering to encourage other patients. She's the perfect example of the new approach to cancer treatment.

Managing Cancer as a Chronic Illness

Oncology is gradually embracing the approach my father started fifty years ago, focusing on adding years of quality to his patients' lives versus destroying tumors at any cost. This concept is managing cancer as a chronic illness. Remember the story of his presenting a case at Memorial Sloan-Kettering—of the patient with active cancer who was living a normal family and work life ten years after diagnosis? Don't miss the irony of this: Andrew D. Seidman, an oncologist at Memorial Sloan-Kettering Cancer Center, has said that metastatic breast cancer is now often treated and experienced like a chronic disease, similar to a novel with different chapters, as the patient's case evolves.[2]

Most patients, when they first come for treatment, ask me to do whatever it takes to get rid of the cancer. It takes a bit of listening and education to show the benefits of focusing on life and not on cancer. I usually ask questions like:

1. Do you want to live longer than the prognosis you were given?
2. Do you want to minimize negative side effects?
3. Would you be pleased if we could slow down the growth of cancer enough so that you could return to your regular activities and only have to come back occasionally for booster treatments?
4. Would you like to try a non-aggressive approach that will help you achieve the first three goals versus aggressive treatments that may or may not work but will certainly have debilitating side effects?

From time to time I encounter a patient who'll tell me to be as aggressive as possible with little regard to side effects, but most people are more interested in living well by controlling cancer than devastating the quality of life while trying to destroy the cancer. My goal for all my patients is to help them live longer and stronger.

Conclusion

At the 2010 Stand Up to Cancer event, Hall-of-Fame center Kareem Abdul-Jabbar said,

> Cancer doesn't care that you scored the most points in NBA history. My whole life, I got up every morning, went to the basketball court, and played my hardest. I knew that whoever scores the most points wins,

then I got cancer. And I learned that cancer is the only game where a tie is a win.[3]

ACTION STEPS

1. Focus on life, not cancer.
2. Set your treatment goals based on the quality of your life, not the destruction of tumors.
3. Remember, when it comes to cancer, a tie is a win.

CANCER VICTOR TIPS

Burga Ratti, Germany
Stage II Invasive Lobular Carcinoma
Victor Since 1987

1. Listen to all the options the oncologist gives for treatment.
2. Take time to evaluate the given options (it took me a few weeks); do not succumb to pressure to decide "right then."
3. Do research to see if there are other treatment plans that you feel to be a better fit for you. I believe the only way is a treatment focusing on body-mind-spirit.
4. Once you've chosen your "way," support your decision wholeheartedly.
5. Do all you can to strengthen your immune system through positive thoughts, health-promoting plant-based foods for body and mind, and simple relaxation techniques. Last but not least: do not give up!

Defining Success
https://vimeo.com/61728408

Chapter 24

The Economics of Cancer

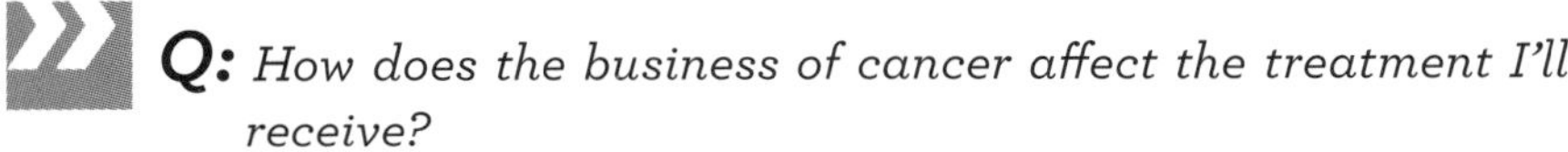

Q: *How does the business of cancer affect the treatment I'll receive?*

A: Present FDA regulations require terribly expensive accruement of clinical data as part of the drug approval process. This results in astronomical prices for new therapies. State-of-the-art technologies and novel medications, effective or not, are priced out of reach for even the wealthy. Insurance companies and Medicare are refusing payment on expensive drugs and thus limiting treatment options. It's no longer always the oncologist who decides the treatment. Now the payers make many of the decisions by pre-approving or denying payment.

The US economy has never been more volatile than it is now. E-businesses can mushroom into multi-billion dollar entities, seemingly overnight, and disappear just as quickly. Global businesses are Goliath in size. For example, a few years back, combined worldwide Walmart revenue hit $1,000,000,000 on Black Friday. Imagine how big a business must be to sell $1 billion of merchandise in one day. Walmart has huge economic impact by generating hundreds of thousands of jobs and managing a retail machine that keeps the wheels of thousands of manufacturers, logistics firms, textile mills, farms, and pharmaceutical companies rolling. Could the economy survive the closure of Walmart?

Amid the current crisis has come a new phenomenon called "Too Big to Fail." The basic concept: were behemoth corporations to go bankrupt, the resultant ripple effect would deal a fatal blow to everything else. It's why President Obama led the charge to increase the national debt in bailing out, subsidizing, or conceding to mega-corporations. Government stepped in when economists advised that we could not withstand large-entity failure in major industries (e.g., auto, agriculture, and petroleum).

The banking industry, one of the most dubious, is intertwined in a codependent relationship with the federal government. Though estimated national debt is $16 trillion and climbing, the "Troubled Asset Relief Program" (TARP) gave Citigroup $2.5 trillion, Morgan Stanley $2 trillion, and Bank of America $1.3 trillion from 2007 to 2010.[1] On the one hand we're pouring money into the banks; on the other we're paying $2.7 trillion annually in *interest*. The president explained the justification this way: "Right now the most important task for us is to stabilize the patient. The economy is badly damaged; it is very sick. So we have to take whatever steps are required to make sure it is stabilized."[2] Fascinating that he used this metaphor to describe our economic condition, and it's not the first time the economy and illness have gone hand and hand.

In 1971, the same year he declared the "War on Cancer," President Nixon took the US off the international gold standard,[3] since which inflation has caused prices to escalate. Since this war began, the cost of cancer has skyrocketed from $15 billion in 1972[4] to an estimated $226.8 billion in 2007.[5] Cancer's mortality rate in the US has decreased only 5% after four decades of research, yet, in the Nixon tradition, the current administration plans to double spending on cancer research.[6]

Though it's impossible to fully understand why cancer treatment is so expensive and so ineffective, it should be clear that economic forces may limit your access to treatment options and that you may have to deal with some obstacles along your path of healing.

Is the Cancer Industry "Too Big to Fail"?

This leads to the notion that cancer has created an industry that generates so many jobs and so much revenue that if the cure were to be found, the business would shut down and the economy would suffer a fatal blow. Conspiracy theorists believe the cure already exists but has been hidden by the government to protect the big pharmaceutical, medical equipment, and hospital corporations.

I found one study estimating that eliminating cancer would bring an increase in healthcare cost of $3,800.00 annually per life-year-gained.[7] This suggests it would cost taxpayers, the government, and insurance companies more if cancer were to be cured than to just let it continue to take almost 600,000 American lives a year.

I choose not to believe that a government conspiracy has concealed the cancer cure. After thirty years of clinical experience and research I can tell you that cancer is far too complex to have "a cure"—there's no silver bullet. Still, I recognize that this disease is big business.

Again, the annual US cost of cancer is more than $226 billion. Only half is related to research and treatment (other elements include out-of-pocket patient expenses, insurance co-payments, and deductibles). Nevertheless, Medicare pays $1.5 billion dollars for radiation therapy and $1.8 billion for chemo every year.[8] And one market study projected that $57 billion would be spent on all types of cancer therapies in 2013.[9]

Further, cancer's cost is terribly underestimated because it does not take into account many hidden costs: childcare, transportation, ostomy supplies, assistive devices, wigs, food, lodging, prostheses, etc.[10] Another huge indirect cost is lost wages;[11] cancer is also the leading cause of all long-term disability (11.8% of all claims).[12] The financial burden on patients can be as distressing and debilitating as the disease itself. The biggest factors in soaring costs are the development of innovative treatments, inflation, population growth, and an aging population.[13]

Each year more than a thousand new drugs are registered with the FDA for testing. Cost is prohibitive. One course with Provenge (for prostate cancer) is $93,000,[14] while 90% of all new FDA-approved cancer drugs cost at least $20,000 for twelve weeks of treatment.[15] The annual increase in oncology drugs is 15% (it's 5% for other drugs).

Take the recent change in first-line standard treatment with fluorouracil administered with leucovorin (FU/LV). The FDA approved a new regimen, adding oxaliplatin to FU/LV. The new combo, referred to as FOLFOX, has resulted in increasing colorectal cancer (CRC) survival by 1.4 months; total average cost in caring for a patient with CRC increased from $60,586 to $107,994.[16] More than $47,000 increased survival by less than a month and a half. (This makes me want to compare drug companies with casinos. The house never loses.)

One study found that the average oncologist salary increased 35.6% from 2000 to 2004 while primary care physicians increased 9.9%.[17] That's been reversing since as the overhead of a private oncology practice has increased, drug costs have soared, and reimbursement (Medicare, insurance companies) has decreased. Eroding profit has caused many oncologists to retire early or close and seek large-hospital employment.[18] This seems again to identify skyrocketing drug costs as the main culprit.

What's Driving Up Drug Costs?

Average cost to develop a cancer drug is $1.2 billion.[19] Companies introduce new patented drugs at sky-high prices to quickly recoup investments and generate profits. Once a patent expires, competing manufacturers can introduce an identical generic drug at a very low cost. The fundamental economic concept is that price is determined by supply and demand; *The New England Journal of Medicine* says there are cases where a manufacturer halts production of generic cancer drugs to protect their name-brand price.[20] Essential chemo drugs have become short on supply. This has given birth to unofficial markets where unregulated vendors can mark up drugs by 3,000%.[21]

With all the evidence in the medical literature, it seems logical to put the lion's share of excessive-cost blame on pharmaceutical companies. Drug makers place it on the exorbitant cost of development. I have a different opinion: the essential flaw is that *everyone is funding the search for the cure.* Only 2% of the NCI budget is dedicated to cancer prevention research. When President Obama signed the American Recovery and Reinvestment Act (2009), the NCI received an infusion of $1.3 billion, yet the 2012 annual proposal didn't even mention increasing prevention.[22]

How to Lower Costs

The best way to lower the cost of cancer is through prevention. Take the EPA's SunWise program, which teaches students how to protect themselves against cancer-provoking damage from overexposure to harmful rays. It was found that for every $1 invested in the program, $2 to $4 would be saved in medical costs and loss of productivity.[23]

Other measures could be cancer-exclusive hospitals, improving treatment planning, and benchmarking centers of excellence.[24] With the first, centers could have better control of resource management and allocation; improved physicians' and nurses' case-management skills could result in better treatment outcomes. The second could bring more efficient treatment, eliminating countless overtime hours. The third would mean other facilities could mimic cost-lowering best practices.

Conclusion

Adam Schickedanz summarized our treatment paradigm: "The U.S. spends far more per person than any other country in the world in treating cancer, without demonstrably superior results."[25] There's no evidence that a patient can put full faith in our treatment delivery system. To be a cancer victor, you must establish your own path toward healing, then make informed decisions and partake of what's available through conventional means while supplementing with alternatives. If you simply do as you're told without thinking things through, you can easily become another statistic. You are not a widget to be put into the medical-profit-generating machine. *You're a cancer victor in the making.*

ACTION STEPS

1. Ask for generic drugs whenever possible. They're the same formula and work as well as brand names but at fractional cost.
2. Do not accept when an insurance company denies payment of an expensive cancer drug. Be the squeaky wheel and continue to contact your insurer until they pay.
3. Expensive drugs are not always most effective. Natural therapies are often cheaper and can be as good or better. In addition to your oncologist, consult a natural health practitioner as well.

CANCER VICTOR TIPS

Mr. Ghazal, Canada
Colorectal Cancer
Victor Since 2008

1. Be aware of how nutrition is related to cancer.
2. Obtain cancer information and be aware of how we can keep it at bay.
3. Meet other people with a similar disease.
4. Be aware of how vitamins work against cancer.
5. Have faith and hope that you can become whole again.

Chapter 25

Limitations and Pitfalls of Science

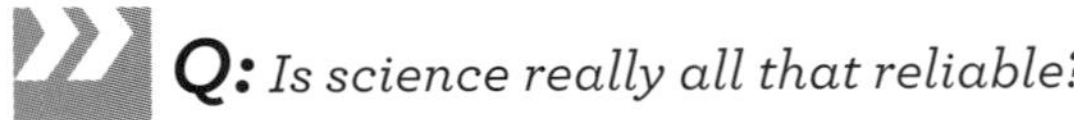

Q: *Is science really all that reliable?*

A: For all the bells and whistles medical science boasts, and its earnest efforts to only practice evidence-based medicine, the fact remains that more people will die of cancer this year than last. The scientific method is not a panacea, and we should be open to alternative scientific methodology tackling cancer.

If we look around we'll see scientific advancements making our lives easier and more productive than ever. We've come to believe that the scientific method, followed correctly, results in good outcomes. Students are given its steps as a recipe when the method actually is just a set of general and practical investigative guidelines that will be modified through trial and error (lots of errors) during research. That is, following the scientific method doesn't necessarily translate into exact science.

• • • • • • • • • • • •

We cannot always rely solely on senses for what may seem obvious patterns in nature. When Copernicus told the scientific community of his time that the earth was circling around the sun, they scorned him; from unmoving ground, observing sunrise to sunset, it was clear the one moving was the sun! His colleagues also had another lien against his theory: if he were right, then Venus would have phases as the moon has. From where they stood, Venus always appeared bright. Copernicus had no explanation for this; he said, "God in time will provide the answer."

A century after his heliocentric theory was discredited, Galileo Galilei, aided by more advanced technology, telescopically saw and then sketched the phases of Venus, and you know the rest of the story. It's true that reality never changes; however, our perception of it does, depending on the tools we have to observe it.

We establish present scientific observations as fact based on systematic and careful study, creating what we call models that can be impressively precise. The problem is when we want to extrapolate (apply) the models to other circumstances or to different conditions. If we become attached to a model, we will be biased and subject to error.

Aristotle scientifically established the static-universe theory. After years of carefully, systematically observing the heavens, he established that the position of all known stars never changed and, hence, concluded that they've been there eternally. This theory was challenged on religious grounds but scientifically stood strong for twenty-two centuries.

Albert Einstein introduced his cosmological equation in 1917 as a modification to his theory of general relativity. His mathematical model showed the universe to be expanding; a staunch believer in a stationary universe, he added the cosmological constant to correct this "fault" and thus satisfy his scientific bias.[1] He even refused to accept the validation of his original equation by other respected scientists. Not until 1931, when he visited Edwin Hubble and saw the stars moving—in other words, the universe expanding—did Einstein come to his senses. Hubble's demonstration of the cosmological redshift proved the original model. A victim of what we call cognitive dissonance, Einstein later called the tweak to his equation the "biggest blunder" of his life.[2]

Theories and Models Change

It's improbable that in modernity theories and models will be upheld for centuries without challenge. There will always be more intelligent researchers with newer toys, more sophisticated observational tools to prove a model at least outdated if not obsolete. But it seems that in medicine generally, and oncology particularly, the models have not been challenged enough.

Not only is there significant researcher's bias, there also is establishment cognitive dissonance that doesn't allow us to see the obstacles we must overcome. It's been said that while in other professions the mistakes are exposed, in medicine they are buried.

In the US, death caused by doctors—our third leading cause (after heart disease and cancer, with 250,000 annually)—is a real problem. Dr. Barbara Starfield found that while US medicine is among the world's most expensive, it's far from the most effective, ranking thirteenth of fifteen nations evaluated.[3] In her assessment Japan ranks #1 in all aspects, chiefly in diagnostic technology. Thus fewer Japanese receive medical treatments; in the US, second only to Japan in technology, diagnostic tests are linked to overtreatment and iatrogenic events.

Often our scientific models are so powerful that they deceive us into thinking we're on the right path due to institutional, governmental, or peer pressure. For instance, the cancer research model has focused on the tumor. It's all been learning about cancer, developing methods to combat tumors, and measuring tumor destruction. Sounds like a good plan, right? But think about it: that focus is on developing a method to establish a model that addresses the tumor, not the patient.

Also, the scientific method is predicated on managing or reducing variables to arrive at a conclusion objectively. There are hundreds of publications on the impact of specific genes or specific receptors within specific cancer cells doing specific malignant things. More than 90% of the grant money is allocated to finding out everything there is to find out on every primary cancer. Meanwhile, only a fraction of cancer patients die from a primary tumor. More than 90% die from secondary tumors, what we call metastasis; less than 10% of research money is spent on this issue! Why? Because metastatic disease just has too many variables.

It's only after this type of basic science that the next model, drug development, comes into action. We start applying the designed chemical to cancer cells "in vitro" (*glass*), in a Petri dish. If cancer cells are killed, the model is extrapolated to an "in vivo" (*living*), done in live animals. If tumors in animals are destroyed, the model is extrapolated to a clinical trial, with actual cancer patients. I mentioned earlier that extrapolation is a massive problem. A review of the "in vivo" result of most anticancer drugs would astonish you—you'd be amazed by the millions and millions of animals we've cured. Conversely, extrapolation to humans has been so dismal that once I proposed to try the drugs that did *not* work on animals to see if they had the reverse effect on people.

Nevertheless, physicians, institutions, the government, and the media flood us with the hyperbole of breakthrough and the progress of evidence-based cancer-therapy development. The medical literature contains report after report showing tumors killed left and right, yet the American Cancer Society's Facts & Figures reports that more cancer patients are expected to die in 2013 than in 2012. Why this dissonance? Once more: philosophically, the establishment's scientific methodology focus is the *tumor*. If the drug destroys tumors, it goes into the books as effective, whether or not patients survive. So we find lots of successes and lots of dead patients (treatment-wise, "successful failures").

Conclusion

At Oasis of Hope we established a model based on a philosophy that focuses on our *patients*. Everything we do is aimed at improving their quality of life; their tumors are secondary. Thousands of patients have come to us after their doctors sent them home to die; years later, they're still alive. X-rays will show tumors here and there, but they couldn't care less; they're enjoying life (even though we're definitely not disappointed if the tumor does go away!). I call these patients "failed successes."

ACTION STEPS

1. The scientific method is inexact; research all models to find the one that fits your needs.
2. Alternative medicine is scientifically based.
3. Conventional oncology has some of the answers but not all. An integrative approach is best to combat cancer.

CANCER VICTOR TIPS

María de la Cruz, México
Breast Cancer
Victor Since 2008

1. Believe in the treatment you're taking, and be positive.
2. Put everything in God's hands and accept His will.
3. Accept help from your family and friends.
4. Follow your doctor's indications for treatment and nutrition.
5. Have faith.

Limitations and Pitfalls of Science
https://vimeo.com/61761526

Chapter 26

Clinical Trials

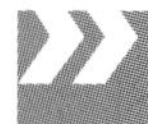

Q: *Are clinical trials the last hope or the best option for me?*

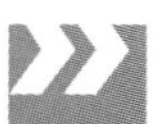

A: There's no question that clinical trials are necessary and good. I don't recommend participating in one that's just rehashing refurbished therapies. Look for truly innovative trials, especially those using non-aggressive elements.

Many medical breakthroughs have resulted by chance discovery. It's well known that penicillin was discovered in London when Alexander Fleming was cleaning up Petri dishes that had sat in a sink for some time.[1] He noticed that a green mold from the *Penicillium notatum* family had killed the staph bacterium in the dish and published a paper in the *British Journal of Experimental Pathology* in 1929. By the end of World War II, hundreds of billions of units of penicillin were being produced at a pharmaceutical grade, which revolutionized infectious disease control.

Penicillin was not the first treatment discovered through mishaps. In 1895 a German physicist, Wilhelm Röntgen, discovered the X-ray quite by chance.[2] He was using a cathode ray tube for experimentation and it produced a fluorescent glow. Shielding the tube with black paper, he observed that a light could still be seen on a screen a few feet away. He then discovered this invisible light could pass through other materials like flesh but couldn't pass through materials like bone and metals.

In the early 1900s it was discovered in France that daily doses of radiation would increase a person's probability of surviving cancer.[3] Soon thereafter it was also learned that over-exposure could lead to cancer; many X-ray technicians ended up getting cancers such as leukemia. This is one example of how helpful agents can also be harmful, and how discovery by chance can lead to great breakthroughs while costing many human lives. And, it's one reason why drug and medical device research became regulated and systematized.

Purposes

In cancer treatment there's far more knowledge about what doesn't work than what does. The need to find safer, more effective treatments drives research and the market for new drugs. The main purposes of clinical trials include finding more effective treatments with fewer adverse side effects and, if possible, more economic than existing therapies. The scientific method of medical discoveries matured throughout the last century, and medical ethics came into play as well. To minimize the possible harm to humans from medicinal experimentation, the FDA developed a protocol for drug and medical apparatus testing and approval. As outlined by the NIH, clinical trials consist of four phases:[4]

- **Phase I:** Researchers test a new drug or treatment in a small group of people for the first time to evaluate its safety, determine a safe dosage range, and identify side effects.
- **Phase II:** The drug or treatment is given to a larger group to see if it's effective and to further evaluate its safety.
- **Phase III:** The drug or treatment is given to large groups to confirm its effectiveness, monitor side effects, compare it to commonly used treatments, and collect info that will allow it to be used safely.
- **Phase IV:** Studies are done after the drug or treatment has been marketed to gather information on the drug's effect in various populations and any side effects associated with long-term use.

Inclusion Criteria

While it can be hard to find data on clinical trials, it can be even harder to be a right match and be accepted. Striving to produce valid data, protocol writers and researchers are very discriminatory about who they'll admit. Access may be limited by any number of criteria, including:

1. Sex
2. Age
3. Type of cancer
4. Stage of cancer
5. Is the experimental treatment applicable to the patient?
6. Is the experimental treatment safe for the patient?
7. Activities of daily living
8. Life expectancy (Is patient expected to live to finish the trial?)

Because inclusion criteria (really, *exclusion* criteria) are formal and stringent, between 44% and 66% of patients who have a specified cancer will not be accepted to clinical trials.[5]

Ethical Issues

Each trial phase presents its own set of ethical questions. The main point is that a physician, first and foremost, must do no harm to her patient.[6] The dilemma is whether it's ethical to recommend that a patient participate in a study with an unproven treatment. This is especially true for phase I trials where goals are not oriented to potential benefits. If it's about safety and dosing, the question is if it's appropriate to expose a patient to unknown potential toxic adverse reactions. Researchers have agreed that full disclosure about the nature of the trial and possible negative side effects must be provided. Patients review and sign a lengthy, comprehensive, and legal informed-consent document.

Once the safe dosage is identified, a phase II study can begin. The new ethical issue is whether to offer an unproven treatment in lieu of treatments already approved.[7] In addition is the question of whether the study's design will generate valid data. Much of the accepted research is based on theories and assumptions derived from historical data, but in many cases this data is far from conclusive. Also, there's no way to assure that the condition of the patients in the current trial matches the condition of those included in studies that make up the historical data.

Phase III trials suffer from similar issues. One common problem is that the data collected from phases I and II is insufficient to validate the phase III design.[8] Have you ever wondered what happened when you hear a new approved cancer drug was later pulled off the market? Many would think a pharmaceutical company irresponsibly pushed a drug through the process.

An explanation probably closer to the truth is that not enough data and evidence was available at each phase of testing, the sample size wasn't large enough or wasn't adequately randomized, the assumptions were incorrect, and/or the trial's design was flawed in another way. In all industries, products are launched and then later recalled once they're used by enough people to detect design flaws. That's the nature of product development, and cancer research is no exception.

The promise, the draw, of a clinical trial is that you may be given the new breakthrough treatment that actually works when nothing else does. But remember, this is an experiment. Some people voluntarily participate with motivating factors that include believing more personal attention and support is given to patients in a trial, hoping for a better outcome with the experimental therapy than with the standard treatment, or feeling pressured by friends/relatives to try this versus giving up.[9] Such reasons aren't enough to convince everyone to participate.

Some don't want burdens[10] like time requirements and reporting. A trial has strict parameters; some won't be able to adjust work schedules or other activities around it. Some also have a negative perception about the process. They may believe trials on humans are unethical or that the results benefit manufacturers, not patients.

Probability of Help

Clinical trials exist for scientific goals of advancing knowledge. Whereas your physician's goal is to help you beat cancer, the researcher wants to find out what works and what doesn't. You may be looking for access to a promising drug because known treatments don't offer much hope, yet keep in mind that trials are simply tests on new drugs whose efficacy and safety are unknown. If you participate, you may be the one who responds. The right mentality is one where you're looking at the greater good of patients who come after you. Whether or not you're helped directly, your participation would help others in the future.

Safety

If you're accepted, your primary concern (and that of the physician overseeing your care) should be your safety. Most important is to build rapport with your nurses. Oncology clinical trial nurses are largely responsible for assuring patient safety as well as documenting and reporting adverse effects.[11] If you ask the right questions, your nurse can be your most important information asset.

Symptoms to look out for include:

- Pain
- Shortness of breath
- Weight loss or gain
- Changes in vital signs
- Nausea
- Headache
- Fever
- Body aches

The tricky thing is that all these symptoms are associated with most oncology treatments. It's up to you to report them and then converse with your nurse to gauge if it's safe for you to continue. Be sure there's an established way for you to communicate with the trial nurse so you can report symptoms. If there isn't a defined channel, don't enter the trial. In addition to your symptoms, doctors and nurses will monitor your blood work, tumor markers, and radiological studies.

Conclusion

There's growing interest and advancements in the scientific community in developing mathematical models that can simulate tumor growth and response to new treatments.[12] These use clinical data to create possible values and parameters to predict potential reduction and change in tumor composition. There may be a day where enough data has been collected on human clinical trials that valid computational models could replace the current system of research and phase trials.

These models may be so sophisticated that they're scientifically credible. For example, a sensitivity analyses model may include tumor dynamics like cell-cycle duration, time interval before a dormant cell dies through necrosis, time needed for necrosis to be complete, time needed for apoptosis completion, apoptosis rate, necrosis rate, fraction of stem cells that perform symmetric division, treatment-specific cell-kill ratio, etc., etc., etc.

The terminology alone creates a cognitive elixir that seduces the most scientific minds. Validity will increase as we gather data; these models may have weighty impact later in our lifetimes. For now, phase trials are the only option for drug and device development.

ACTION STEPS

1. Talk to your oncologist about trials for which you may be eligible.
2. If you choose to participate, look for phase III studies where safety and effective doses are already defined.
3. If you participate, adopt the belief that whether or not you receive personal benefits, you are benefiting future cancer patients.

CANCER VICTOR TIPS

Jose Elpidio Eloy, Dominican Republic
Prostate Cancer
Victor Since 2008

1. Go to Oasis of Hope; no other place treats people with such compassion.
2. Always be positive. This will help you help yourself.
3. Let your food be your main medicine, always.
4. Let chemo and other conventional therapies be your last option.
5. Read and research everything you can before you make decisions.

Clinical Trials
https://vimeo.com/61763168

Chapter 27

Cancer Research

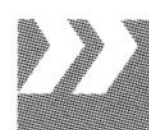

Q: *Will cancer researchers find the cure?*

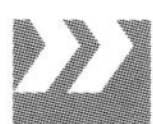

A: With the present philosophy, I think not. Nothing on the horizon is close to a cure. The best hope of making a dent is implementing comprehensive metabolic therapies with a multi-prong approach that attacks cancer from all flanks.

Albert Einstein said insanity is doing the same thing over and over but expecting different results.[1] I believe that for the last forty years this is what researchers have been doing in search of the cure. In chapter 21 I explained how the absolute incident rates and death rates clearly show that the many billions of dollars haven't reduced the number diagnosed, annual deaths caused, or lifetime probability of being diagnosed. Survivability improvements have mostly resulted from early detection. The US has never had more deaths due to cancer than we do now.

You may find a report that seems to indicate the cancer death rate dropping by 20% from 1991 to 2009.[2] A closer look at how that statistic was derived shows that the improvement happened in three cancers: prostate, lung, and breast. But the reduction didn't result from research or better treatment. Here's why there was a decrease in death, with each:

- Most prostate cancers found via PSA screening are chronic diseases that never cause death. Due to early detection, many now are over-treated. Men who didn't need medical intervention are suffering consequences like incontinence or impotence.
- Fewer are dying of lung cancer because public education has been effective in motivating people to quit smoking.

- The breast cancer death rate is dropping as doctors are wising up and putting fewer women on hormone replacement therapy (known to cause breast cancer) and as fewer women are smoking.

A Different Path

I could share plenty about ineffectiveness, but rather than outlining shortcomings of research I'd like to propose a new research paradigm.

Networked Team Effort vs. Isolated Approach

I applaud the research community's shift away from independent research centers. In an emerging trend, multiple research and treatment centers in different countries are sharing data.[3] By involving treating physicians in the process, there may be a way to overcome the lack of participation by groups who tend to avoid participating in clinical trials.[4]

New integrated networks of doctors, researchers, patients, hospitals, labs, and government agencies are forming; info-sharing could speed up the research process. And some success is starting to show. For example, the childhood acute lymphoblastic leukemia five-year survival rate has increased from 15% in 1969 to nearly 80% today.

Research Natural Elements vs. Develop and Test Drugs

The last ten years have been much more promising for natural therapies. Scientists have been discovering how nutrients from different foods and herbs can reprogram malignant-cell behavior. These elements may not directly kill cancer cells, but they can change the treatment outcome and help people overcome cancer.

The body of evidence for the anti-cancer power of nutrients supports the argument that we should shift some of our time away from testing pharmaceuticals and devote more effort to researching natural elements.

Test Comprehensive Protocols vs. Single-Drug Testing

A new tendency to test drugs in combination is taking research in the right direction but still falls into the same *drug*-testing trap. I believe we'd make more progress if we funded more *patient*-centered studies. That some programs in France (and other nations) make sure the patient is at the center of every decision[5] may be one reason France is producing many exciting treatment protocols.

Once more: clinical trials are designed to determine if a drug is safe, what the dosage should be, and if it destroys tumors. What if trials were designed holistically that involved multiple therapies to meet all needs of the patients to help them live longer and stronger? The argument against testing protocols is that we'd never know what drug actually worked. *More lives would be saved.* Shouldn't that be the goal?

Focus on Metastasis vs. Study Primary Tumors

Early stage primary tumors are highly treatable; later tumors that result from spread are called metastatic. Nearly 100% of cancer research is done on primary tumors, yet almost all deaths attribute to metastasis. Research on effective ways to treat and manage metastasis likely would cause the death rate from all cancer to decline dramatically.

Prevention vs. Cure

Again, the NCI directs less than 2% of its annual research budget at prevention (see chapter 24). Benjamin Franklin rightly said, "An ounce of prevention is worth a pound of cure,"[6] and nowhere is this more true than with cancer. Much money would be better spent on programs to motivate lifestyle change in children. We know that people who eat plenty of fruits and vegetables[7]—in general, have a high-in-fiber, low-in-animal-proteins diet—substantially reduce their risk for many cancers, and can improve their risk factors even more by exercising several times a week.[8-10] Whether or not adults will make the necessary changes, the best hope for a cancer-free world lies in showing children the right way from birth.

Life Extension vs. Tumor Eradication

When a patient is first diagnosed with cancer, the instinct is to get rid of it as quickly as possible. But, unlike a bad tooth, "tumor removal" does not mean "cured." Cancer, a problem of the immune system, results from the breakdown of multiple body functions. Most treatment focuses on destroying the tumor; while aggressive chemo almost always destroys a tumor initially, it's frequent that a recurrence will bring back a tumor no longer affected by the same therapy. Cancer is constantly mutating.

For this reason, we need a more comprehensive treatment approach, aiming less at tumor eradication and more at life extension and quality.

The Payoff

In our world stars and celebs make tens (or hundreds) of millions of dollars while schoolteachers make thousands. Everything rises and falls on financial incentive. In fact, many drugs known to be effective aren't made because too little money would be made to warrant the investment. With rare diseases like chronic lymphocytic leukemia, there's not a wide enough need for pharmaceutical firms to allocate development monies.[11]

But before I start in on corporate evils, let me ask: why do you leave home and go to work? Like me, you need to earn and provide. If the job didn't pay enough to cover expenses, would you continue with it merely from moral goodness? Ultimately, without making ends meet, you'd be obligated to make a change so you could provide for your family's needs.

Many people brand Big Pharma as the evil profit-at-any-cost force that cares nothing for people. Yet the cost to take a drug through the FDA clinical-trial process is $485,000,000–$800,000,000![12] After all formula-development research, labs equipped to manufacture lots for testing, and education, promotion, and distribution for getting the drug to patients, each new market-entering cancer med has over $1.8 *billion* of investment to be recovered before there's a penny of profit.[13] The purpose of a patent is to provide a time where no competitor can introduce a generic form, allowing the inventor to recoup the initial investment. This also is why using new drugs can yield *monthly* costs of up to $100,000.

To change the R&D process, we'll need to change clinical-trial and patent processes. Researchers, drug companies, health institutions, and physicians need to be rewarded not for tumor reduction, but for patient survival. ObamaCare's two thousand pages of legislation is said to have wording to the effect that doctors will be compensated by how their patients fare. It would be glorious if things worked out this way. My concern is that the plan will take us as close as possible to a socialized medical system, which works against cancer patients without significant means. Every nation with this system has extremely limited availability of new drugs, wherein people of means go to private clinics to acquire the treatments.

Conclusion

I think major changes in the drug industry within our lifetime are improbable. Hence, it's even more crucial that you're willing to think unconventionally and seek out info for yourself on integrating alternative therapies with plenty of patient testimonials supporting their claims.

ACTION STEPS

1. There's an abundance of information on natural medicine. Search for it and incorporate it as best you can.
2. Find a forward-thinking doctor who practices patient-centered medicine.
3. Focus not on tumor eradication but on living longer and stronger.

CANCER VICTOR TIPS

Paul Champoux, Michigan
Bladder Cancer
Victor Since 2008

1. Ask the Supreme Healer, the Lord Jesus Christ, for healing mercy, by undeserved grace alone.
2. Take and follow a protocol of therapies at Oasis of Hope, then always follow their regimen thereafter as a permanent lifestyle change.
3. Greatly reduce animal protein intake, especially red meats and dairy. Eat more fish, beans, nuts, organic vegetables, oats, and whole grains.
4. Develop a regular, progressively increased program (in length and intensity) of aerobic exercise.
5. Use a targeted, broad, doctor-recommended range of vitamin, mineral, and herbal supplements and medications.

Cancer Research
https://vimeo.com/61822466

Chapter 28

Alternative Cancer Treatments

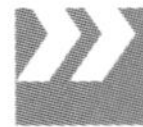

Q: *Do any alternative cancer treatments really work?*

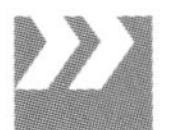

A: Yes. Many alternatives are effective when administered correctly. For best results, many cancers require an integrative approach.

Billy Best was sixteen when his life was derailed by a cancer diagnosis.[1] Chemotherapy for Hodgkin's lymphoma at Boston's Dana-Farber Cancer Institute made him sicker and weaker with each treatment. Having recently witnessed his aunt's breast-cancer chemo experience—she became very weak and ill, and died—he decided not to go that route. He grabbed his skateboard and split; he'd gone as far as Houston when his parents convinced him to come home to Massachusetts, promising he wouldn't have to resume chemo. Authorities were looking into putting him in foster care so he would have to continue when his parents took him to Canada for alternative therapies including 714X and Essiac tea.

Alternative treatment worked for Billy. Soon after he went into remission, he accepted our invitation to come to Oasis of Hope and share his story with our patients. He was wise beyond his years; he stayed a couple of weeks, breathing hope into our patients. To date, he continues to be in good health, taking a few ounces of Essiac every day and two twenty-one-day cycles of 714X per year.[2]

Before my father, there really wasn't anybody known for alternative cancer therapy in Mexico. He put both alternative treatment and Mexico on the medical map; Oasis of Hope became *the* destination for alternative medicine, and now hundreds of such cancer centers tout thousands of different therapies.

FRANCISCO CONTRERAS, MD *and* DANIEL E. KENNEDY, MC

I've found that every single treatment has at least one success story like Billy Best. Now, a case study of one isn't sufficient for a therapy to be FDA-approved or physician-respected. But, at any rate, alternatives are largely dismissed. Doctors who use them are often investigated by the FDA or simply labeled quacks, frauds, or charlatans, as in the case of Dr. Stanislaw R. Burzynski.[3]

The case for alternative cancer therapy has been tarnished by stories of high-profile individuals who opted for such treatments and didn't recover, like Steve Jobs, who avoided surgery and chose a macrobiotic diet.[4] People criticize his choice but fail to realize he outlived his prognosis, which may not have happened with conventional medicine. At the same time, those like Suzanne Somers, who treated her breast cancer with mistletoe[5] extract instead of chemo, surgery, and radiation, are living proof that natural medicine has every bit as much possibility of helping a person beat cancer. The difference may come down to quality of life. Natural therapies are rarely debilitating; chemo and radiation almost always cause severe negative side effects.

A 2002 NIH survey found that one third of the US population has used some form of natural medicine, and people who have cancer are increasingly aware that conventional treatment may not be enough. Let me share a few definitions from the NCI's online dictionary of medical terms. Then I'll introduce some classic alternative cancer treatments.

Definitions and Treatments

Alternative Medicine.[6] Treatments that are used instead of standard (conventional; currently accepted and widely used) treatments. Standard treatments are based on scientific research results, while less research has been done for most types of alternative medicine. Alternative medicine may include special diets, megadose vitamins, herbal preparations, special teas, and magnet therapy. For example, a special diet may be used instead of anti-cancer drugs as a treatment for cancer.

Complementary Medicine.[7] Treatments not considered standard that are used along with standard treatments. These include acupuncture, dietary supplements, massage therapy, hypnosis, spiritual healing, and meditation. For example, acupuncture may be used with certain drugs to help lessen pain or nausea and vomiting.

Integrative Medicine.[8] Combination of standard treatment with complementary and alternative (CAM) therapies that have been shown to be safe and to work. CAM therapies treat the mind, body, and spirit.

Complementary and Alternative Medicine.[9] Treatment forms used in addition to (complementary)/instead of (alternative) standard treatments.

Conventional Medicine.[10] A system in which medical doctors and other healthcare professionals (e.g., nurses, pharmacists, therapists) treat symptoms and diseases using drugs, radiation, or surgery. Also called allopathic medicine, biomedicine, mainstream medicine, orthodox medicine, or Western medicine.

In light of these definitions, all the below alternative treatments fall into the Complementary and Alternative Medicine (CAM) category, which means they have insufficient clinical data to make medical claims of being effective cancer treatments.

714X

714X, a camphor compound mixed with nitrogen, ammonium salts, sodium chloride, and ethanol,[11] was developed by Gaston Naessens, who believes cancer is a result of immune system dysfunction. 714X is either injected or inhaled; Naessens claims its active agents attack cancer cells and boost the immune system. No publications have indicated that 714X is unsafe to use. Reports of its efficacy are anecdotal.

Gerson Therapy

Developed by Dr. Max Gerson to address toxicity and lack of nutrients in the body,[12] this therapy isn't only for cancer. As it's aimed at physical detox and providing nutrients needed to restore the immune system to proper function, people with heart disease, arthritis, diabetes, and other illnesses have turned to it. Gerson Therapy is an organic, high-fiber, vegetarian, low-sugar, low-sodium diet; Gerson's daughter Charlotte has championed it for decades. Success stories are anecdotal, but hundreds gladly testify to how this therapy healed them of cancer, and I believe it could be a worthwhile addition to almost any cancer treatment protocol. It was our honor to host the Gerson Clinic for a number of years, and we witnessed many favorable results.

Issels Therapy

Dr. Josef Issels developed a comprehensive immunotherapy that utilizes cancer vaccines, cytokines, and cell protocols to boost the body's self-healing ability.[13] Issels was well known for injecting Coley's toxins into his patients to cause a fever that would bolster their immune systems. Oasis of Hope has hosted the Issels Clinic for more than ten years, and we've seen a high success rate. We've also noted many similarities between Issels' approach and ours.

Essiac Herbal Extract

Essiac herbal extract contains burdock root, sheep sorrel, slippery elm bark, and Turkish rhubarb. No clinical trials have been conducted, but clinical data confirm that its herbs do have estrogenic, cytotoxic, anti-estrogenic, anti-tumor, anti-inflammatory, anti-mutagenic, and anti-oxidant properties. There are no reports that Essiac has caused tumors in women with breast cancer to grow, but one in vitro study concluded that it can cause breast cancer cells to grow.[14]

Black Salve

The various "black salves" sold on the market contain zinc chloride and bloodroot.[15] Proponents claim it goes deep beneath the skin and draws out cancer. There's no clinical data on black salve's efficacy or safety; it's corrosive in nature and if used improperly can lead to skin damage and deformation. Many patients say their spot of skin cancer was completely removed using only the salve, and they have the scars they say proves it. My opinion is that a treatment being natural doesn't mean it should be used without professional supervision. Black salve may be effective; it may be dangerous. If you wish to use it, seek out a naturopath who has experience with it to supervise your treatment.

Hoxsey Therapy

Another classic alternative also is named after its inventor.[16] John Hoxsey is said to have first used this combination of herbs, mixed into a tonic and salve, to cure the cancer on his horse; his great-grandson, Harry Hoxsey, sought to promote and popularize the therapy in the twentieth century. No scientific data supports its efficacy or safety.

Rife Frequency Machine

Every atom vibrates at a precise frequency. Frequency medicine asserts that the specific frequencies of malignant cells can be identified and exposed to another frequency that will destroy the tumor. It may be legend, but many alternative practitioners believe that the frequency machine Royal Rife invented was curing cancers in the 1930s.[17] Those original machines no longer exist; no one believes any similar machines are nearly as effective. I embrace the theory of frequency medicine but have yet to find an effective frequency medical device.

DMSO

Dimethylsulfoxide (DMSO) is said to promote better blood flow, protect nerve cells from injury, and reduce inflammation. One recent multi-centric study concluded,

> The vast number of experimental and clinical studies has shown DMSO could be a useful agent to treat pain of different causes and genesis. Our neurobioenergetic model of cancer development strongly suggests that DMSO can be used as excitatory modulator to manage several factors associated with cancer pain genesis. More significantly, DMSO also positively influences cellular energy metabolism and tissue regeneration, thus it could be the therapeutic agent of choice for patients with side effects of cancer therapies such as chemotherapy, radiation and diagnostic/therapeutic surgeries.[18]

DMSO is well tolerated but has not produced results superior to other treatments that are part of my protocols.

Laetrile

My father is the poster child for laetrile, a pharmaceutical extract from apricot kernels. Maybe the most controversial alternative cancer therapy, laetrile has a cyanide radical that's neutralized (rendered harmless) by the rhodanese enzyme in healthy cells;[19] cancer cells, deficient of rhodanese, succumb to the cyanide. In a number of clinical trials, results seem to skew toward the opinion of whoever is conducting; individual case studies do point to laetrile's efficacy and safety.[20] We've used amygdalin, its natural form, with tens of thousands of patients and consider it an effective adjuvant (but not standalone) cancer therapy.

Shark Cartilage

Shark cartilage, a powerful immune booster and anti-inflammatory, is an effective anti-angiogenesis agent. That is, it inhibits formation of new blood vessels,[21] which tumors need to feed themselves. I believe it's a good addition to a treatment support program, though I wouldn't recommend it as a stand-alone cancer therapy.

Guava and Asparagus

About once a year there's a huge online buzz about a natural cancer cure—usually it's some extract from somewhere exotic. Most of these have some validity as containing nutrients that provide benefits to the immune system and other parts of the body, but never has one really been the answer. I'm presenting two of them here because they've been studied at length on cancer cells with published results.

The most recent natural wonder, guava, has the active components ursolic acid, oleanolic acid, arjunolic acid, glucuronic acid, saponin combined with oleanolic acid, morin-3-O- -L-lyxopyranoside and morin-3-O- -L-arabinopyranoside, pentane-2-thiol, and many flavonoids.[22] Guava leaf extract has a potent antioxidant capacity and so is a powerful free-radical scavenger; it also has been found to induce apoptosis in cancer cells. Researchers understand much of how and why guava's components have anti-cancer qualities, and they've shown in vitro its ability to destroy human prostate cancer cell lines. These initial studies warrant further investigation as preliminary reports are promising.

Extract from asparagus root is being studied in vitro and in mice-embedded human cancers; numerous results are showing how it can inhibit growth of leukemia HL-60 cells, breast cancer cells, and liver cancer cells.[23] Asparagus extract contains components that modulate the immune system and hormones as well as inhibit the production and activity of inflammatory cytokines interleukin (IL)-1 and tumor necrosis factor (TNF) by macrophages.

I will continue following the research on natural plant extracts from guava and asparagus. It's exciting to discover that God put a natural pharmacy on earth with nutrients that can prevent and cure any and all disease. This reminds me of Ezekiel 47:12, which, within a vision of His unimaginably magnificent blessing, says "the fruit will be for food and the leaves for healing."[24]

Conclusion

I've had to become comfortable between a rock and a hard place (conventional and alternative medicine, respectively). I'm a conventionally trained surgical oncologist, yet I provide body, mind, and spirit therapies with an emphasis on natural medicine. Alternative doctors dismiss me for utilizing chemo, radiation, and surgery. Conventional doctors have publicly criticized me. But when one conventional oncologist at the World Congress in Canada challenged me, asking, "So what kind of medicine do you practice—is it conventional or alternative?" I answered that *my intention is to practice good medicine.* My criteria are to offer whatever treatment has a scientific basis with evidence that it has the potential to be helpful and not harmful. "Integrative medicine" best describes what I do at Oasis of Hope. I believe it offers you the best hope as well.

ACTION STEPS

1. Be open to possibly integrating alternative and complementary medicine into your treatment plan.
2. Natural medicine is powerful. Be sure to work with an integrative doctor who will oversee your treatment with alternative or complementary treatments.
3. Don't follow fads. Work with a physician who's studied the mechanisms of, and knows how to administer, natural therapies.

CANCER VICTOR TIPS

Vera Congdon, Louisiana
Infiltrative Ductal-High-Grade Adenocarcinoma w/ER
Victor Since 2006

1. Eat organic, drink fresh veggie juice, and eliminate meats.
2. Exercise daily and breathe deeply. Cancer cells hate oxygen.
3. Laugh a lot, and believe the report of the Lord (see Habakkuk 3:2).
4. Have no doubt or unbelief in God's healing power.
5. It is easier to trust God than to be fearful.

Alternative Cancer Treatments
https://vimeo.com/61903784

Chapter 29

Overcoming Cancer Genes

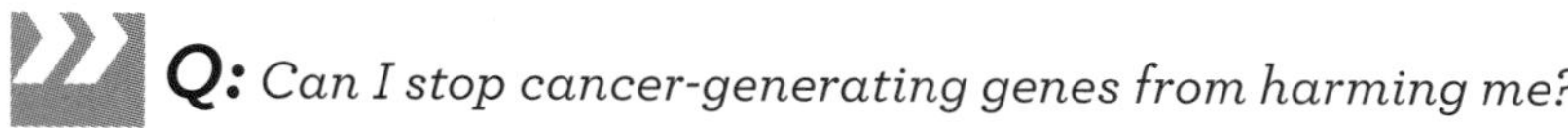

Q: *Can I stop cancer-generating genes from harming me?*

A: Since most generational cancer baggage is in the epigenetic realm, the answer is yes. Genetic alterations are reversible through lifestyle changes.

Epigenetic marks (see chapter 14) are chemical tags that switch vital genes off or on and contribute to cancer's development. Researchers have been finding more and more active food components (nutrients, phytochemicals, dietary chemicals) that can influence the three major marks: DNA methylation, histone modifications, and chromatin remodeling. For this reason experts believe foods, rather than drugs, will be the cancer therapies of the future.

Using Foods to Neutralize Epigenetic Marks

Though there's a lot to learn about epigenetic marks and how to neutralize them, certain patterns are being observed—such as, malignant tumors in general are linked to low methylation levels in specific genes, though some genes promote cancer through hypermethylation. In other words, methylation can fight and help cancer at the same time! Can you increase methylation in some genes and decrease it in others? Apparently yes; you just have to know which foods to give. For instance, one study that showed that cancer can be induced by severe dietary methyl deficiency and then reversed by dietary methyl supplementation.[1]

Dr. Mingzhu Fang found that tea polyphenols, genistein from soybean, or isothiocyanates from plant foods inhibit the development of cancer by reducing DNA hypermethylation status in cancer-associated genes.[2] Dr. Roderick H. Dashwood has done a study tracing the effect on gene expression of broccoli's sulforaphane, first in the Petri dish, then in mouse experiments and finally in human tests of patients with colon and prostate cancers. In the animal models, sulforaphane therapy reduced tumors by 50%. Patients who took a single serving of sulforaphane-rich broccoli sprouts had a dramatic level of HDAC (a cancer-inducing epigenetic marker) inhibition immediately following the vegetable meal.[3]

One study on thirty-four healthy premenopausal women evaluated the effect of supplementing (40 mg or 140 mg) with daily genistein, a soy isoflavone, through one menstrual cycle on systemic estrogen and breast-specific gene methylation. After the treatment the women went through nipple aspiration to obtain intraductal cells to measure specific estrogenic markers, changes in cytology, and methylation assessment of five different cancer-related genes. First, daily supplementation increased serum levels of genistein; second, genistein has a direct antiestrogenic effect; third, the increased serum levels of genistein induced a dose-specific change in gene methylation in two breast-cancer related genes.[4]

Dr. Elio Riboli is leading a massive study (520,000 people from ten European countries) designed to investigate relationships between diet, nutritional status, lifestyle, and environmental factors and the incidence of cancer (and other chronic diseases) that may reveal links between methylation modifiers and other epigenetic marks. This study is called EPIC (European Prospective Investigation into Cancer and Nutrition).[5]

I am encouraged for all of the recent studies revealing the healing powers of foods at the DNA level. For years, Oasis of Hope has been using food as medicine based on its activity through metabolic signaling pathways. And newer studies suggest these foods contain nutrients that may also be reprogramming our cancer patients' gene expression. This could be another reason our patient survival rates are frequently better than the conventional-approach results. (We give some nutrients as nutraceuticals; others are present in the food we provide.)

As for food-active components that reprogram epigenetic marks:

- *Folic acid* is in leafy vegetables, peas, beans, sunflower seeds.
- *Choline* comes from lettuce, peanuts, eggs.

- *Methionine* is in spinach, garlic, Brazil nuts, kidney beans, tofu.
- *Organosulfur* is a garlic compound.
- *Butyrate* is a compound produced in the intestine when dietary fiber is fermented.
- *Biotin* is found abundantly in Swiss chard.
- *Lipoic acid* is in spinach, broccoli, potatoes, yams, carrots, beets.
- *Epigallocatechin gallate* (EGCG) is a polyphenol in green tea extract.
- *Genistein* comes from soy.
- *Resveratrol compound* is found largely in the skins of red grapes.
- *Curcumin* is in turmeric.

Conclusion

An epigenetic diet's health benefits are enormous, for they have the potential to modify gene expression to fight cancer. The more we learn on this, the better we'll be able to address malignancies and other diseases.

ACTION STEPS

1. Learn more about how to reprogram your genes to work for you.
2. Immediately start consuming the foods listed above.
3. Look for nutritionists and doctors who understand epigenomics.

CANCER VICTOR TIPS

Deedy Carrier, Florida
Stage IV Lung Cancer
Victor Since 2010

1. Believe and trust God for your healing. The Bible is alive and active; stand firm on His promises, knowing that He is good and faithful. Find Christians who believe in healing and have them pray over you.

2. Surround yourself with positive people who will fill each day with encouragement and laughter. Choose to enjoy the good things in life, every day, and do not let negative thoughts captivate your mind.
3. Find good books about nutrition and cancer. And live actively—make time to exercise as much as possible. It will help you feel better!
4. Take time to relax and heal by minimizing commitments and tasks. It's necessary to eliminate what makes you "busy" so that you can focus on things that bring healing. I've greatly benefited from massages, family time, naps, walks on the beach, detox bath, and my new puppy.
5. Have doctors and health care professionals who work together on "your team" to support the treatment plan you've chosen.

Overcoming Cancer Genes
https://vimeo.com/61906899

Chapter 30

Immunotherapies

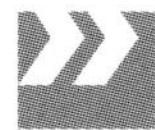
Q: *How can I improve my immune system while undergoing cancer treatments?*

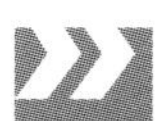
A: One of the biggest failures of conventional therapies is that they're immune-suppressive. But many counteractions can protect, stimulate, and improve your immune system in the treatment process. I highly recommend elements and therapies like nutrition, prayer, meditation, laughter, music, and worship.

In military strategy it's sometimes the covert operation rather than the full frontal assault that determines the outcome. One case in point was with Osama bin Laden. The many thousands of soldiers deployed came up empty-handed, yet through a network of intelligence gathering and a highly trained team of Navy Seals, the al-Qaeda leader was taken down with relatively little incident.

Hollywood has really embraced the sniper, making many movies like *Sniper*[1] (1, 2 and 3) starring Tom Berenger or the somewhat more recent *Shooter*[2] starring Mark Wahlberg. Maybe these films are popular because a sniper often is more effective than a nuclear bomb; he can go deep behind enemy lines and take out a target of interest without harming civilians. Many tyrants have met their demise due to a sniper's precision.

Snipers never work alone—they always go out in a team of two. The partner is the spotter, responsible for locating the target, estimating distance, and calculating wind factor. Weighing all facets, he provides the adjustments the sniper needs to succeed with the first shot; the sniper rarely has the chance of a second without giving away their position.

The human immune system has cells that are similar to sniper and spotter. Dendritic cells are similar to a spotter in seeking out malignant and other unhealthy cells. Once they spot them, they send signals to activate NK (natural killer) cells to exterminate the cancerous cell. The NK cells are precise and, much like a sniper, will not harm a healthy cell.

Cancer can only proliferate in a person whose immune system is functioning incorrectly. My first goal as an oncologist is to get my patient's immune system working again because, as the most effective cancer killer we know, it will help extinguish malignant cells and help diminish risk of recurrence. Let me tell you about one of God's greatest gifts to you, your onboard cancer-killer team.

Your Internal Cancer-Killer Squad

Last year I was driving, listening to talk radio, when an ad from LA's most famous cancer center caught my ear. It said something about being on the absolute cutting edge in treatment. Tagline: "Imagine, we use your immune system to kill cancer." As we've seen, this approach has long been in use, and I was surprised the ad was promoting it as innovative, but I applaud this center for starting to use such effective therapies.

The human body possesses an amazing ability to protect itself from all kinds of harm and is constantly engaged in neutralizing internal and external danger. The immune system is a group of mechanisms that protects against disease by identifying and killing pathogens, germs, mutated cells, and tumors. Most importantly, it can distinguish between dangerous elements and healthy cells.[3]

With all my patients I prescribe agents that can aid the immune system's ability to attack cancer by optimizing the function of natural killer cells (NK) and cytotoxic T-cells (T_c). NK cells can kill a broad range of cancer cells; T_c cells target cancer cells that express specific proteins not produced by healthy tissues. Though immune cells rarely can destroy large tumors, they might kill the small nests of tumor cells that give rise to new metastases or that can cause a recurrence of cancer following a remission. Therefore, boosting activity of NK cells and T_c cells is our first piece of immune-stimulation therapy. Let me share about some of the agents I recommend.

Melatonin

One immuno-supporter is the hormone melatonin, once daily before bedtime. Multiple clinical studies show it tends to have a favorable, statistically significant impact on survival in patients with advanced cancer.[4-6] The chief reason may be an immuno-stimulant effect that boosts NK-cell and T_c-cell activity; the effect is indirect because melatonin acts on dendritic cells (which function as antigen-presenters for T_c cells), amplifying their capacity to stimulate NK cells and T_c cells. Melatonin boosts dendritic cells' ability to produce interleukin-2, which helps cancer-attacking immune cells reach maturity.[7-9]

Probiotics

Another key immuno-supportive set, probiotics, are capsules that introduce live healthy bacteria into the gastrointestinal (GI) tract. They have enteric coating, which protects them from stomach acid so they can pass through to the intestines. Included in this supplement are strains of lactobacilli and bifidobacteria that can stimulate the immune system with polysaccharides (complex carbohydrates, in their cell walls) that cause dendritic cells to encourage growth and activation of NK cells and T_c cells.[10-14] Dendritic cells recognize the bacterial polysaccharides as foreign material made by invading bacteria and respond appropriately. Scientific studies have concluded that probiotics may reduce the proliferation of tumor cells in some types of malignancies, including colo-rectal cancer.[15]

Selenium

Selenium, which sparks an increase in the capacity of stimulated NK cells and T_c cells to express receptors for interleukin-2,[16-18] is an essential growth factor of the immune cells that attack and kill cancers. In other words, when NK cells and T_c cells express receptors for interleukin-2, they grow in greater abundance. Selenium also therapeutically induces malignant-cell apoptosis (programmed death).[19]

Cimetidine

The anti-ulcer drug cimetidine is immuno-supportively included in CMIT protocols (see chapter 50) primarily due to firm evidence that it can reduce risk of metastasis in many cancers. There's also evidence that it has immuno-stimulant activity for NK cells and T_c cells.[20-22] Furthermore, cimetidine may reduce metastatic spread by inhibiting endothelial expression of a cell adhesion molecule called E-selectin.[23]

• • • • • • • • • • • • •

These agents comprise one aspect of immune-stimulation therapies. The other involves measures intended to counteract the defensive actions tumors use to survive. Cancers often evade immune destruction by evolving mechanisms—called *immuno-suppressive factors*—that attack and either kill immune cells or reduce their tumor-destructive capacities. By counteracting these factors we can maximize the intensity of the body's immune response.

Metronomic/Low-Dose Chemotherapy

One way cancer cells suppress the immune system is with T-reg cells: special lymphocytes that colonize tumors and kill or disable attacking immune cells by producing immuno-suppressive factors. Metronomic chemo is extremely useful for controlling T-reg cells, which are exquisitely sensitive to being killed by small doses of cytotoxic drugs. In fact, the doses are too small to harm other immune cells or cause notable side effects.[24] Here's a case where chemotherapy can help *boost* immune defense! Studies indicate that in some cancer types, low-dose chemo is not toxic and yet is as effective as high-dose chemo (which is aggressive, produces side effects, and damages the immune system).[25-26]

Diclofenac

Many tumors express an enzyme, Cox-2, that produces immuno-suppressive compounds called prostaglandins. The anti-inflammatory "safe drug" diclofenac blocks their production by inhibiting production of Cox-2. The drug's action effectively blocks the tumor's defense mechanism, thereby counteracting immuno-suppression.

Caffeine

Another tumor-produced immuno-suppressor, especially in poorly oxygenated regions, is adenosine.[27-28] Doctors have long known that caffeine's energizing effects are evidence of its ability to block the activation of adenosine receptors in the brain. Evidently, caffeine has the same potential in tumors, offsetting adenosine's immuno-suppressive activity.[27] It may also act as an interceptor that will protect DNA from invasion and mutation.[28] That's why, for patients who tolerate coffee well, we recommend several cups daily. (Please avoid sugar and cream!)

Spirulina

The moderately oxidative environment in many tumors is extremely toxic to NK cells and T_c cells, impairing their tumor-killing capacities or even killing them.[29-31] Most such oxidative stress is bred by a specific enzyme complex.[32-33] Phycocyanobilin, a key phytonutrient found in spirulina, functions as a potent inhibitor of this complex, counteracting the tumor's defense by cutting at the root of oxidative stress.[34] Moreover, spirulina contains cell-wall polysaccharides that stimulate immuno-supportive dendritic cells;[35-36] it can act directly on some cancer cells, slowing growth and spread, and it interferes with the angiogenic process.[31,37-38] As it thus appears to work in at least four complementary ways to slow tumor growth and support the immune system, I include dietary spirulina as part of my patients' at-home treatment program.

Conclusion

By bolstering the immune system, you can improve your body's ability to avoid damage from infectious agents and mutated cells. Plus, by blocking the mechanisms tumors use to suppress the immune system, you can enjoy the maximum benefit yours provides and increase the speed and strength with which it responds to the perceived threat of cancer. Right now, your immune system needs to be your top priority.

ACTION STEPS

1. Consult an integrative practitioner or naturopath who can help you build your immune system.
2. Ask your physician about the proper use of melatonin, selenium, spirulina, and the other nutraceuticals outlined above.
3. Investigate the potential benefits of low-dose chemotherapy.

CANCER VICTOR TIPS

Lori Billeter, Arizona
Infiltrating Ductal Carcinoma, Grade 2, HER2-Negative
Victor Since 2008

1. Pray fervently for God's strength to carry you through. "God has not given us a spirit of fear, but of power and of love and of a sound mind" (2 Timothy 1:7 NKJV). Draw close to God. He will not fail you.
2. Have a ready plan of action. I chose the aggressive (raw, vegan) Hallelujah Diet. Go online to research it. I also went immediately to Oasis of Hope for a three-day evaluation . . . my second opinion.
3. Research! Do your homework!! Don't rely on just the doctors' opinions. There are natural options other than chemo, radiation, and surgery. Keep a notebook of all your research and reports.
4. I chose a lumpectomy . . . nothing else. Then I went to Oasis of Hope for their treatment plan. Journal your journey and keep a prayer blog so that others know how to pray with you.
5. Take *all* the supplements they advise. I still do.

Immunotherapies
https://vimeo.com/61909235

Chapter 31

Cancer Vaccines

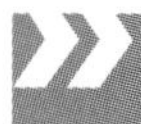

Q: *Will there ever be a vaccine for cancer?*

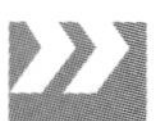

A: I don't think so. To date, two anti-virus vaccines are known to significantly increase risk of cancer. The recently FDA-approved cervical cancer vaccine is really a vaccine against the human papilloma virus (HPV). I do believe we can develop immune therapies to awaken cancer-fighting elements like dendritic cells. Such vaccines soon will become a more common part of cancer treatment.

In *Health in the 21st Century: Will Doctors Survive?*[1] I laid out a strong argument against massive, compulsory vaccination. I'm not questioning whether the vaccines work; rather, for twenty-plus years I've been saying it's unclear whether the benefits outweigh the risks in some environments and when safety cannot be secured. What may be needed in parts of Africa or Latin America may not be best in the US or Europe. As Daniel A. Salmon stated, concluding a 2006 study, compulsive vaccination risk "might not be acceptable in some countries where high coverage has been achieved through other approaches or efforts, such as in Sweden, Norway, Denmark, the Netherlands, and the UK."[2]

Vaccines and Safety

While vaccines can save countless lives in poor, undernourished, disease-infested communities, they can also provoke havoc in affluent groups where incidence, morbidity, and mortality for aimed-at diseases are extremely low.

For example, hundreds of soldiers have rejected anthrax vaccination due to its link to Gulf War Syndrome; in 1994 a Senate committee found this vaccine was being considered as a possible cause, yet more than a hundred studies avoided weighing this important factor.[3] Also, the incidence of autism has skyrocketed recently, and despite fervent efforts by the vaccine industry to prove there's no link between the two, after a decade of pressure from the National Childhood Vaccine Injury Act (NCVIA), in 1999 the FDA, in conjunction with the U.S. Public Health Service and the American Academy of Pediatrics, ceased to license thimerosal-containing vaccines and the MMR (measles, mumps, and rubella) vaccine because of their strong link with autism.[4] The 2012 CDC report indicates that even though thimerosal was removed from vaccines, autism rates continue to climb,[5] which continues to inspire doubt as to whether vaccines truly are safe. Regardless, with *all* medications, one must weigh potential benefit against known risks.

Vaccines, the Immune System, and Cancer

With that off my chest . . . will there be an anti-cancer vaccine?

To qualify my answer, I need to give a quick overview of the way our immune system works in relation to vaccines. We've come a long way since Edward Jenner's successful 1796 use of cowpox material to create immunity to smallpox,[6] Louis Pasteur's 1885 rabies vaccine,[7] and the 1930s dawn of bacteriology with rapid developments of antitoxins and vaccines against diphtheria, tetanus, anthrax, cholera, plague, typhoid, tuberculosis, and more. Smallpox inoculation, or variolation, actually started in China seven centuries before Jenner and was also practiced in Africa and Turkey before it spread to Europe and the Americas. Many scholars propose vaccination as a top-ten public health achievement of the last century, and even those with concerns agree. Vaccination has saved millions, making pests of the Dark Ages a thing of the past; the hope is that it will nullify even-more-deadly pests expected in the future.

What separates Oasis of Hope from other cancer centers is not that we offer alternative options or even integrative therapies but that we aim our efforts at providing resources to our patients for them to heal themselves, and the most vital entity to achieve this is the immune system. Vaccines are at the heart of this concept, and it's high time the oncological scientific community pays attention to this facet of anti-cancer strategy, especially because its most-oft-used tools—chemo, radiation and surgery—all cause profound immune-system insult.

A vaccine's aim is to boost the immune system's natural ability to protect against foreign invaders like microbes *and also* internal invaders like mutated, malignant cells. Our defense mechanism consists of a complex network of organs, tissues, and specialized cells that work in unison to defend us from outer and inner attacks. One of this system's most amazing features is that after destroying a foreign body (bacteria or virus) it "remembers" the aggressor and, should the microbe invade again, prevents another infection. A vaccine infects the body in a controlled way with harmless (killed or weakened) versions of microbes to reduce the natural and lethal risk of such infection. This controlled infection causes a vaccine-induced memory that enables the immune system to act quickly against the microbes used to make the vaccine to prevent infections. Vaccination then is, conceptually, a preventive tool.

Because vaccine development has been founded on this principle, to date there are only three FDA-approved cancer-preventive vaccines using antigens from microbes that cause/contribute to malignant development. In essence these are aimed primarily at preventing infection from viruses; if the infection is avoided, then, secondarily, a cancer may be prevented.

The Hepatitis B Virus (HBV) vaccine was the first FDA-approved and successfully marketed for cancer prevention.[8] Chronic HBV infection can lead to liver cancer, which is why today most children in the US are HBV-vaccinated shortly after birth. But the most targeted bug right now is the human papillomavirus (HPV), a family of about a hundred different types. Most known HPV types cause no symptoms to humans; some can cause warts, and a few can increase risk of developing several cancers. The FDA approved the vaccine Gardasil in 2006 for females aged 9 to 26 for prevention of HPV types 16 and 18, found to cause about 70% of all cases of cervical cancer worldwide and also some vaginal, vulvar, anal, penile, and throat cancers.[9] Two additional types (6, 11) do not cause cervical cancer but were added for causing about 90% of all genital wart cases. As it addresses four HPV types, Gardasil is a quadrivalent vaccine; in 2010 the FDA also approved it for males aged 9 to 26 to prevent anal cancer and precancerous anal lesions (types 16, 18), and genital warts (6, 11). The Cervarix vaccine, approved in 2009 for females aged 9 to 25 to prevent cervical cancer, is bivalent (addresses only types 16 and 18).[10]

At least seventeen other HPV types are responsible for the remaining 30% of cervical cancer cases, and as of now there's no vaccine for them. These three vaccines are textbook examples of exposing much of the population for the actions of a smaller portion of society. HBV is only prevalent among drug addicts and gays, and HPV amid the promiscuous.

Vaccines: Not Just for Prevention

The immune system's role in defending us against disease-causing microbes is well established, but some researchers finally are concluding that it also has great potential to protect the body against threats posed by certain damaged, diseased, or abnormal cells, including cancer cells. And so we're investigating this approach for using vaccines to treat and not just to prevent. Paul Naylor said that "therapeutic cancer vaccines have the potential to generate a long lasting immune response that will destroy tumor cells with specificity and safety, in contrast to many other current cancer therapies," yet to date clinical success has been limited if not absent due to many challenges.[11] And Dr. Lijin Li believes the new DNA sequencing platforms will revolutionize medicine and that cancer genome sequencing has opened the door toward personalized medicine.[12]

Cancer vaccines belong to a class of substances known as biological response modifiers and aim to boost or restore the immune system's ability to fight malignancies, in particular by stimulating white blood cells (leukocytes). These play the main role in immune responses through carrying out tasks required to cleanse the body from disease-causing microbes and abnormal cells and through their wide range of functions.

Some types of leukocytes defend the body through general immune protection, patrolling the circulation for foreign invaders and diseased, damaged, or dead cells. But lymphocytes, one of the five types, provide targeted protection against specific threats, be it infectious or from aberrant cells like cancer. This entity from the white-blood-cell family has two groups: B lymphocytes (or B cells), named for the bone marrow, where they're produced, and T lymphocytes (T cells), also produced in the bone marrow but named for the thymus, where they mature.

B cells make antibodies that inactivate and help destroy foreign invaders or abnormal cells. Their specificity comes from their capacity to remember prior encounters, be it through former bouts, infections, or vaccination. T cells are cytotoxic; they actually kill cells or microbes by releasing chemicals or prompting apoptosis, and so they're also known as killer T cells. B and T cells are the main actors in the theater of war against disease, yet they're only able to do their jobs effectively with excellent supporting actors. Those roles are filled by other types: helper T cells, which help activate killer T cells, and dendritic cells, which enable killer T cells to recognize specific threats.

Microbes are completely foreign; our immune system has no problem recognizing them. *Malignant cells* are ours, mutated but not recognized straightforwardly as foe; thus the need for a "finger pointer" called a dendritic or presenter cell. (These lymphocytes are so crucial that I've dedicated the next chapter to them—read on.) Cancer vaccines are designed to work by activating B and killer T cells and directing them to recognize and act against specific cancer types with one or more specific or nonspecific antigens. Biological therapies include interferons, interleukins, colony-stimulating factors, monoclonal antibodies, gene therapy, vaccines, and nonspecific immunomodulating agents.

At Oasis of Hope we've been working for many years with a number of biological response modifiers. The antigens used can occur naturally in the body and be stimulated or can be produced in the lab. The aim of immunostimulating therapies is to alter interaction between the body's immune defenses and cancer cells, to cause a shock to the system in order to boost, direct, or restore the body's ability to fight and kill cancer. One is allogeneic lymphocyte therapy, wherein killer T cells are harvested from a young, healthy, unrelated donor and infused intravenously to a patient. This vaccine-type therapy increases the patient's own production of T and dendritic cells to specifically fight his own cancer. We're likewise investigating interleukin-2 in dosages that don't provoke terrible side effects. I'll expound on these two immune therapies in chapter 32.

Also, we're in the research stages of administrating a macrophage activating factor (MAF) through a functional change in the Gc protein (Vitamin D-binding protein), thus called GcMAF—a lymphokine that prepares macrophages to become cytotoxic to tumors. Macrophages are phagocytes that, when activated, will more effectively kill cancer cells.[13]

Conclusion

A vaccine that can wipe cancer from the earth is not yet in sight, but doors are opening to new horizons in the quest for therapeutic vaccines, and we're positioned to take advantage of the breakthroughs.

ACTION STEPS

1. Keep an open mind and ear to new developments in the realm of cancer treatment vaccines and biological response modifiers.
2. Look for research facilities planning (or already administering, through clinical trials) elements like interleukin-2 and GcMAF.
3. Consult experts who specialize in immune therapies.

CANCER VICTOR TIPS

Kimberly Schoof, Washington
Stage IVa Squamous Cell Carcinoma (Tonsil) & Stage IV Squamous Cell Carcinoma (Tongue) with Metastasis to the Lung
Victor Since 2005

1. Pray! Have faith that God will get you through this. Trust in Him.
2. Don't panic. Keep a positive attitude and know you *can* get through it.
3. Immediately stop eating sugar and change your whole diet as needed.
4. Get rid of all stress. Make sure you get plenty of sleep.
5. Find the clinic that can do the best for you.

Cancer Vaccines
https://vimeo.com/61914605

Chapter 32

Dendritic Cells

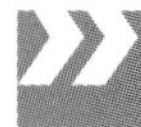 **Q:** *Should I pay any attention to the dendritic-cell hype?*

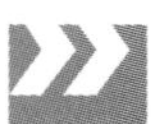 **A:** I believe that activation of the dendritic-cell system can powerfully boost the immune system's capacity to destroy tumors.

There's great potential for using dendritic cells in cancer treatment. Still, if you seek answers in the growing body of evidence that's gaining weight at a faster rate than the US populace, you may be dispirited by the dissonance between enthusiastic scientific rhetoric and the meager advances in practical applications of this immune system subdivision's capabilities. The government has spent hundreds of millions of research dollars for such a find to finally hit the real-world battleground, and yet there's so little to show for it. No question the realm of dendritic cells is complicated; nonetheless, there should be some way we can help patients with it. Well, not all is disappointment! Please read on.

Presenters

In 1868 Paul Langerhans discovered the neuron-resembling skin cells known as dendrites, which have branched projections (from the Greek *déndron*, "tree"). "Langerhans Cells" remained an enigma for over a century before Ralph M. Steinman and his collaborators recognized their function and significance. Their pioneering work demonstrated that these cells belong to the immune system and christened them "dendritic cells" to differentiate them from the nervous system cells known as dendrites.[1] Steinman received the Albert Lasker Basic Medical Research Award in 2007 and the Nobel Prize in Physiology or Medicine in 2011. Today, dendritic cells are positioned as the master regulators of immunity.

Dendritic cells, our first line of defense, are present in tissues in contact with the external environment, such as the skin and the inner lining of the nose, lungs, stomach, and intestines. Their main function is to act as messengers between our innate and our learned immunities. In other words, they present or introduce stored antigens to other cells of the immune system so they can produce the specific antibodies for an all-out attack against any and all foreign bodies. Dendritic cells function as antigen-presenting cells and so also are known as "presenter cells."

Dendritic cells store and maintain the memory files for each of the millions of antigens encountered during life so they're available for protection at a moment's notice. Antigens, substances or particles that provoke an immune response, provoke production of antibodies and so initially were known as "antibody generators." Antibodies—proteins of the immunoglobulin superfamily—are also known as immunoglobulins, and we have millions of these because they're incredibly precise and specific; one antibody for every threat-type ever encountered so that each binds to one specific antigen in the way that a given key opens one specific lock.

Our health depends on our capacity to produce antibodies capable of neutralizing antigens from the external environment (non-self) or formed within the body (self). Our immune system identifies and attacks as foreign invaders "non-self" antigens like bacteria, viruses, and other microorganisms or parts of them (and the toxins they produce); also, non-microbial exogenous antigens like pollen, egg white, and proteins from transplanted tissues, organs, or transfused blood cells. Our normal cells, through the metabolic process, decay, or other mechanisms, also produce antigens, but the immune system usually tolerates these "self" antigens and refrains from attacking; when not, an autoimmune disease (arthritis, type 1 diabetes, multiple sclerosis, lupus, etc.) is unleashed.

Dendritic cells store a well-organized inventory of millions of "keys" acquired through past encounters. When an old enemy threatens, the cell retrieves the specific key and presents it to a B-cell, which has millions of "locks" and chooses the correct one to unlock the antidote, a massive production of antibodies that either identifies and neutralizes the foreign object or "tags" it for destruction by the immune system!

Dendritic Vaccines

If dendritic cells are so phenomenal, why do they allow cancerous cells to thrive? Because cancer cells are basically ours—mutated, yes, but ours, and the antigens they generate are "self," ones our normal cells also make. These "self" antigens can become treacherous; first because our immune system tolerates them, and second because in comparison to normal cell production they're produced in enormous amounts. So, even when the dendritic cells acknowledge the threat of overabundance of these antigens, their numbers are insufficient to deliver a sufficiently loud and clear message for a potent immune attack on cancer.

Several researchers have reported that cancer patients are deficient in dendritic cell count, a finding that motivated investigators to develop solutions.[2] Advances on the early 1990s led to the ability to generate dendritic cells in the lab and opened the door to a new attack: dendritic cell therapy. This technology involves harvesting white blood cells from a patient and processing them in the lab to produce dendritic cells in high amounts; they're returned to the patient to provoke a massive dendritic cell influx to optimally activate the immune system against the tumor(s).

So far the results are not encouraging. The most likely reasons:

- That the increased number of dendritic cells is flooding the system with antigens that are not tumor-specific.
- Even if specific tumor antigens are encountered, they're part of "self," that is, not sufficiently foreign for the immune system to generate antibodies.
- If antibodies are produced, they are insufficient to neutralize the massive tumor production of antigens.

Research at Stanford under Dr. Edgar Engleman has paved the way for the development of drugs that address the three reasons for failure: the conception of "monoclonal antibodies."[3] Thus it's now possible to clone a specific antibody in the lab, which bypasses the dendritic cell "self" limitation in quality and quantity. Through a method called recombinant DNA, gene sequences are used for molecular cloning.

Several pharmaceutical labs can select a specific antigen, isolate the generating gene from the dendritic cell, transfer this gene to bacteria, and clone the bacteria to the nth degree to produce huge quantities of the antibody.

Examples are Herceptin (Trastuzumab), used mainly to treat breast cancers, Rituxan (Rituximab), for lymphomas and leukemias, and Avastin (Bevacizumab), for various cancers including colorectal, lung, breast, glioblastoma, kidney, and ovarian.

Unfortunately, again, monoclonal antigens have been only partially and temporarily effective, prolonging the life of cancer patients by three to four months at a cost of approximately $10,000 a month. Why?

- Tumors rely on the production of multiple antigens.
- Tumors find a way to avoid or shield against the antigens via suppressor cells, inflammatory type II T-cells, and regulatory T-cells (Tregs), all of which prevent the function of antibodies.[4]

In short, monoclonal antibodies are a narrow-spectrum therapy. But Engleman's group was the first to develop a therapeutic dendritic-cell vaccine, a targeted, broad-spectrum immune therapy that aims to expose dendritic cells to tumor-specific antigens extracted from a patient's cancer. Researchers applied this method to humans with encouraging results against lymphomas and concluded that dendritic-cell vaccination can induce immune responses and durable tumor regression.[5] The group later increased the number of patients to reaffirm the vaccine's potential and published results that paved the way for this anti-cancer therapy.[6]

In a 2007 lecture Engleman stated that more such clinical trials are virtually impossible to repeat in state-sponsored research because of new FDA regulation. In the 1990s the cost to prepare and test for purity (that only dendritic cells are in the preparation) and sterility (contamination free) was $500 to $600. With the FDA involved, the cost soared to $30,000, even though not one sample of the original test was impure or contaminated with the methodology used in the mentioned studies.[7]

In 2010 the FDA approved Provenge (Sipuleucel-T), the first cancer vaccine to fight tumors in the prostate—in fact, the first cancer vaccine approved for use in humans.[8] This customized immunotherapy sensitizes each patient's immune system to his own tumor. It's available only in fifty treatment centers FDA-approved to harvest dendritic cells; then, antigens from the tumor are isolated and incorporated into the dendritic cells, along with an immune system booster. These combined procedures form the "vaccine," then administered back into the bloodstream.

More dendritic vaccines are in the works for many other types of cancers. Dendreon, which owns the patent, reported that the procedure costs about $93,000 per patient. And the dendritic vaccine extended the lives of the patients with advanced prostate cancer an average of four months when compared to a placebo.[9] You read that correctly: a $93,000 treatment for a four-month life extension. I believe if we gave a patient $93,000 to spend in Cancun he would live longer and enjoy it a lot more.

Obstacles to Overcome

Dendritic cells make up a key part of our incredible immune defense mechanism. How can we effectively take advantage of them for cancer patients? Let me assure you, some treatment centers are leveraging the power of these cells. So let's review the main obstacles dendritic cells encounter to limit their practical therapeutic anti-tumor potential:

- The dendritic cell count
- The specificity of antibodies that affect only one antigen (tumors count on myriad antigens to thrive)
- The fact that "self" antigens are tolerated, effectively suppressing the dendritic-cell immune response

We address these critical issues with the following proven methods.

Ultraviolet Light Irradiation

Dendritic cells represent an ideal therapeutic target for anti-tumor application, and cancer patients usually have a low dendritic-cell count; so, therapies to increase them in patients is paramount. We stimulate their production by exposing blood cells to ultraviolet light, extracting about 200 cc of blood and re-infusing it after irradiation. This method, extracorporeal photopheresis, has been considered an efficient therapy for treating malignancies and autoimmune diseases.[10] Researchers have been studying the effects of photopheresis on dendritic-cell biology due to their role in initiating specific immune responses.[11] It's been proven that UV irradiation promotes the transformation of monocytes into immature dendritic cells; they're like the reserves in the armed forces. In their immature state dendritic cells are localized in the peripheral tissues, waiting to be called upon. Once they come in contact with antigens and/or "danger" signals (e.g., microbes or malignant cytokines), dendritic cells initiate their maturation process and migrate to regional lymph nodes where they activate and mobilize immune attacking cells.[12]

Allogeneic Effect

Having addressed quantity, we must establish a way to induce dendritic cells to attack the host tumor with a broad-spectrum arsenal. How can we do this affordably? *Not* all dendritic-cell therapies are economically unreachable. Dr. Masaru Kondo developed a less complicated and more reasonable immunotherapy with an allogeneic lymphocyte infusion. "Allogeneic" means the lymphocytes are harvested from a donor (young, healthy, and unrelated). Over four hundred deemed-hopeless patients with stage IV cancers of all sorts were treated; tumor reduction by more than 50% resulted in 20% to 30% of them.[13]

Kondo's work was severely criticized, first, because the results were deemed too good to be true, and, second, because he was unable to explain the mode of action of the "allogeneic effect" for reducing tumor load. This effective therapy stayed under the rug for twenty-five years until a group led by Dr. Ephraim Fuchs discerned Kondo's mode of action,[14] defining it as an immune response that promotes T-cell cytotoxicity, including tumoricidal activity, by an infusion of allogeneic lymphocytes that trigger the following immune response:

1. Mobilization of dendritic cells, boosting antigen-presenting activity
2. Activation of B-cells, with broad-spectrum antibody production
3. Activation of cytotoxic T lymphocytes (CTLs), which directly attack and kill cancer cells
4. Activation of NK cells, which also attack many cancer cells.

Using mice in their study model, they "show[ed] that treatment of . . . allogeneic donor lymphocyte infusion induces regression of established tumors with minimal toxicity in models of both hematologic and solid cancers, even though the donor cells are eventually rejected by the host immune system."[15]

Mini-Dose Chemo

All of this is for naught if we cannot limit the mechanisms that prevent autoimmune disorders. Both Kondo and Fuchs used mini-dose chemotherapy, a few days prior to allogeneic lymphocyte infusion, to reduce regulatory T cells (Tregs) and so leave the way unimpeded for the attacking cells to destroy tumors.

Conclusion

Much focus has been on making vaccines that leverage dendritic cells, but results have been very expensive, not very effective vaccines. Another tack has led to relatively inexpensive, highly effective anti-cancer treatment with dendritic cells. Combining three approaches—increase dendritic-cell count, provoke broad-spectrum immune attack, and skew immune-regulating mechanisms—has improved clinical efficacy of cancer immunotherapy in patients with metastatic disease at Oasis of Hope.

ACTION STEPS

1. Make sure you're abreast of new developments while being informed of the ones that are practical and already in current use.
2. While vaccines are only given in very specialized centers, there are other means of stimulating the immune system effectively.
3. The info about this is technical and complicated even for most doctors; consult with experts for answers to your questions.

CANCER VICTOR TIPS

Kari Dinges, New Jersey
Stage III Breast Cancer
Victor Since 2008

1. Look into all options before making treatment decisions; don't rush.
2. *You* have to be convinced that the treatment course you choose is your best option. Be *sold* on it!
3. Treat cancer like a burglar. Don't just scare it away—be vigilant in keeping it away.

4. "An ounce of prevention is worth a pound of cure." Amen!
5. Place hope not in a cure but in God. "Be of good courage, and he shall strengthen your heart, all ye that hope in the Lord" (Psalm 31:24 KJV)!

Dendritic Cells
https://vimeo.com/61916384

Chapter 33

Multi-Disciplinary Team

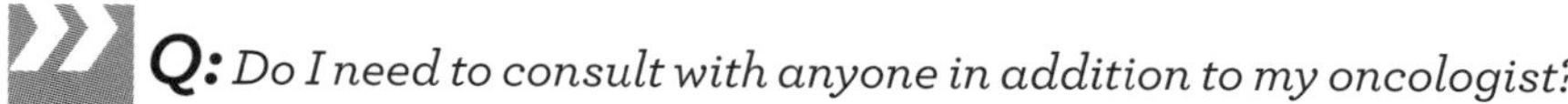

Q: *Do I need to consult with anyone in addition to my oncologist?*

A: Cancer is a multitude of diseases; it requires the attention and collaboration of multiple medical specialists. More than a physical ailment, cancer negatively affects emotional well-being and stresses spiritual foundations. An effective multi-disciplinary team (MDT) is one that includes emotional and spiritual care.

In ancient times, people who were ill would call upon the elders to pray for them and anoint them with oil. They would confess the healing promises of God. They would eat foods that heal, and a physician would give them herbal remedies including teas and poultices. Team efforts ministered to body, soul, and spirit.

When my father, Dr. Ernesto Contreras, Sr., studied in the late 1930s, medical science was undergoing a technological revolution, with the art of healing being purposefully excised. He was instructed to avoid making friendships with patients to avoid emotional attachment and so maintain ability to diagnose objectively. His total focus was to be on lab work, pathology, and radiology reports. Emotional and spiritual support was left behind. Doctors became specialists of illness in the body.

After graduating, he specialized in pathology and oncology, receiving training in pediatric pathology and serving in several hospitals. He became concerned when he noted that 30% of all tissue he examined was healthy; three of ten surgeries were unneeded. (Studies within the last *year* indicate that one in five of all procedures and tests are unnecessary and that medical errors are responsible for 100,000 US hospital deaths annually.[1]) His conclusion: doctors needed to stop hiding behind lab work and start including patients in the diagnosis process. As he started to see his oncology patients, he discovered that even the doctor-patient relationship was a healing agent. Talking with them at length, he confirmed his belief that patients need more than a body mechanic.

The Total Care Approach

Dr. Contreras, Sr. cofounded the Association of Oncologists and the Association of Pathologists in the 1950s and decided he would address both groups with his vision of treating the whole body-soul-spirit patient. There were no standing ovations; his memberships both were terminated. Yet even though they weren't ready for a holistic approach, he found his patients intuitively knew they needed comprehensive care. He turned his efforts from trying to convince others to developing a treatment approach that would meet their needs. He dubbed this "the Total Care Approach."

He founded our hospital and put in place a multi-disciplinary team including oncologists, general and family medicine specialists, internists, radiologists, physical therapists, nurses, nutritionists, food preparers, emotional counselors, spiritual counselors, health educators, patient care reps, and follow-up care staff. Again, cancer is a complex disease that affects all our systems; body, soul, and spirit are interconnected, and total health is only possible when physical, emotional, and spiritual health are in balanced harmony. He was one of the first to put multiple health practices all under one roof, working together to help the patient. He also was one of few doctors to include his patient on the healing team and to solicit patient opinions when developing the course of treatment.

Team Medicine

A study on multi-disciplinary team (MDT) treatment of gastro-esophageal cancer found improvements in both staging and treatment management.[2] Of the patients without MDT, 9% were under-treated, 20% over-treated, and 18% offered inappropriate treatment. Among MDT-treated patients, only 2% were under-treated and 19% over-treated.

A number of such models are being used in a few US cancer care centers. In the "sequential model," a treatment coordinator interviews the patient by phone and then schedules her to see each specialist (e.g., radiologist, clinical oncologist, surgical oncologist, pathologist) in logical sequence.[3] The benefit is efficiency for physicians and less time wasted for patients on return visits due to missing tests or procedures. However, this model does not create a cooperative team that shares information and experience for the patient's benefit. It simply streamlines care and hence falls short of the true power of a multi-disciplinary team.

The "concurrent model" adds to the sequential a group meeting of all doctors involved in the patient's care. The attending physician presents the case and the medical info and gets feedback and input from all the others. A study on multi-disciplinary care concluded that 90% of physicians perceived its value and 90% of patients believed they were benefited.[4] Cancer centers also frequently offer orientations to familiarize patients with the multi-disciplinary team and increase their self-efficacy.[5]

Oasis of Hope uses the concurrent approach with the additions of mind and spirit counselors, nutritionists, and physical therapists. This model's advantage is that each discipline is working together and both avoid contraindications and create synergy.

The Oasis of Hope Multi-Disciplinary Team

Here's a quick overview of the MDT we've developed to utilize the total care approach.

- We provide roundtrip transportation between the airport in San Diego and our facility in Tijuana. Our goal is to help people feel they've arrived at their second home when they get off the plane. As they get into our shuttle, they receive a personalized tablet that is their connection to many resources for cancer care, including a welcome video to watch on the twenty-minute drive to Oasis of Hope.
- Sunday evening we have a welcome event, new-patient orientation: tour of the facility, overview of the treatment schedule, tea and organic snacks, and questions from newcomers.
- For each patient's exam and evaluation, we review records from previous care and conduct a comprehensive oncology physical exam.

- We order new lab work, radiological studies, and pathology studies. All info is compiled for presentation to the MDT physicians' meeting.
- Oncologist meets with patient and recommends the oncology regimen to be integrated into the cancer treatment protocol as a part of our metabolic therapy.
- MDT discusses all aspects of care for our patient. Each specialist contributes to the treatment program; the attending physician integrates all the therapies into a personal treatment plan.
- Attending physician meets with patient and explains treatment plan. Patient is invited to ask questions, make suggestions, and be part of decisions before we initiate treatment. Patient can access plan and explanation of each therapy on his personalized tablet, thus there is no worry about neglecting or forgetting vital information.
- Nurses begin to administer daily treatment.
- Each morning our pastor leads with devotions and worship music.
- Doctors and staff give daily lectures to explain the what, how, and why of each treatment. There's time for questions and answers, and each video session is available on the tablet for future reference.
- Activities to promote emotional healing include support groups, art therapy, and lectures.
- Patients receive education and cooking classes from our nutritionist for learning how to integrate healing foods into their lifestyle.
- Sessions with our physical therapist teach our patients how to exercise and increase oxygenation, range of motion, and lymph movement. This addition can also be helpful for pain management.
- One of the week's highlights is laughter therapy. Search YouTube for Oasis of Hope laughter therapy and enjoy our therapist in action.
- Cooking classes (also on tablet) teach patients and companions quick and easy ways to make delicious meals without oil or unhealthy ingredients while maintaining the foods' integrity.
- Patients are invited to the healing room each week for individual prayer therapy, a confidential opportunity for deep spiritual healing.
- Thrice daily we serve healing foods: high in anti-cancer nutrients, low on the glycemic index, organic, pesticide-free, and gluten-free.
- Dr. Contreras or our pastor shares the healing power of God's Word at our Sunday service.

- We never say good-bye to our patients because we partner with each for life. At a weekly farewell event we encourage them to exchange contact info, and we say, ""“Farewell, until we meet again.”
- We’re staffed and designed to follow up with our patients. We make regular contact and provide support formally for five years, and then for life for those who choose to continue in connection.

Conclusion

Having examined the benefits and efficacy of integrated total care, let’s continue looking at how to connect and communicate with others to make the most of our opportunities for balanced and complete health.

ACTION STEPS

1. Make sure you have more than an oncologist to help you. Consider adding a nutritionist and others to your treatment team.
2. Consider being treated at a comprehensive cancer center that supports patients with care provided by a multi-disciplinary team.
3. Form an MDT home care team involving food prep, local support group, coordinator of meds/appointments, and prayer partner.

CANCER VICTOR TIPS

Esperanza Kazuga, México
Breast Cancer
Victor Since 2003

1. I recommend that you go to Oasis of Hope.
2. Take a holistic approach to healing: body, soul, and spirit.
3. Change your diet to vegetarian.
4. Take time to listen to what your body wants to say.
5. Don’t be afraid: God is with you.

Multi-Disciplinary Team
https://vimeo.com/62383973

Chapter 34

Social Network

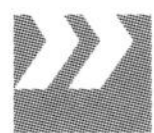

Q: *What should I do to get the support I need?*

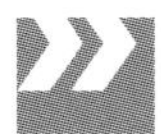

A: Build a team that goes beyond physicians. Involve family and friends to help you to be compliant to your therapy and to keep informed of treatment options. You can also help your team by being a source of health information for them and an ambassador for a healthy preventive lifestyle.

Humans were designed to be socially interdependent. Most have an emotional need for friendships and social interaction. We express our desire for connection through, for example, shared gaming, messaging and comments, and social surveying (learning what friends and family are up to).[1] It's the driving force behind social networking sites (SNS) and the explanation for why Facebook has more than a billion active users.[2]

There's a growing trend for health practitioners to share info on social networking sites.[3] (Check us out on Twitter: @DrContreras and @PastorDKennedy.) Cancer support groups are springing up online too. More than six hundred breast cancer groups on Facebook, formed to raise awareness, raise funds, promote products and services, and provide patient and caregiver support, have more than a million members.[4]

SNS are a start toward the support cancer patients need but are hardly sufficient—*virtual help for real life can only go so far.* Patients face many psychosocial issues that can cause chronic stress and emotional distress, counterproductive to the healing process. Many report feelings of anxiety and depression; loneliness affects 50% of cancer patients.[5] Those with less support have higher incidence of negative symptoms and report lower quality of life.[6] Most medical lawsuits point to a breakdown of communication, another huge issue for people facing cancer.[7] Also common when a person is diagnosed is to isolate socially.

Many people find it exceedingly difficult to talk to friends and family about the cancer-related difficulties, and the future, that they face.[8] But social support is the right course of action. Consider the benefits.

Effective Social Support

A social network is the combination of support and resources that can be provided through relationships. For patients, these usually are based in family, friends, peers, and acquaintances through organizations like churches. Each network is unique, depending on the number of contacts, how often the person interacts with them, and the social roles of each relationship.[9] Good social support helps a patient maintain a positive attitude, increase hope, and improve motivation to actually fight cancer.[10] Family support is key in helping patients diminish feelings of loneliness; friend and family support also acts as a buffer from stress. And a caregiver can help in the communication process between doctor and patient and diminish confusion; he or she also can help remember and document details. Improved communication can result in both improved treatment experience and improved quality of life.

• • • • • • • • • • • •

The following short list, for caregivers, is a concise guide of what not to do. These behaviors aren't supportive[11] and may even be damaging.

- Don't become socially disengaged or distant.
- Don't force quick fixes. Cancer requires consistent, long-haul support.
- Don't compel a positive outlook. Be encouraging, not coercive.
- Don't minimize the importance of the patient's concerns.
- Don't blame, criticize, or bestow guilt.

H.O.P.E. Team

Probably nobody has a cancer support team assembled when they're first diagnosed. But there's no doubting the importance of organizing your social network and wrapping support around yourself. Here is an acronym, using the word *HOPE,* to help you build your support group:

H	Helpers	Accept help for everyday needs: shopping, cleaning, companionship, transport, food prep, donations. . . .
O	Oncologist	Pick an oncologist you can trust; engage him/her in personal conversation so that he/she makes an emotional investment in the relationship with you.
P	Physicians, nurses, other practitioners	Assemble a multi-disciplinary team; include general practitioner, nurses, nutritionist, naturopath, chiropractor, fitness trainer, massage therapist.
E	Emotional and spiritual counselors	Individual counseling, spiritual care, and groups are a priceless support source that can help you manage anxiety, depression, anger, guilt, and stress.

Conclusion

God did not design us to be alone, and when we're facing true challenges we need others as much as ever. Ask Him to give you courage and wisdom in approaching people, and, in any areas where your relationships are lacking, make your current situation an opportunity for initiating and building healthy two-way bonds with others.

ACTION STEPS

1. Make (don't break) connections. Engage others. Ask for help.
2. Do a mental survey of all your contacts; determine who has skills and a disposition to help, then invite them onto your team.
3. You'd help friends and family if they had cancer; let them help you.

CANCER VICTOR TIPS

Lizz Garcia-Nicholson, California
Breast Cancer
Victor Since 2011

1. No matter what you're told, God is the only one with your "stop date," and He has your life *all* under control!
2. Be in a state of forgiveness to whomever has hurt you; rebuke the spirits of fear, negativity, anger, and worry. (All of those bring up your cortisol levels, which are dangerous when elevated.)
3. Eat an organic, fungal-free alkaline diet along with alkaline water. Take on a good cardio exercise regime (jogging, spinning, cycling, power-walking, etc.).
4. Always follow what your naturopathic doctor or team has planned for your success—they really want you well! Work with them and educate yourself to build up the strongest immune system possible.
5. Above all: *Laugh, Laugh, Laugh!* Science has shown this releases endorphins (great medicine physically, mentally, and spiritually).

Social Network
https://vimeo.com/67691691

Chapter 35

Biopsies

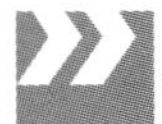

Q: *Are biopsies dangerous?*

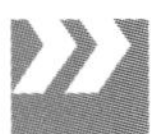

A: All surgical procedures have risks. The gain of determining the cancer's type and nature trumps all risks, for it allows doctors to design your best therapy.

In all aspects of life we take risks, and of these there's no question biopsies have their share. What's central with risks in general is that we evaluate them against actual and potential benefits. There are risks and costs to whatever we do; sometimes the cost of inaction is greater. Many patients fear a biopsy can cause their cancer to spread, and yes, this is possible—but it's extremely improbable. From thirty-five years of surgical oncology I can count on one hand the cases where, as a biopsy's direct effect, a tumor invaded the procedural area or caused any metastasis to other organs or lymph nodes.

In most patients cancerous cells are always circulating; there is no evidence of correlation between increase of metastasis or deterioration of survival related to biopsies or surgical procedures. For instance, the cure rate for early cervical carcinoma is almost 100% with surgical removal of the cervix or uterus. "Cure" inherently means there's no recurrence or invasion to any other tissue. The same goes for early stages of nearly any other cancer that can be removed surgically.

Any surgical procedure is an insult to the immune system; this can indeed aid a malignancy to take advantage of the immune suppression and, in advanced stages, a patient may experience tumor dissemination after surgery. For that reason, at Oasis of Hope we administer immune-stimulating nutraceuticals before and after every surgical procedure, no matter how small, including needle biopsies.

Benefits of biopsies far outweigh their risk. For instance, a study by Dr. Marco Greco showed that development of lymph node metastasis to the axilla after breast biopsies was only 2% in low-risk patients (tumors < 3 cm) and 6.7% in high-risk patients (tumors > 3 cm). He said, "Many, possibly all, of these metastases would be present before any medical attention, but undetectable clinically."[1] More aggressive breast cancers can give rise to occult (undetectable) blood-borne metastases very early on, thus many or most such metastases will have been pre-existing. The same considerations apply to other cancers with high cure rates.

It's true that doctors easily admonish patients to have biopsies done. Though I agree with the caution of Joaquín Setantí to "Be wary of the man who urges an action in which he himself incurs no risk,"[2] I do believe that to best treat a patient it's critical that we establish the most complete diagnosis possible, and a biopsy is the ultimate diagnosis.

• • • • • • • • • • • •

Albucasis, an eleventh-century physician, reportedly was one of the first to develop diagnostic biopsies,[3] but not till 1879 did Ernest Besnier introduce to the medical community the neologism "biopsy," from the Greek *bio* ("life") and *opsia* ("to see"). Biopsy is removal and examination of a sample of tissue from a living body for diagnostic purposes.

Generally, a pathologist examines the tissue under a microscope; it also can be analyzed chemically. Depending on the site and extension of the disease, biopsies may be done under local or general anesthesia. The following are the most commonly performed types.

Fine-needle aspiration biopsy. A very thin needle is placed into lump or suspicious area to remove small sample of fluid and/or tissue. No incision (cut) necessary.

Core needle biopsy. A large needle is guided into lump or suspicious area to remove a tissue cylinder (core). No incision necessary.

Vacuum-assisted biopsy. Basically a core biopsy assisted by a suction device to obtain better samples.

Image-guided biopsies:

Stereotactic biopsy. Imaging finds exact location of tumor or suspicious area and creates 3D view for better approach to lesion.

Guided biopsy. Ultrasound, MRI, CT, or fluoroscopy guides the needle.

Endoscopic biopsy. Uses any kind of scope to reach the diseased area (digestive, respiratory, urinary tracts, abdomen, or joints).

Surgical biopsy (or open biopsy). Surgeon removes part or all of a lump or suspicious area through an incision into the diseased area.

Incisional biopsy. A small part of the lump is removed.

Excisional biopsy. Entire lump is removed.

Cytological biopsy. If there is only liquid (no tumors), it can be obtained through a needle; pathologist will obtain cells to determine if they're benign or malignant. Cells can be obtained too by washing lactation ducts from breast nipple or by brushing bronchia. The most common cytological test is the Papanicolaou test (Pap smear). Bone marrow tissue can also be harvested to diagnose blood-borne diseases.

• • • • • • • • • • • •

These are the techniques to obtain the samples; the second leg of the process is their preparation. The sample may be chemically treated or frozen and sliced into thin sections to be placed on glass slides that may be stained to enhance and contrast the cells under a microscope. Now a pathologist can evaluate the biopsy—the third leg—and provide an interpretation or result. Microscope potency has evolved tremendously in recent decades, yet pathologists develop the skill of cell observation through many years of practice. They learn the normal structure of all organs and tissues and all possible pathological structures including hundreds of types of cancers. For instance, they're able to determine from a lung biopsy if the original tumor comes from the lung or if it's a metastasis from the breast or the colon. Not only that, they also determine the cancer's aggression. The grade is sometimes expressed as a number on a scale of 1 to 4. Grade 1 (low-grade) cancers are generally least aggressive and grade 4 (high-grade) are generally most aggressive.

Special Tests

Other tests on cancer cells can help to guide treatment choices. It is now possible to determine the cells' immunological activity so that with immunohistochemistry tests we can know if a tumor is binding to a certain antigen that can be unbound and stopped. A number of these markers help pathologists to distinguish members of one difficult-to-diagnose cancer family. Breast cancer has two main members, one that arises from the milk ducts and one that comes from the breast tissue itself. Immunostaining for e-cadherin tells DCIS (ductal carcinoma in situ: stains positive) from LCIS (lobular carcinoma in situ: does not stain positive). Of the immunohistochemical markers that pathologists use to fine-tune interpretations, these are the most common:

- Estrogen/progesterone staining (breast cancer hormone dependency)
- CD15 and CD30 (Hodgkin's disease)
- Alpha-fetoprotein: for hepatocellular carcinoma
- CD117: for gastrointestinal stromal tumors (GIST)
- CD10: for renal cell carcinoma and acute lymphoblastic leukemia
- CD20 for B-cell lymphomas
- CD3 for T-cell lymphomas

As with all medical testing, there's room for error here—not so much as in other specialties (e.g., imaging), but still mistakes are possible. Thus we must be sure to take results with caution. While denial in general isn't in our best interest, when in doubt, seek a second opinion.

For instance, pathology expert Jonathan Epstein reviewed the biopsy slides of 6,171 patients referred to Johns Hopkins medical institutions for cancer treatments and found that eighty-six (1.4%) had significantly wrong diagnoses that would have led to unnecessary or inappropriate treatment. He said that while this percentage is low, when put into perspective it meant that at Johns Hopkins alone about one cancer patient a week would have a wrong diagnosis, and nationwide this conservatively could add up to thirty thousand mistakes a year. Epstein added: "If I were a patient and was diagnosed with a malignancy, I would get a second opinion before undergoing any major surgery, chemotherapy or radiation. And if I had a negative biopsy on an organ that's known to have a higher rate of error I'd also get a second opinion."[4]

Conclusion

Biopsies do not spread cancer. All surgical procedures suppress the immune system, which opens up the opportunity for cancer to spread. Do natural therapies to boost the immune system before and after any surgical procedure to minimize risk of spread. Remember, biopsies are our closest confirmation of being absolutely certain, but there is a margin of error. I believe everyone should get a second opinion.

ACTION STEPS

1. Establish the most complete diagnosis possible to design the best therapy to address a disease, especially cancer.
2. Be assertive in discussing all aspects of a biopsy with your doctor.
3. Make sure you understand the results, and, if in doubt, do not be shy in seeking a second or third opinion.

CANCER VICTOR TIPS

Lovolia C. Isaac, South Carolina
Breast Cancer and Bone Cancer
Victor Since 2005

1. Adopt a plant-based diet.
2. Eliminate all added sugar, processed food, dairy products, and meat.
3. Reduce the amount of stress. Put yourself first.
4. Think positive; there is hope.
5. Get plenty of exercise and rest.

Biopsies
https://vimeo.com/62386938

Chapter 36

Imaging

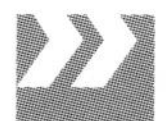

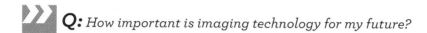

Q: *How important is imaging technology for my future?*

A: Imaging is both the most effective tool to establish the size and stage of your disease and also the means by which to evaluate results.

Images are *important.* Consider that God addressed their power in commanding (for worship), "You must not make for yourself an idol of any kind or an image of anything in the heavens or on the earth or in the sea."[1] John Lennon showed he grasped the significance of imaging with his wardrobe, branding, and the song "Imagine."[2] I would have loved if he'd substituted for the first line, "Imagine there's no cancer."

Vision is essential to success. And imaging—the capture, projection, and interpretation of an object—is integral to beating cancer.

Study of Human Anatomy

Understanding the human body is at the center of the art of healing. Looking inside the body, since ancient times, has been key to advancing medicine, but access presented obstacles. Through much of history the anatomy was accessible only to warriors who cut their foe asunder. Lack of technology and scientific method constrained early doctors, and religious restrictions (pagan, Islamic, Christian) hindered medicine's advance for more than a millennium.

In the second century, in all aspects of life, the known world was either ruled or led by the Roman Empire. In AD 169, when the Antonine Plague broke out, Caesar Marcus Aurelius summoned Galen, the Greek who'd made his mark in Rome humbling doctors less trained and even less able.[3] During his tenure as court physician Galen became the Empire's most celebrated physician and wrote extensively on theories and innovations that dominated the next twelve centuries of Western medical thinking. But human dissection was banned in Rome, and many of his theories were wrong because they were based on the anatomy of apes and other animals. His only exposure to human anatomy had come when as a young doctor he'd cared for injured gladiators.

In the sixteenth century, Andreas Vesalius changed the direction of medical sciences by convincing authorities that dissecting cadavers was central to training and research. This effort culminated in 1543 in his most important work, *On the Fabric of the Human Body*.[4] After centuries of anatomical misdirection, at last a new era of progress exploded.

Birth and Modernization of Imaging

Three hundred and fifty years later, a revolutionary discovery propelled advancements further. In 1895 Wilhelm Röntgen was working with electromagnetic radiation wavelengths when he accidentally discovered a cast image that was not deflected by magnetic fields and penetrated many kinds of matter.[5] With no clue what these wavelengths were, he called them X, or X-rays; his colleagues called them Röntgen rays.

A week later he took an X-ray film of his wife's hand. The photo circulated in both scientific and nonscientific circles, astounding everyone because it clearly revealed her hand bones with her wedding ring. Anna Bertha Röntgen's image was the first medical X-ray. To date, in German-speaking countries, X-rays are still called Röntgen.

This invention's applications were apparent not only to the medical field but to others too. The Foot-o-scope, an X-ray fluoroscope machine developed to visualize the foot inside the shoe and assess how well it fit, was in stores in some countries from the 1920s to the 1970s.[6] It began disappearing as awareness of radiation hazards became known.

The last hundred-plus years have brought a cascade of innovations that defy human comprehension. And today we can invade the privacy of the human body's innermost recesses with startling precision aided by imaging toys that would amaze physicians from just a generation past. X-ray machines are now digitalized; the different-size films have been replaced by sensors that transfer captured images to a computer, and software helps us "doctor" them for optimal interpretation.

There are all kinds of fluoroscopes; these X-ray machines allow us to view a specific part of the body "live." They're used for many purposes, such as to evaluate transit of part or all of the digestive tract, to help place a catheter in an exact spot, to perform angioplasty, and to insert intra-coronary stints for avoiding bypass surgery.

CT Scan

The most used X-ray device, the Computer Tomography (CT) scan, provides images of the body in "slices," allowing us to pinpoint size and location of any anatomical aberrations, especially tumors. With helicoidal technology, the patient is filmed with a camera moving spirally around him, giving high-quality, high-quantity images that then are processed by the CT's computer to construct 3D images we can rotate and color to establish the scope of the problem and, hopefully, a correct diagnosis.

It's now possible, thanks to advanced software, to analyze the status of our coronary arteries without catheterization or contrast materials; more and more cardiologists are using this non-invasive, less risk-prone procedure to evaluate cardiac patients. Many gastroenterologists in Europe relieve their patients by ordering virtual colonoscopies.

PET/CT Scan

Following five decades of multi-disciplinary cooperation by chemists, physicists, computer analysts, and physicians, Positron Emission Tomography (PET) now diagnoses diseases by measuring differences in energy consumption. To measure tissue activity, the patient is injected with a glucose radioactive tracer; as malignant cells multiply much faster than normal or benign tissue, they need a lot more sugar to generate the energy needed, thus the glucose tracer concentrates more in malignant tumors. The PET will "light up" cancerous (but not benign) tumors.

The images—functional rather than anatomical—aren't easy to view, so they're joined to an imaging study. The combined PET/CT scan provides the radiologist an active (metabolic) *and* an anatomical lesion. The tracer's standardized uptake value (SUV) measures the metabolic activity; the SUV of normal cells is 1, and an SUV of 2.5 or greater indicates abnormally high energy consumption that could indicate malignancy or other diseases. A

PET/CT can uncover tumors earlier, as this activity can show even before a tumor is visible on a CT scan.

MRI

Other imaging studies use different electromagnetic waves. On one, yet another Nobel Prize-winner, scientists from the fields of mathematics, physics, and chemistry provided knowledge and inventions over a hundred-year period that culminated in what we now know as magnetic resonance imaging (MRI), also known as nuclear magnetic resonance (NMR). This technology has evolved into a clinical tool capable, for instance, of real time in-utero cardiac imaging of a fetus, and of imaging a single cell. A powerful magnet generates the waves that produce the images; no X-rays are involved, thus it's completely nontoxic to a patient.

Ultrasound

Another nontoxic tool is also known as sonography because the energy that generates the images—sound waves of twenty thousand or more vibrations per second—is far above the frequency heard by the human ear (thus, "ultrasound"). Karl Theodore Dussik introduced ultrasonic research to the medical field in 1942; in the 1950s Ian Donald developed practical technology and applications for ultrasound as a diagnostic tool. Ultrasound machines use a transducer to emit the waves through our bodies and, because every cell of every tissue is different, they will produce a specific echo when they collide and thus generate images depicting organs and tissues with their abnormalities (hence ultrasound is also called echography). Sound waves are innocuous, so they're widely used to examine the health and development of unborn babies and to analyze heart disease, bone structure, and cancer. They're even used for muscle healing and tooth cleansing.

If you're a Trekkie like me, you know that the original *Star Trek* takes place in the twenty-third century. Captain Kirk's famous *communicator*, by the way, was Martin Cooper's inspiration to develop the personal cell phone while working for Motorola in the 1970s. Kirk's medical officer, "Bones" McCoy, used a *tricorder* (multifunction handheld device) for sensor scanning, data analysis, and diagnostics, which has inspired development of yet another device. Mobisante paired the *communicator* with the *tricorder* to come up with a mobile ultrasound, basically a software app. A physician can connect an ultrasound transducer to a smartphone's USB port and view a patient's insides on the screen. This affordable, mobile technology can be of tremendous help for making fast and proper diagnosis onsite. Mobile Ultrasound is available now as a prototype and, according to experts, is the stethoscope of the near future.

Misdiagnosis

Still, as technology changes our lives and advances bring benefits, we must keep weighing risks. At the 2010 meeting of the Radiological Society of North America (RSNA), the world's largest medical conference, James Brice gave an impacting presentation titled "To err is human; analysis finds radiologists very human" on the high incidence of interpretation errors in imaging studies.[7] Also, Young W. Kim and his colleagues had analyzed 656 imaging exams from two military hospitals spanning seven-plus years. They identified 1,279 errors and reported that nearly a third of the diagnoses were missed on the first exam *and* weren't recognized on subsequent radiological exams. Upon review of the medical literature, Kim said that there are errors daily in 3% to 4% of all studies due simply to dictation mistakes.[8]

So misdiagnosis perseveres as medicine's Achilles' heel. Diagnostic errors are the leading cause of malpractice litigation, accounting for twice as many claims as medication errors. Dr. Leonard Berlin reports that radiologists have become the specialists most frequently named in suits involving breast cancer and that mammography has become the most prevalent procedure involved in malpractice suits against radiologists. Furthermore, breast cancer misdiagnosis is the most prevalent condition precipitating medical malpractice lawsuits against all physicians: "The radiology literature is replete with articles that document error rates among competent radiologists in the interpretation of mammograms."[9]

For thousands of women who'd been told nothing was wrong, on second inspection tumors are found. Studies show that 30% to 70% of breast cancers detected at follow-up mammography are retrospectively seen on first mammograms as showing normal findings. At the other extreme are women over-treated because of screening mammography. In a peer-reviewed study published in the ultra-prestigious *New England Journal of Medicine*, and then in *Medical Benefits*, Dr. Archie Bleyer stated that mammograms caused more than a million US women over the past three decades to be diagnosed with early stage breast cancers that would not have proved fatal if left undetected and untreated.[10]

• • • • • • • • • • • • •

Dr. Kim identified these main reasons for radiologist's mistakes:

- Failure to diagnose or under-reading (not seeing abnormality): 42%
- Failure to thoroughly examine anatomy after seeing abnormalities relevant to a primary diagnosis: 22%
- Faulty interpretation: 9%
- Failure to notice pathology in peripheral or unexpected locations; tunnel vision; missing pathology in first or last image in a series: 7%
- Over-reliance on prior radiology report: 6%
- Lack of comparisons with prior studies: 5%

Kim says that, despite all the modernization in imaging technology, his findings "are similar to those of published reports on radiology error rates going back to the 1940s."[11] Dr. Antonio Pinto reports comparable results in Europe.[12]

In turn, to reduce their liability, radiologists and doctors order more and more tests not because they're necessary but to appease lawyers, tremendously increasing the cost of care. These reports remind me of the words of Pulitzer-winning writer Russell Wayne Baker: "An educated person is one who has learned that information almost always turns out to be at best incomplete and very often false, misleading, fictitious, mendacious—just dead wrong."[13]

One factor compounding the failures is communication of results to colleagues and patients. In my opinion, the most devastating factor in imaging testing is the delivery of bad news. Most doctors do this without delicacy; many share shattering results coldly or dismissively, leaving behind feelings of hopelessness. I believe a medical report is like a meal—food is important, but presentation is imperative, and a well-presented plate makes all the difference in the experience. As John Maxwell said, "People do not care how much you know until they know how much you care."[14] We should be sure to deliver bad news in the most positive way and at the correct time. There's no need to lie, ever, but we must present the message with care and with hope.

Conclusion

As a surgical oncologist, I'm the first to sing the praises of imaging. I look daily at images from available technologies for help making treatment decisions and maintaining a conservative approach to surgery. Imaging equipment also allows minimally invasive procedures. But please regard imaging as an art; not a science; radiologists are trained to *interpret.* They "see" what others cannot. Images are shadows and contrasts, and the radiologist must determine what's going on in all of the nuances. This is one reason we do blood work and biopsies as well—we seek to put together an effective diagnosis and treatment plan by corroborating radiology, pathology, and laboratory results.

ACTION STEPS

1. Inform yourself about advancements in imaging technology.
2. Ask your doctor if a study would help in therapy decision-making.
3. Make sure your medical team is up to date on imaging advances.

CANCER VICTOR TIPS

Sharon Martinson, Minnesota
Ovarian Cancer
Victor Since 2009

1. Be open-minded about non-traditional treatments.
2. Accept that God is in charge and has a plan for you.
3. Get as much prayer support as you can.
4. Do your own research rather than accepting what one doctor says.
5. Eat the best diet you can.

Imaging
https://vimeo.com/62446199

Chapter 37

Nanotechnology

Q: *Is nanomedicine science fiction, or is this novel methodology really available?*

A: Some nano-applications are available today, but the greatest breakthroughs are still to come. In my opinion, nanotechnology will improve drug delivery directly to tumors so the patient will no longer endure (or will endure far less of) the negative side effects or collateral damage to healthy cells from toxic chemotherapies. Nanotechnology will also revolutionize diagnostic techniques.

The era of the tiny is here to stay; the "new industrial revolution" is believed to come from minuscule particles in all sciences and all aspects of life. From packaging to agriculture, the business of the very small, already a trillion-dollar industry, is measured in *nanometers* (*nm*), derived from the Greek *nano* ("dwarf"). Before the electronic microscope, we had no idea of the smallness of this unit of measure; there are one billion nanometers to a meter. If you shrunk to a nanometer's height, your average neighbor would be almost five billion feet tall—standing on earth, his head would be about four times farther away than the moon.

Or think about this: a red blood cell measures 7,000 nanometers; a typical virus 75 nm; the DNA helix 2 nm; a sugar molecule 1 nm. An *atom* is a bit smaller—three to five of those fit into a nanometer. In a sense, it truly is a small, small world. And this technology's impact is not only quantitative; more importantly, it also is qualitative. Now it's possible for us to manipulate matter on an atomic scale.

While in many other industries (mainly engineering) this technology is thriving, it has been slow to impact medical applications due to the incredible complexities of biology and the challenges of ensuring safety. And yet the pursuit is relentless. An ancient but effective strategy Homer depicted in the *Odyssey*[1] is being developed twenty-nine centuries later by strategists desperate to penetrate cancer barriers that, like the wall of Troy, have been impenetrable. Odysseus tried unsuccessfully for ten years to overcome that protective wall. Pretending to sail away, he left a gift in token of accepted defeat (as was customary). After being brought inside, agents hidden inside the enormous, infamous Trojan Horse opened the city's gates to their own army, and . . . the rest is legend.

Medical Trojan Horse

Researchers believe that through the development of nanoparticles, nanocarriers of anti-cancer drugs can, like Trojan horses, cross some of the up-to-now impenetrable biological barriers and specifically target cancer cells, achieving therapeutic concentrations within a tumor. These targeted therapies would not harm healthy cells, reducing the toxic side effects of typical chemo drugs. Welcome to the world of nanomedicine, more specifically of *nano-oncology*; the application of nanobiotechnology to cancer management is now cancer research's most important chapter.

In "Nanotechnology and Drug Delivery: An Update in Oncology," Dr. Tait Jones states,

> The field of nanotechnology has exploded in recent years with diverse arrays of applications. This customizable approach has raised the possibility of drug delivery systems capable of multiple, simultaneous functions, including applications in diagnostics, imaging, and therapy which is paving the way to improved early detection methods, more effective therapy, and better survivorship for cancer patients.[2]

There's little doubt nanoparticulate pharmaceutical carriers are the future in the field of drug delivery, including liposomes, polymeric micelles, microcapsules, quantum dots, nanoparticles, and dendrimers.

Next-generation smart drugs will have features that can be designed to function in an orchestrated order, simultaneously or sequentially, depending on specific needs. They're being designed to resolve the main challenges of past and present drug delivery systems, and they could revolutionize diagnosis, targeting tumors much earlier than ever thought possible. Nanodevices can be used to:[3]

1. Detect sub-microscopic cancer cells at an early stage.
2. Provide effective concentration in the body for a prolonged period. Presently, most drugs are given in very high dosages to deliver the effect for the time needed, increasing risk of damage.
3. Activate the treatment once the specific target is reached or invaded. The nanocarriers will *know* exactly where to go and when to release the anti-tumor agent.
4. Deliver noxious agents to the target cells and release the entrapped drug depending on abnormal-tissue differences (like temperature of pH values inside their cells).
5. Assess effectiveness. The nanocarriers will have a traceable element to evaluate the accumulation and distribution of the drug within the target to evaluate the therapy's outcome through imaging.

• • • • • • • • • • • • •

If you think this is too good to be true . . . well, it is. We're still years away. But some progress has been made since the first nanocarriers were developed decades ago. They were initially formed as carriers for vaccines and chemo agents; many are still in the research phase, a testament to the challenges inherent to such a sophisticated modality.

In 1995, doxorubicin, with lipid droplets called nanoliposomes, became the first FDA-approved nano-drug. Unfortunately it was still quite toxic. Not till 2005 did the FDA approve another nanochemo, Abraxane (paclitaxel), used in treatment of breast cancer, usually given after other cancer meds have been tried—and also very toxic.[4]

In 2010 Dr. Murali Yallapu published a study in which he lamented that clinical trials are slow to come by and promoted the use of polymer micelle nanotechnology-based chemotherapies (for ovarian cancer) that can minimize the very toxic side effects caused by present treatments. He says the technology is already ripe, that both the structural aspects and the production methods are in place to proceed with human trials.[5] He's not alone in believing that nano-oncology has come of age and should be implemented. Dr. Ritu Dhankhar gives rational approaches for targeting breast cancer with nanotechnology's potential in managing it.[6] And Dr. Manjul Tiwari notes that across the surface of many cancer cells is a protein healthy cells typically do not express as strongly. By conjugating gold nanoparticles to an antibody, his team was able to get them to attach to the cancer cells. Such technology "[m]ay help us unravel the inner workings of a cancer cell and produce better treatments."[7]

How We Can Use Nanotechnology Now

While nanochemo is an exciting proposition, it'll be a while before these drugs come to the rescue in a nano-toxic presentation. Though researchers aren't slowing down, and many scientific papers have established theories and proved hypotheses, it's practical applications that patients and doctors in the trenches are eager and ready for.

Still, while nanodrugs are being developed and tested, I believe we can use this technology with another soon-available practical approach. I'm working to develop nanocarriers for nutrients, where safety is of no issue. Yes, we're designed to uptake nutrients from food by our digestive system for daily needs, but malignant tumors create a singular environment with singular requirements that normal metabolism does not supply. That's *why* drug delivery to these areas is difficult.

Study after study reports that we can derail the metabolic pathways of malignant cells via signaling transduction, with an array of nutrients, in lab and animal models, causing production-blockage of essential proteins for cancer's survival—efficiently and inexpensively combating it without pain. Why such meager results in patients so far? For the same reason chemo has failed: lack of effective delivery to the tumor's environs in the concentrations needed. Nutrient nanocarriers could be the answer.

To date, at Oasis of Hope we're combating cancer with nutrients in high doses, hoping these elements will reach the tumor. Nanotechnology could remove guesswork from the equation and provide the ideal nutrient delivery systems to target tumor sites and choke cancer. One example is the profoundly, profusely researched curcumin. Dozens of publications tout its anti-tumoral, radio-sensibilizing, chemo-sensibilizing activities against various aggressive and recurrent cancers (e.g., leukemias, lymphomas, multiple myeloma, melanoma, and brain, breast, skin, lung, prostate, ovarian, gastrointestinal, pancreatic, colorectal epithelial, and liver cancers). Curcumin has attracted much attention for its potent anti-proliferative, anti-invasive, and apoptotic effects on cancer cells through multiple molecular mechanisms.

The one problem: Poor systemic bioavailability and high metabolic instability. That is, curcumin is poorly absorbed by our digestive system, and once it's absorbed its phytochemicals degrade rapidly; hence what little reaches the tumor barely threatens it. We're researching the design of more stable curcumin formulations, packaging them in nanocarriers that will deliver it to targeted sites in effective quantity and quality. These will be practical and potent weapons in an oncologist's arsenal.

More and more researchers and clinicians are joining the effort to inspire people to change their diets to reduce cancer risk. We're thankful, but there's much more to be done. While supplementation has been a controversial subject for decades, the scientific evidence is overwhelming in favor of supplementing nutrients to those obtained by dietary efforts. Now some scientists are pushing the envelope and designing next-generation supplements through nanotechnology to improve delivery.

Dr. Imtiaz Siddiqui recently introduced *nanochemoprevention*, using naturally occurring phytochemicals capable of impeding carcinogenesis at one or more levels. He says nanotechnology can enhance the outcome of prevention through this potent supplementation delivery system;[8] the reason for limited success in human studies (compared to overwhelming lab success) is inefficient systemic delivery and bioavailability of these chemopreventive agents.

To prove the hypothesis, his research group developed nanoparticles of epigallocatechin-3-gallate (EGCG), a phytochemical found abundantly in green tea. The *Nano-EGCG carrier* was found to retain biological effectiveness with over tenfold dose advantage, exerting its pro-apoptotic, cell-growth-inhibitory, angiogenic-inhibitory effects compared to non-nano-encapsulated EGCG.[9] Since oral consumption is the most desirable and acceptable delivery form, such studies establish a foundation for using nanoparticle-mediated delivery of natural products to enhance the bioavailability of active agents—thus their great disease-preventing potential, especially against cancer.

Conclusion

Through years of research we've found better and better ways to improve delivery systems, and our encouraging results show it. For today and for the future, we are decisively pursuing nanotechnology to enhance the power of nutrition. It may take some time before this technology is readily available, but with this knowledge there are some things you can incorporate into your cancer battle plan today.

ACTION STEPS

1. Learn cooking methods that don't destroy foods' critical nutrients.
2. Research ways of enhancing nutrient absorption by your digestive system. For instance, piperine, a derivative of black pepper, increases the absorption of curcumin twentyfold!
3. Find specialists who integrate nutrients to treat cancer; you'll be amazed by the results.

CANCER VICTOR TIPS

K. L., Poland
Breast Cancer
Victor Since 1982

1. Don't panic. Be around positive people.
2. Get informed and consider your options.
3. Get good counsel.
4. Get information on alternative treatments.
5. Don't let doctors intimidate you.

Nanotechnology
https://vimeo.com/62447524

Chapter 38

The Mechanics of Hyperthermia

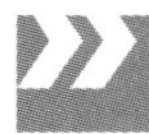

Q: *How do cancer cells respond to heat?*

A: Cancerous tissues are very susceptible. Heat can destroy cell membranes, effectively killing the cell. Heat also changes tumors' microenvironment, making them more vulnerable to agents like chemo, radiation, or even vitamin C.

Since time immemorial we've used heat to calm our ailments, from warm-water-soaked towels on superficial wounds to hot water bottles for tummyaches to microwave-heated wheat-packs for stiff muscles. One effective way to speed up healing of the flu is to cause profuse sweating. Heat also has been used to treat complicated conditions for millennia.

The Egyptian priest/physician Imhotep used natural human heat in fever form by infecting patients before surgically removing tumors in 2600 BC.[1] In *Hyperthermia in Cancer Treatment: A Primer*, Gian F. Baronzio tells of doctors in the Roman Empire using heat to treat breast masses and ancient Indian practitioners applying regional and whole-body hyperthermia.[2] To end all discussion about fever therapy's effectiveness, the Greek physician Parminides, in 500 BC, said, "Give me a chance to create a fever, and I will cure any disease."[3]

Fever Therapy

While intentionally infecting a patient to provoke hyperthermia or fever sounds counterintuitive, it long was integral to cancer therapy. Into the nineteenth century doctors applied dressings contaminated with erysipelas, gangrene, or syphilis to ulcerated tumors to deliberately infect. The first to introduce the scientific method to fever as a therapy was William Coley in the early 1890s. Reviewing records of patients with bone sarcomas, he saw that one who'd undergone three surgeries on an egg-sized cheek sarcoma was deemed terminal when it kept growing. After the third surgery he'd become severely infected with erysipelas, with concomitant high fever bouts. The record showed he survived the infection; and, incredibly, each bout of fever reduced the tumor size until the sarcoma disappeared. Coley thought it too good to be true, so he tracked down the patient, personally examined the large scar, and was astonished that, seven years after his discharge, he was in perfect health.

It was obvious to Coley that the fever was an immunological reaction to the infection and that this boost to the immune system was the reason for the sarcoma's regression. This prompted him to develop a concoction to provoke fever in others. They were considered terminal, so he infected his next ten sarcoma patients with erysipelas. In 1891 he published his first experience, noting that while in some patients the treatment worked and the cancer regressed, in most the infection itself was fatal. This type of study is what we would call now "proof of concept."[4]

To reduce the risk of fatal infections, Coley decided to administer killed erysipelas to promote fever without actually infecting the patient. He called this the "Mixed Bacterial Vaccine," but the remedy became known as "Coley's toxins" or "Coley's Vaccine" The first patient to receive it had an advanced sarcoma with abdominal and pelvic metastasis. He experienced a complete regression of the sarcoma and its metastasis and lived twenty-six more years before a fatal heart attack.

Coley was world renowned and was considered to have successfully treated more sarcoma patients than any other physician in his time. Some colleagues started using his vaccine to successfully treat other cancer types including carcinomas, lymphomas, and melanomas.[5] Other specialists and textbook authors recommended it also. For instance, the 1931 edition of *Modern Operative Surgery* recommends that "after amputation, prophylactic injections of Coley's fluid should be given in doses sufficient to cause a sharp febrile reaction."[6]

For over forty years Coley and others used these toxins to treat patients with a variety of cancers. His daughter, Helen Coley Nauts, subsequently compiled and published eleven different retrospective site-specific reviews of the progress notes concerning all these known cases. She and her colleagues documented 896 cases with inoperable soft-tissue sarcomas treated with Coley vaccine as of 1969; they found the five-year survival rate was significantly determined by the strength of the hyperthermia achieved. The rate for patients whose fevers averaged 38–40°C (100.4°–104°F) during treatment was 60%, but 20% with those who averaged temperatures of 38°C or less—that is, little or no fever at all.[7–8]

Progress on other fronts ultimately doomed this effective therapy. First, the rise of asepsis and sterile techniques as well as the evolution of antibiotics came strongly into play. Infecting patients purposely became passé and considered counter to the new school of surgery that wanted to ensure it didn't revert to the barber surgeons. Second, chemo and radiation therapy emerged as the cancer treatment mainstays. Third, the FDA began regulating more heavily and stringently after the thalidomide disaster that finally forced its removal from the market in 1962.

Researchers banked on pharmacological advances to standardize drugs for safety and efficacy (Coley's vaccine at the time would have been impossible to standardize), hoping chemo and radiation therapy would eventually result in high cure rates. Of course we're still waiting—fifty-plus years, billions of dollars, and millions of cancer deaths later. But some researchers continue looking at how to use the vaccine. In 2012 a study on pancreatic cancer cell lines concluded, "Coley's Toxin still holds promise for further preclinical analyses that could finally contribute to a successful treatment regimen in vivo."[9] *Not everything old is inferior!*

Backward-Stepping Advancements

Physicians largely cast aside modulating the immune system to combat cancer by relying on antibiotics to treat bacterial infection, and quite successfully. Yet Coley emphasized that fever was the key to his treatment; tumor regression was directly proportional to the vigor of the fever achieved. Today patient comfort is paramount; we do not allow fever's post-surgical symptoms (sign of a critical immune contribution to the healing process) and routinely administer antipyretics (anti-fever meds). To add insult to injury, after most surgical tumor removals we start chemo and radiation—potent immunosuppressors.

Some researchers believe the overuse of antibiotics, chemo, and radiation has caused the sharp fall in spontaneous cancer remissions often observed in the past as associated with acute infection. Drs. John Ruckdeschel and S. D. Codish reviewed the medical charts of patients who developed empyema, an infection with pus production, after lung cancer surgery and compared five-year survival against patients who had no infectious complications after the same procedure. Though 50% of the infected patients survived five years, only 18% of the uninfected patients did.[10] An unexpected effect of clean surgeries and effective antibiotic therapy *is* partial impairment of the immune system's ability to fight cancer. But establishment of more effective therapies was expected to overcome or surpass the results of such an antiquated approach.

In 1999 Dr. Mary Ann Richardson and colleagues decided to review and compare Coley's results against results with modern therapies. Given the massive medical and surgical advances, they expected that any group receiving state-of-the-art therapies to have better survival than those given obsolete treatment. The comparison data obtained from the NCI's SEER program showed the ten-year survival rates of patients given costly contemporary chemo/radiation therapies were not better than for those treated by Coley's toxins.[11] Development of the most advanced cancer therapies did not meet, much less exceed, the expectation of the billions of dollars invested to debunk the century-old vaccine.

Coley theorized that the fever facilitated a total healing experience wherein the immune system played a role, that also there was some sort of tissue detoxification, and that the heat actually liquefied the cancer cells. Yet he died without ever knowing the mechanism behind his vaccine. The tools were not really available at that time; now we know precisely the mechanisms that kill cancer cells through hyperthermia.

There's no question in my mind that fever is a lot more than a rise in body temperature. Febrile thermogenesis is an immunological reaction conducive to restore healing due to mechanisms like the triggering of a multitude of cytokine cascades (tumor necrosis factor [TNF], interleukins, interferons) and the enhancement of leucocyte proliferation, maturation, and activation. Hyperthermia alone has significant anti-tumor effects.

I've concentrated elsewhere on immune system mechanisms, so here I'll focus on pure heat's effects on cancer and normal tissues. First, let me succinctly detail our body's mechanisms for temperature control.

Regulating Temperature

Pulse, respiration, and body temp measures are our "vital signs" for, at their normal ranges, our cells and thus our organs function best. This is *homeostasis*: a dynamic state of stability between internal and external environments. The most tightly regulated of the three is core body temp, a function called thermoregulation. We have a remarkable ability to hold between 36.5°C and 37.5°C (97.7°F–99.5°F) regardless of external temperature. At the height of summer or in the coldest of winters, our body temp variations can be measured by a few tenths of a degree.

Our bodies regulate temperature similar to how a thermostat turns on and off our home's AC and heating units. The hypothalamus, our thermostat, responds to a multitude of temperature receptors (sensors) throughout the body (mainly skin). For instance, if you get into a Jacuzzi, those skin sensors will send signals to the hypothalamus, which will instruct the skin to sweat more to cool the body. Variations beyond tenths of degrees can cause severe complications. During surgery, anesthesiologists medically protect patients from hypothermia because anesthesia and surgery commonly cause core temp drops of 1°C to 3°C that, unmanaged, may result in impaired coagulation, prolonged drug action, and negative postoperative nitrogen balance; these medical procedures interfere with thermoregulation.

If the external temperature drops and the skin temp drops below 37°C, our body thermoregulates by the following mechanisms:

- Vasoconstriction (to decrease the flow of heat to the skin)
- Cessation of sweating (to diminish heat loss from evaporation)
- Shivering (to increase heat production in the muscles)
- Secreting norepinephrine, epinephrine, and thyroxine (to increase heat production).

Hyperthermia—significant elevation of body temp—also can cause havoc, causing proteins to break down and harming cell membranes, which are proteins, to the point of melting. Damaged membranes have an impaired capacity to control permeability; things that should stay out of the cell will come in, and things that should be in will come out. This can cause cell death leading to organ insufficiency and eventually death.

To prevent this, the hypothalamus instructs our body to lose temperature by the following mechanisms:

- Vasodilation (to increase circulation, which works as a cooler)
- Increased sweat production (to evaporate some of the heat)
- Reduced production of norepinephrine, epinephrine, and thyroxine (to reduce heat production).

Taking all of this into consideration, let's explore how heat can destroy cancer cells and leave normal cells undamaged. The Coley's-fever-therapy experiences verified that this is so, but what we want to know is the degree to which hyperthermia therapies are effective and practical.

How Heat Can Kill Cancer

What Coley proved is that cancer cells are more sensitive to heat than normal cells. We can exploit this fact to selectively kill malignant cells without, or at least with limited damage to, healthy cells and realize the true potential of hyperthermia as a therapy to destroy tumors.

However, the notion that healthy cells withstand heat better than malignant cells is incorrect. Again, heat denatures proteins; cellular membranes of benign and malignant cells have the same proteins. In fact, lab tests in vitro show that normal and cancer cells have the same membrane responses to hyperthermia. So why are cancerous cells more susceptible to heat? Because *their cooling system is deficient.*

The late Dr. Harry H. LeVeen measured the blood perfusion of tumors with an isotope technique and reported it as only 2% to 15% in comparison to the normal surrounding tissue. As to the reason, he said, "The heated tissue is cooled by the circulation of blood, which carries away the heat. Impaired perfusion, as in cancers, impedes cooling."[12]

In chapter 8 I shared that tumor vasculature—vast but aberrant, irregular (heterogeneous), and disorganized—promotes an unfavorable microenvironment inside cancerous tumors (e.g., low oxygen, low pH). This protects cancer from effects of oxidative therapies like radiation and many chemo agents because oxygen is needed for such agents to oxidize the malignant cells. Abundant scientific evidence shows that heating animal and human cells to 40°C or 42°C (104°F–107.6°F, moderate hyperthermia) changes malignant cells' microenvironment, making them vulnerable to direct apoptosis or conventional oxidative therapies.

So the main cooling system of malignant cells cannot dissipate the protein-denaturing effect of abnormally high temperature. The cooling thermoregulation mechanism of normal cells is intact. Some studies show that hyperthermia increases blood flow to heated areas, but while perfusion in tumors is doubled, in normal tissues it increases tenfold.[13] Hyperthermia, then, may directly kill cancerous cells or at least maim them to become more susceptible to other anti-tumor agents.

Heat's effect is directly related to *temperature* and to *time of exposure*. Even a few minutes of extreme heat can cause death; moderate hyperthermia for a prolonged time can also be lethal. There are many biochemical consequences to the cell's heat-shock response, so let's look at how this works. In the frame of therapeutic hyperthermia, heat can directly kill cancer cells. Several studies have shown in animals with malignant tumors and in human cancer patients that at temps around 42°C (107.6°F) for thirty minutes, cancer cells, compared to normal cells, die at an exponential rate. Also proven is that heat slows cell division by inhibiting DNA repair and by heat-induced cytotoxicity.[14] Again, blood flow and oxygenation are tremendously increased in cancer cells during and even days after hyperthermia exposure. Their oxygen concentration is further increased through consuming less oxygen than normal cells.

Dr. Chang W. Song measured the magnitude of increase in tumor oxygenation before and after temps to at least 42°C or 43°C. He reported,

> It is often impossible to uniformly raise the temperature of human tumors to this level using the hyperthermia devices currently available. However, it is relatively easy to raise the temperature of human tumors into the range of 39°C to 42°C, which is a temperature that can improve tumor oxygenation for up to 1–2 days."[15]

Mild hyperthermia plainly has great potential; hopefully more research will develop even better ways to deliver effective anti-tumor temps.

Heat not only increases oxygen content, which makes cancer cells more radiation-sensitive, it also enhances medication delivery by increasing cell membranes' pore size for entry of large-molecule chemo- and immunotherapeutic agents (molecular weight above 1,000 Daltons), such as monoclonal antibodies and liposome-encapsulated drugs.

Even when hyperthermia is induced mechanically, instead of via fever, there still is a significant natural immune response similar to the one experienced with a real fever. Hyperthermia activates natural killer (NK) cells, macrophages, and other components of the immune system.[16]

Therapeutic Hyperthermia Is Not Easy

If the case for hyperthermia to kill cancer cells is so strong, why isn't it widely used? How can it be that even in the alternative movement so few cancer centers are applying it? Some centers in Germany and Mexico offer hyperthermia, with some success, but thus far expectations haven't been met. Why the disappointing results?

We conducted a clinical trial with whole-body hyperthermia, with conflicting results. We found it to effectively diminish tumor activity, yet compliance to the whole protocol was scant due to patients' intolerance or physical impossibility to participate. In short, we discontinued our project because we found that the criteria of exclusion were too high—too many patients couldn't take part—and that the therapy is overly labor-intensive—the patients had to be anesthetized and monitored for hours, making the process quite expensive in comparison to other therapies that are as effective or even more effective. However, due to recent advances in hyperthermia devices, and sedation rather than anesthesia, we're now designing a new protocol to evaluate efficacy, practicality, and cost.

(Briefly: the aforementioned devices include infrared hyperthermia domes, or thermal chambers, where only the head is left out [the brain is ultra-sensitive to heat]. Also, there are [electric] blankets with inductive coils, and warm-water blankets with in-woven plastic tubing to heat the patient from the shoulders down. Hot tubs [warm-water immersion] likewise can achieve higher temperatures to the body and not the head.)

Properly controlled trials on artificially induced hyperthermia began in the 1970s. By the late 1980s and early 1990s, most outcomes were disappointing; researchers deemed the cytotoxic results unsatisfactory. Yet most also concluded that heat therapy improves the efficacy, as an adjuvant, of radiotherapy because, once more, hyperthermia strongly intensifies blood flow and oxygen concentration in malignant cells.

Still, despite so much evidence, very few radiation oncologists are actually combining the two therapies. Why?

First, most patients who seek alternatives have advanced disease (stage IV) with metastasis in several organs. The patients included in clinical trials have received multiple aggressive therapies without success and thus generally enter whole-body hyperthermia in poor health and with massive tumor activity.

Second, often it's impossible to uniformly raise the temp of human tumors to 40°C or 42°C, especially when they're scattered throughout different organs (the liver handles heat very differently from the bones). This is true even when the most contemporary devices are used and the technique is administered flawlessly. Every metastasis is unique; the disorganized vasculatures may be not so disorganized in some areas of the tumors, thus dissipating the heat similarly to benign tissue.

One challenge in all hyperthermia therapies is delivering sufficient heat to targeted tumors. The temp must be high enough and sustained long enough to damage or kill the cancer cells. The patient's temp must be monitored at all times to reduce risk of damaging healthy tissues and to avoid side effects. The goal is to maintain around 42°C (108°F), the upper limit compatible with life. The most common side effects, which, at most, last only hours, are nausea, vomiting, and diarrhea; however, if temps are too high or too prolonged, serious (though rare) side effects including coagulation problems or heart and other major organ failure can be initiated that cause death. Hyperthermia therapy should be undertaken only under very experienced health providers.

• • • • • • • • • • • • •

While the direct anti-tumor efficacy of whole-body hyperthermia is questionable, its debilitating effect on malignant cells is not. There is sufficient data to assert that it leaves malignant cells pregnant with oxygen and prey to other oxidizing agents like ionizing radiation, some chemotherapies, vitamin C, laetrile, or insulin potentiation therapy (IPT).

Internationally recognized radiation oncologist Carlos A. Perez, in *Principles and Practice of Radiation Oncology*, says that joining radiation and hyperthermia increases radiation's effectiveness significantly. The complete response (tumor fully gone) rate of radiation alone is 30%, but for patients receiving combo therapy the rate rose dramatically to 70%.[17]

In a prospective, randomized trial Dr. Jacoba Van Der Zee and colleagues treated 114 patients with locally advanced cervical cancer;[18] half with radiation alone, the other half with radiation and hyperthermia. In the former group, 57% achieved complete tumor eradication; in the latter group it was 83%. The researchers noted that radiation toxicity was not enhanced by hyperthermia, and survivability was statistically significant too. After three years of follow-up, 27% of the radiated patients were alive; 51% of the combined-treatment patients were alive.[19]

Most clinical trials have been with advanced cancer patients where standard therapies have failed, yet Dr. James Haim I. Bicher published the results of a study in early stage patients (forty with breast cancer, seventeen with head and neck tumors, fifteen with prostate cancer) who refused conventional treatments like surgery and radiotherapy. All were treated with thermoradiotherapy and followed for five years. Complete response rate was 82% for breast patients, 88% for head/neck tumors, and 93% for prostate patients. Projected five-year survival (cure) rates were 80%, 88%, and 87%, respectively;[20] the results were comparable to if not better than conventional therapy alone. Furthermore, because of the synergism between radiation and hyperthermia, the radiation dose was reduced considerably, and Bicher adds that side effects were less than with curative radiation therapy alone.[21] This offers another option for a much less aggressive approach to early detected breast, head, neck, and prostate cancers in particular and other tumors in general.

Conclusion

Hyperthermia is picking up steam, and, as we improve devices and techniques, more effective and affordable protocols *will* be available. Next chapter I'll discuss some of the more viable options for heat therapies.

ACTION STEPS

1. When you have a fever, don't stop it; manage it. It may kill some malignant cells, and it will boost your immune system.
2. Keep your eye open for treatment options that include some form of hyperthermia.
3. Hyperthermia is serious and delicate. If you do it, make sure your treating physician is experienced and has a good reputation.

CANCER VICTOR TIPS

Chuck Bender, California

Prostate Cancer
Victor Since 1999

1. Never give up or give in. Prayer is a big healing factor.
2. Learn as much as you can about your type of cancer.
3. Explore all types of treatment for your cancer.
4. Remember, "You are what you eat." Junk in produces junk out.
5. Before you make a final decision on treatment, visit Oasis of Hope.

The Mechanics of Hyperthermia
https://vimeo.com/62449244

Chapter 39

The Today and Tomorrow of Hyperthermia

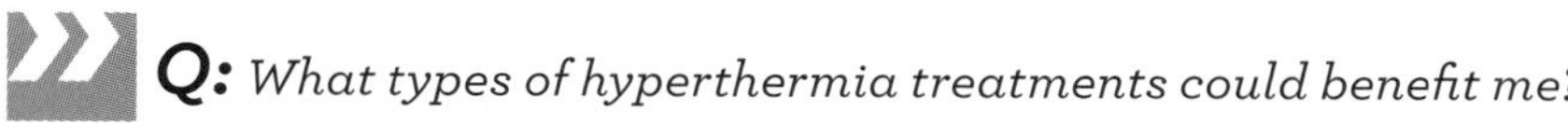

Q: *What types of hyperthermia treatments could benefit me?*

A: It could be whole-body, regional, or local, depending on tumor-type, location, and the spread of disease. In most cases, regional or local is most practical.

Regional Hyperthermia

While it's exceedingly hard to uniformly increase tumor temperature with whole-body hyperthermia, especially with metastases in various organs, it's relatively easy to raise the temp of single or regional tumors into the desired range. Again, most studies are in combination with radiation, chemo, or other anti-tumor agents because heating tumors increases their oxygen concentration, which can last twenty-four to forty-eight hours.[1] But this type of hyperthermia has its own merits as an anti-cancer therapy, and I believe more studies should be done. The following example is one of the few animal research studies I found.

Dr. David S. Muckle conducted an experiment on mice in 1974 to test the hypothesis of heat's selective inhibitory effect on cancer cells and its application to human neoplasms. The finding for regional and for whole-body treatment was that up to 42°C had a powerful anti-tumor effect, causing marked necrosis of tumor cells with 80% to 95% reduction in tumor volume. But Muckle noted that regional hyperthermia had a significant advantage: 50% of the animals receiving it survived, while only 30% survived of those given whole-body.[2] In a control group, the mice inoculated with tumors but untreated all died.

Regional or local hyperthermia aims to increase the temp of the tumor's area (or if possible the tumor itself) to kill it directly with heat or sensitize it to other anti-tumor agents without damaging surrounding tissue. Some devices for this use microwave, radio frequency, ultrasound energy, or magnetic hyperthermia; each has a different method to raise the temp of the area or tumor, from direct application to a surface tumor (superficial or deep-tissue hyperthermia) to the use of needles or probes (interstitial hyperthermia). To improve efficacy of chemo for peritoneal carcinomatosis, where the intestinal lining and the whole abdomen is cancer-riddled, the chemotherapy itself is heated and directly injected into the abdominal cavity during surgery or through a percutaneous catheter. This is called hyperthermic peritoneal perfusion (CHPP) or hyperthermic intraperitoneal chemotherapy (HIPEC).

Because only a region or a tumor is the target, higher temps (under 44°C) can be achieved, in comparison to the under 42°C limit in whole-body treatment. Again, rise of temp and time of exposure are vital, but in this modality there is practically no chance of severe side effects.

The most important hyperthermia program in the US is led by Duke University Medical Center jointly with North Carolina State University. The program of this multidisciplinary team of clinicians, engineers, and physicists includes the latest in monitoring techniques to ensure that tumors are correctly heated while normal tissue is protected. To achieve this they have a hybrid machine with the most advanced heat source and temp measurement device (a GE Healthcare 1.5 Tesla MRI system). It provides a tumor's 3D shape, size, and location and dynamic control over heat delivery. I hope that they soon will provide published results.

Radiofrequency Ablation

The most common hyperthermia utilized today, radiofrequency ablation (RFA), uses completely localized, very high temps. The innovator Harry H. LeVeen (see chapter 38) strongly endorsed this method; he did research with superheated ultrasound waves in animals, eradicating tumors altogether without damaging surrounding tissue. Then, upon studying twenty-one human patients with malignant tumors, he reported that RFA produced tissue necrosis or substantial cancer regression in them all.[3] His therapy had elevated temps by 5°C to 9.5°C above that of healthy tissue, and after these results he was sure RFA would be the fourth cancer therapy after surgery, radiation, and chemo. While it's now established, it's far from being utilized as he envisioned.

RFA's high-energy radio waves produce temps between 50°C (122°F) and 100°C (212°F), delivered through a needle-like probe into the tumor to reach ablation. Ablation is the surgical excision or amputation of a body part or tissue. In RFA, tumor excision is achieved by killing the cancer cells, coagulating its proteins, and destroying the blood vessels—a virtual cooking. The probe determines the hyperthermia's reach and limit; to date the largest area that can be ablated is a 5-cm-diameter sphere. The control is such that a couple *millimeters* outside this sphere of heat the normal tissue is absolutely unaffected. Exposure ranges between ten and thirty minutes, depending on tumor size. Ultrasound, MRI, or CT scans are used to guide and place the probe.

RFA's limitation is obvious: tumors larger than five centimeters (two inches) across won't be cooked completely. Theoretically, any tumor reachable by a probe could be treated, but the most commonly targeted are in the liver, kidneys, and lungs, as sufficient data proves efficacy there. (If there are many tumors, RFA is not indicated.) More areas are being researched. LeVeen published his results in 1976; though we still don't have long-term post-RFA outcomes, preliminary results are encouraging.

With RFA we can treat tumors that can't be surgically removed due to location or poor health. RFA isn't cheap, but it's affordable compared to new drugs; it also can be an outpatient procedure and can be used in conjunction with radiation, chemo, surgery, and alternative agents.

Help Is Within Reach

There are now nanoparticles that can create high-enough temps after electromagnetic activation. Efficacy of this modality, called magnetic thermal ablation, to destroy malignant tumors depends on maintaining constant therapeutic hyperthermia throughout the targeted tissue while keeping healthy tissues at a safe temp. There are several publications at the investigational level; this promising treatment may soon be available.

Camilo García-Jimeno of the University of Barcelona, in conjunction with scientists in Mexico City, is investigating the temperature increment produced by different concentrations of magnetic nanoparticles using tissue-mimicking materials (phantoms). They placed temp sensors inside and outside phantom tumors and assessed the effect of heat produced. They were able to prove they could achieve therapeutic temps in targeted areas while the temp where there were no nanoparticles was unaltered.[4]

Regarding the phantom studies, the better way to understand how things work is with a clinical trial on real subjects. Dr. Ingrid Hilger studied animals inoculated with human breast cancer to evaluate feasibility of magnetic thermal ablation, administering hyperthermic nanoparticles and then exposing the animals to alternating magnetic fields, like electricity, to activate the nanoparticles.[5] Monitored during the four-minute therapy were the temp of the tumors and temp of the animals' rectums; heat dosage obtained in the tumors ranged between 40°C and 262°C, while the rectal temp was unaffected. In all cases, the tumors showed signs of coagulation and necrosis. The conclusion was that the therapy safely and effectively generates cancer-killing heat.[6]

Whereas that study was with a single intratumor administration of hyperthermic nanoparticles, another infused the tumor continuously with the heat-generating particles. The antitumor effect was reported to be greater with continuous infusion (compared to single injections).[7]

• • • • • • • • • • • • •

Hyperthermic nanotechnology works, but because the particles may travel in the body, away from the tumor, with activating energy working throughout, normal tissues or organs could be ablated. Thus, there's much debate and caution about going to the next phase, clinical trials.

A group led by Dr. Heike Richter has made a magnetorelaxometry device to non-invasively localize and quantify magnetic nanoparticles for thermal ablation. The methodology to evaluate its efficacy is the same as for the previous two; the researchers concluded that it's effective to monitor pre-activation nanoparticle accumulation and to measure post-activation, electromagnetic energy-generated heat for cancer therapy.[8]

Conclusion

It's time to move forward with hyperthermic nanotechnology. Unfortunately, though some NCI clinical trials are underway, probably it will be years before any patient receives this therapy. In the meantime, RFA and other regional hyperthermic therapies are yielding success in many cases and are worth discussing with your physician.

ACTION STEPS

1. Ask your physician if you're a candidate for regional hyperthermia.
2. Talk to your oncologist about RFA as an alternative to surgery.
3. Consider seeking treatment at centers with hyperthermic options.

CANCER VICTOR TIPS

Marilyn Gaster, Nebraska
Endometrial Carcinoma
Victor Since 2011

1. Read your Bible daily and pray..
2. Memorize Scriptures that encourage.
3. Sing hymns and spiritual songs that uplift.
4. Share with others how God is encouraging you.
5. Pray for other cancer patients and encourage them.

The Today and Tomorrow of Hyperthermia
https://vimeo.com/62467795

Chapter 40

Stick Up for Yourself

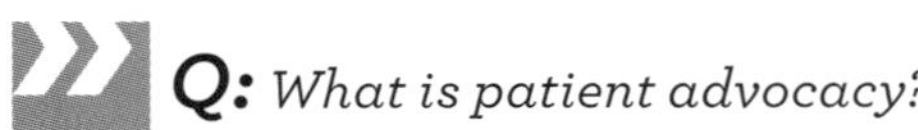

Q: *What is patient advocacy?*

A: Patient advocacy consists of skills to help you ensure you get the care you need. Do not let yourself be intimidated by doctors. Be informed, and let it be known you will make your own treatment decisions based on physician recommendations. This is both your right and your responsibility.

The Learning Channel has some ridiculous shows. ("Honey Boo Boo," anyone?) As a professional and an educator, I don't quickly acknowledge viewing anything on it. But I admit I've been drawn in a time or two. Once I watched "Extreme Couponing,"[1] on which people collect coupons to try purchasing more than $1,000 of groceries for less than $10.

It's amazing, the lengths to which people go to get free stuff. This episode featured a woman jumping into dumpsters to dig for coupons. Many "extreme couponers" preorder items, go to the checkout stand with ten-plus full carts, and stand for hours as the cashier rifles through countless vouchers. Onlookers shake their heads in disbelief.

Some criticize the thrifty for being compulsive, yet manufacturers are offering deals, and the average consumer makes no effort to benefit from what's available. Cashiers make no effort to let people know about the savings they're forgoing. It's up to the shopper to find the bargains.

Today, in untold areas of life, there are many resources available to help, but it's up to people to find them and insist on getting the benefit. This chapter is about patient advocacy; or, to make it more personal, self-advocacy.

Jesus Christ, who knew the power of this trait, told a parable to his disciples about always praying and never giving up:

> "There was a judge in a certain city," he said, "who neither feared God nor cared about people. A widow of that city came to him repeatedly, saying, 'Give me justice in this dispute with my enemy.' The judge ignored her for a while, but finally he said to himself, 'I don't fear God or care about people, but this woman is driving me crazy. I'm going to see that she gets justice, because she is wearing me out with her constant requests!'"[2]

Jesus brilliantly conveyed stories everyone can identify with, can learn a life lesson from, in just a few sentences. He was letting us know in this case that God wants us to learn and employ self-advocacy skills.

If you have cancer, can you rely on your doctors to look out for your best interests in every instance? Maybe, some of the time. I believe most people who go into medicine do so with an altruistic intention. Yet in oncology, after losing some patients, it's difficult to invest emotionally.

Many practitioners begin to go about their days in a routine fashion. But for you, nothing is routine. The doctor has many patients; all the cases are important. But for you, no other case is as important. I'm not suggesting you should lose faith in your doctor. I'm saying you can't sit back and think he or she will figure everything out for you. Become your own advocate and you'll be astounded by the opportunities you can open up for yourself. I strongly urge you to embrace the belief that no one will represent your best interests better than you.

Self-Advocacy Training

A study found that among even highly educated people, fewer than half can communicate their needs adequately.[3] Cancer advocacy training will help you find your voice in a way that will help you in every care aspect. Many free resources are online, like support groups facilitated by oncology social workers, audio training programs, and articles on advocacy. Search with keywords: *cancer self-advocacy, cancer advocacy training, online cancer support group*, etc. One resource, the "Cancer Survival Toolbox®," teaches communication skills, information seeking, decision making, problem solving, self-advocacy, and negotiating.[4] These skills can help you get the best care and access to new therapies.

At cancer.org, the American Cancer Society website, you can find *patient bills of rights* (there are more than one.)[5] They include:

1. Information for patients
2. Choice of providers and plans
3. Access to emergency services
4. Taking part in treatment decisions
5. Respect and non-discrimination
6. Confidentiality (privacy of health information)
7. Complaints and appeals
8. Consumer responsibilities.

I highly encourage you to read the explanation of each bill listed at this site. Enter "Patient Bill of Rights" in its search box.

Also, more and more patient organizations are forming to create awareness and influence the government, drug companies, physicians, and healthcare institutions.[6] You may strengthen your voice and the voice of others by seeking out a local patient rights group.

New Medications

The distance, measured in time, between new discoveries in cancer research and administration of the new drugs to patients can be years or even decades. What's most unfortunate is that sometimes the positive findings from clinical trials never trickle down from institutions to patients. Plenty of drugs are written off as not viable by oncologists who haven't even tried them. Continue asking your oncologist to look for info on new drugs that could help you. A few questions may grant you access to a whole set of options you never knew existed.

Access to Tests

A study with 414 elderly patients, which sought to ascertain why they weren't being given access to cancer screening tests,[7] concluded that many doctors used their own criterion, such as old age, to determine whether or not they would use a test with a patient. You may not be elderly, yet you have no idea why your doctor may or not utilize some tests with you unless you ask. Patients who show initiative and some assertiveness can overcome some oncologists' predispositions that might have limited access to tests and other helpful resources.

Drug Reimbursements

Insurance companies and Medicare have tables that indicate what drugs they'll reimburse an oncologist for each specific cancer type. Often the tables aren't up to date or simply don't include more expensive meds. If your doctor prescribes something the insurer doesn't approve, and he isn't reimbursed, you'll be responsible for payment, and he will bill you.

Few people know that insurance refusing to pay doesn't mean you can't submit the bill directly. Insurance companies have no problem refusing to reimburse a doctor. *You're* the client; *you* pay the premiums. Insist long enough, and you may get reimbursed because the insurer doesn't want the general public knowing they aren't taking care of their clients. Stick up for yourself, especially with your insurance company.

Conclusion

If a doctor recommends a very aggressive treatment that offers little help, you can refuse it. There are numerous reasons some people choose not to take a recommended treatment, such as low success rate, harsh side effects, patient seeking out alternative treatment, or patient wants more time with family.[8] Be your best advocate. Seek wise counsel. If you conclude that a treatment isn't in your best interest, explore alternatives and opinions. You have the right to say no to your doctor.

ACTION STEPS

1. Get involved in a cancer support group.
2. Do some training in self-advocacy.
3. Consider joining a cancer patients' rights group.

CANCER VICTOR TIPS

Batya Segal, Jerusalem, Israel
Breast Cancer
Victor Since 2005

1. *Eat healthy.* Eat food as close as possible to its natural form: fruits, vegetables, nuts, legumes. Eliminate these "whites" from your diet—white flour, white rice, white sugar, white dairy products.
2. *Work out.* Physical activity is inseparable from health. Exercise at least thirty minutes daily. Place it on your list of tasks. Sweat is good!
3. *Surround yourself with positive, happy people.* Make sure you spend time with people who are a good influence on you.
4. *Volunteer.* People who volunteer and give out from themselves are happy indeed. Since I started volunteering and giving from our own resources to the needy, I've found a deep joy and satisfaction.
5. *"Rejoice in the Lord always"* (Philippians 4:4 NIV). This is a command. And remember, joy will bring healing to your body: "The joy of the Lord is your strength" (Nehemiah 8:10 NIV). Reflect joy and happiness in all circumstances.
6. *Forgive and move on.* Be certain you're holding no resentment against anyone. A heart clean of condemnation and resentfulness is the best cure! Where possible, be at peace with everyone, even your enemies.
7. *Worship; read the Word.* Worshiping God is the highest expression of our faith. Reading His Word is medicine to our bodies.

Note: We invite you to view and support the wonderful ministries of Batya and her husband Barry at visionforisrael.com and josephstorehouse.co.uk.

Stick Up for Yourself
https://vimeo.com/62627463

Chapter 41

Exercise!

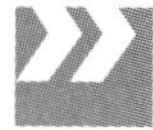

Q: *How beneficial is it for me to exercise—do I need to limit my physical exertion?*

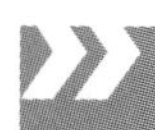

A: Many studies prove an exercising cancer patient will fare much better than non-exercisers. The one limitation: your physical status. If you can move, move!

The road is long to Major League Baseball's World Series. All told, from the time the best of the best report to spring training, players grind out around two hundred games, each team working day after day after day against twenty-nine others for more than eight months to get a shot at the championship. Only a few people have had the joy of playing in the Series; just a handful can say they pitched the game that clinched the title. Two others, ever, have done so in their first postseason start. Jon Lester did just this with the Boston Red Sox in 2007.

It was a fantastic triumph on its own. But considering that as a rookie in 2006 the twenty-two-year-old had been diagnosed with non-Hodgkin's lymphoma, it was awe-inspiring.[1] Lester missed the end of the season, underwent off-season chemotherapy, and fought his way back to the mound in mid-2007. After winning the Series, he threw a no-hitter for the Sox the following May. And he's been going strong since, averaging thirty-two starts, fifteen wins, and more than two hundred innings a year while posting a sub-3.50 ERA in five of six subsequent seasons.

Lester seems on his way to yet another fine year. Through 2013's first third, against six wins he'd taken only one loss, which didn't come until May 20. By the time you read this you may know whether Boston got back to the Series. Regardless, this man's biggest victory has been over cancer. I imagine he had magnificent physicians, effective treatment, and a tremendous fighting spirit, but for certain he had another factor working to his advantage as well, one lots of people overlook—*exercise.*

• • • • • • • • • • • • •

If you're forming a multi-disciplinary team (see chapter 33), maybe you've thought already about an oncologist, an integrative doctor, a nutritionist, a counselor, a pastor. What about a physical trainer, though, or a physical therapist? Let me share about exercise as a beneficial and necessary part of your cancer battle plan.

In chapter 2 I explained that controlling insulin and insulin growth factor-1 (IGF-1), two hormones that directly correlate to the incidence of some cancers, is a foundational anti-cancer facet. R. James Barnard demonstrated that prostate cancer growth was significantly stunted by reducing insulin and IGF-1 levels in the blood through a quasi-vegan diet coupled with a regimen known as the Pritikin program,[2–3] clearly showing the combined impact of diet supplemented by regular aerobic activity.

The influence of exercise in the context of cancer treatment likewise is robustly illustrated in studies of women with breast cancers, which are decidedly sensitive to insulin activity. Women with high levels have far poorer prognoses than those with low levels.[4–5] Other studies also reveal that daily aerobic exercise improves insulin sensitivity with effective risk reduction for breast and colorectal cancer mortality of 50% or more.[6–8]

Benefits, Benefits, Benefits

Further, aerobic exercise before and during cytotoxic treatment (e.g., chemo or radiation) favorably impacts immune-system functions. The most-complained-about side effect, cancer-related fatigue (CRF), affects more than 70% of patients physically and/or psychologically.[9] Regular exercise helps counteract this malady and so improves quality of life.[10–11]

What's more, if you're in treatment, or have been, you know first-hand the unpleasantness of nausea. Know this: among the findings of a 2012 study, patients participating in an exercise program reported a reduction in nausea—in most cases to zero![12] Moderate exercise during treatment also frequently results in reduction of nausea intensity.[13]

Oncologists must closely monitor skeletal complications, and herein I've found another exercise benefit for patients with bone metastasis. Resistance training can delay or even prevent such impediments and hence add years of life.[14] I do advise entering a supervised program with a trainer specializing in oncology fitness, to reduce fracture risk.

Cancer and its treatment can break a person down. Exercise can help you increase or recuperate your strength and fitness. Patients who exercise regularly increase their stamina, their ability to walk or run for longer durations, and also increase their flexibility.[15] Most people believe exercise is good, but many also incorrectly believe they can't exercise during treatment. When you overcome this barrier and get moving, you stand to get stronger and fitter; you may get into better shape than before you were diagnosed, for now you're focused on living longer and stronger.

Most people instinctively know that exercise effectively lowers anxiety and stress.[16] This holds true for people facing cancer. The American Psychological Association says 44% of us are stressed to the point of exhaustion;[17] add cancer to the mix and that percentage can double. As Judith Orloff states, enjoying life directly couples with feeling energetic.[18]

Types and Options: A Few Suggestions

I urge patients to do as much regular aerobic exercise as possible. This means supporting your own weight and for roughly thirty minutes moving nonstop on a brisk walk, for example, or on equipment like stair-climbers, elliptical gliders, and treadmills. Other enjoyable forms include neuromuscular electrical stimulation (transmission of an electrical charge to contract muscle groups) and whole-body vibration[19] through devices like the "Turbo Charger." These implements can greatly aid those with limitations on movement or respiration. Rebounding, another easy and inexpensive exercise, also stimulates the movement of the lymph, a key way to detoxify your body, especially during any type of chemotherapy.

Conclusion

Between 70% and 80% of oncologists agree that science supports the benefits of exercise for their patients,[20] and, on average, 75% of men and 80% of women facing cancer are interested in working with a fitness counselor during and after treatment.[21] The empirical evidence indicates that exercise is effective throughout treatment and afterward, helping to reduce CRF, anxiety, nausea, and stress. It also increases strength, stamina, flexibility, and quality of life. All these benefits are available and inexpensive as a powerful adjuvant to cancer therapy. You want to be well; I hope you will begin getting or continue keeping your life in motion.

ACTION STEPS

1. Choose a trainer and/or program to teach you how to integrate exercise into your treatment regimen.
2. Take a brisk thirty-minute walk at least four times per week.
3. Consider exercising during (not only after) your treatment course.

CANCER VICTOR TIPS

Laura Sandoval, México
Stage 3b Colon Cancer
Victor Since 2009

1. Change your diet to be mostly vegetarian and natural. But don't let this change increase your stress.
2. Do the things you love with the people you love. Be as active as you possibly can within the limits of your condition.
3. Don't allow negative thoughts; you need a positive attitude. Prayer and Bible reading are best medicine against fear, doubt, and sadness.
4. Nourish the right emotions: Love, laugh, share, hug . . . hug a lot. When you need one, don't be afraid to ask for it.
5. Most important: If you don't have a personal relationship with God, draw near to Him now; give Him your life and your circumstances. Jesus Christ, our eternal hope, is the answer to all our needs. If you have a relationship with God, make it your life's most important part.

Exercise!
https://vimeo.com/62470095

Chapter 42

Ethics in Oncology

Q: *How can oncology ethics affect my access to treatment?*

A: Most innovative therapies ethically are only allowed after "proven" therapies have been exhausted. This is fine when the "proven" are truly effective, but chemotherapy's efficacy may only provide a few more months of survival with very low quality of life. More patients with poor prognoses should be given access to innovative therapies at first intervention, not as a last resort.

Sarah Sackett-Hutcheson was just eleven when diagnosed with cancer. She was paying close attention at the top children's cancer center in Texas as her oncologists explained about the diagnosis, prognosis, and the recommended treatment course that would include chemo. But then, rather than go forward with the experts' prescriptions, she said she wished to pursue natural, non-toxic therapy in an uplifting environment with doctors who would pray with her. *She refused treatment.*

The physicians were stunned. This posed a major dilemma: Does a child, with parental support, have the right to make personal medical decisions that differ from what top-of-the-line doctors are convinced would be in her best interests? The oncologists contacted child protective services, who took the family to court. The state made their case—the case the state believed was Sarah's best hope. And she defended her right to seek the care she believed in.

The judge ruled for Sarah, stipulating that she submit regular lab and radiology reports; if her condition deteriorated, the court would remand her to the care of the Houston physicians to undergo chemo.

Sarah became my father's patient. She was healed completely. She and her husband have a son and are senior pastors at Wapiti Valley Church. (And she's the cancer victor featured in this chapter.)

• • • • • • • • • • • • •

Not all such dilemmas have storybook endings. Facing cancer, you want to be able to trust that the doctors have your best interest in mind and will respect your opinions, decisions, and privacy while providing the latest and greatest treatment to help you become a victor. Yet at the same time oncologists and health professionals are navigating an ethics minefield that may or may not impede their ability to care adequately for patients. I hope this chapter will make you aware of the issues facing you and your doctors and nurses, and empower you to circumnavigate the obstacles and stay on the path toward healing. Let it motivate you toward self-advocacy and help *you* determine what's in your best interest.

Oncology, one of medicine's most complex fields, entails thousands of treatment decisions for each patient. It's not diagnosing, looking up the right *Physicians Desk Reference*[1] prescription, and administering therapy—patients, family members, doctors, nurses, administrators, researchers, technicians, medical boards, insurers, Medicare, billing companies, drug manufacturers, and more all must make choices upon choices. Each decision made is passed through an ethics filter, be it conscious or unconscious, and with myriad variables the differences between right and wrong aren't always easy to delineate. Peter Thall even suggested that, in this context, "Any discussion of ethics . . . is purely a matter of opinion. The question of whether or not a particular behavior is ethical hinges on what the individual engaging in that behavior knows, which in turn must rest on that individual's beliefs."[2] Let's take a look at some issues that could significantly impact the care you receive.

Medical Economics

Many hospitals face great pressure to factor in the financial impact of the treatments they make available due to rising costs resulting from technological advances, drug company influence, spiking malpractice premiums, Medicare cutbacks, increasing insurers' power, and changing healthcare legislation.[3] Each patient must ask, "Is the treatment being offered the best existing option, or only the best option approved by the insurance company, hospital administration, Medicare, or Medicaid?"

The "Stark Law" makes it illegal for a physician to refer a patient to any healthcare provider in exchange for monetary gain.[4] It's unthinkable that a doctor would send you for a CT Scan just because thereby he'd receive a kickback. But it's not so difficult to imagine that a hospital would use incentives to try influencing a doctor to refer patients to that hospital. Guidelines are also in place for the pharmaceutical industry to self-regulate promotional efforts that could lead to influencing physicians prescribing habits, and many schools for doctors and for pharmacists regulate interaction between their residents and drug manufacturers.[5] These and other legislative and procedural mandates are intended to remove any economic motivation from doctors so that they can make referrals and treatment plans based on the patient's best interest.

Now, clinical studies conclude that chemo offers no improvement in treatment outcomes to patients diagnosed with malignant melanoma, and yet it's routinely administered. When doctors and nurses were asked, "Would you advise your relative with advanced melanoma to accept treatment?" almost 100% said yes.[6] Asked why, their common answers included to give hope, to ease the illness process, to increase the chance for a cure, to do more than nothing, and for purposes of research.

Regarding new therapies, again, there's a huge gap between cancer research and cancer treatment. Years can pass from when data is published to when a promising therapy becomes widely used, and each oncologist has his or her way of deciding on a treatment's value. Ethical issues we face when evaluating therapies include personal experience vs. clinical data, statistical significance, clinical relevance, objectivity of results involving a pharma-sponsored study, and whether insurance companies would reimburse for a therapy if it was prescribed.[7]

Doctors and researchers constantly look over data. They have the responsibility to determine when there's sufficient evidence to warrant a change in treatment approach for specific cancers as well as ongoing clinical trials.[8] An oncologist has to consider all the known data and choose whether to prescribe the generally accepted treatment, utilize a promising treatment without a long track record, or recommend that the patient have no treatment at all.[9] The pressure involved may slow down the process of adopting new treatments; it's critical that you learn as much as you can about research breakthroughs, for therapies that could potentially help you may not make it through your doctor's mental filter.

Communication and Allocation

Studies indicate that poor communication between doctors and patients leads to malpractice claims.[10] Health practitioners struggle to communicate because the success/failure realities of cancer treatment can be emotionally devastating. Caregivers often want to avoid taking away a patient's hope. Ask questions frequently, and work on developing a trust relationship with your health providers. Open up communication, and help your treatment team share vital information with you.

Administrators frequently make tough decisions based on keeping the hospital in business.[11] When finances are tight, hospitals may be understaffed. Medical procedures may be postponed or even cancelled. Expensive drugs may be substituted for more affordable drugs even though the oncologist wishes to give his patient a newer, more effective treatment. Resource-allocation choices are being made in every industry as a normal practice. You don't want your treatment options determined by administrators. Be sure to ask your oncologist what the absolute best treatment is for you. Then do your best to get your insurer to pay for it.

Conclusion

There's much going on around you as you seek to become a cancer victor. Even though you should be the one receiving all the care and support, it's in your best interest to be supportive of your oncologist and nurses. Ethically, they cannot express to you what they deal with. Just know they're managing many difficult issues. Express gratitude and respect for them. Be affirming and encouraging. A personal connection with your doctors and nurses can motivate them to fight harder for you.

ACTION STEPS

1. Do not blindly accept treatment. Ask frequently about what your oncologist is prescribing to ensure it's the best possible therapy.
2. Be supportive and affirming to your oncologist and nurses.
3. Ask your doctor to share the latest data on new treatments, how they may or may not benefit you, and why he or she would or would not recommend them to you.

CANCER VICTOR TIPS

Sarah Sackett-Hutcheson, Wyoming
Lymphoma, Non-Hodgkins, Large Cell, B-cell
Victor Since 1991

1. Faith is *everything* during the battle with cancer. Knowing that God is in complete control of the situation gives such comfort and peace.
2. Always make sure you get a second opinion on your diagnosis at a different location from where the first was given.
3. Find an oncologist you can trust completely!
4. Keep away from negativity; stay positive, and surround yourself with optimistic people.
5. Eat unprocessed, fresh foods, especially raw fruits and veggies.

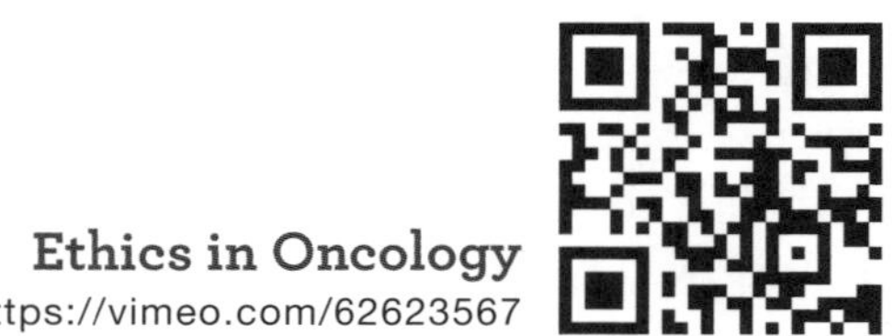

Chapter 43

The Healing Power of the Doctor-Patient Relationship

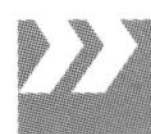

Q: *Does my doctor's attitude matter, or only her knowledge?*

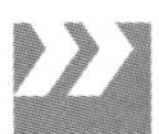

A: I believe one of the reasons we're presently losing the war on cancer is that oncologist negativity transmits hopelessness to patients. An encouraging, fighting, and willing attitude from your physician goes a long way.

Turn back the clock to the 1800s, to a small country town with a one-room schoolhouse and a church where everyone gathered, including the doctor. He was a beloved community member, more like a family member. He knew everyone; they all knew, loved, and trusted him. He almost didn't need a kitchen, for he'd make rounds to care for people in their homes, and they'd share their meals with him. He was familiar with every aspect of family life and would draw upon that knowledge as he diagnosed and treated. His greatest medicine was a combination of caring and compassion. He was not a medical scientist; he was a healer.

Somewhere along the way, the warm hometown doctor was replaced by the sterile institutional physician. The disconnect between doctors and patients makes one think of Kafka's *Country Doctor*,[1] about a practitioner unable to rise above the absurdity of his own existence to reach beyond paradox and paradigm to truly feel, and care, and help.

• • • • • • • • • • • • •

Technological advances are heralded as the patient's medical hope. It's intriguing to see how much a doctor can do through a smartphone. With "telemedicine," patients access doctors and specialists from around the world 24/7 through online "clinics." With some services, a monthly fee allows so many questions per month you can ask a doctor. Others offer a consultation by fee. But you may not get the same doctor, and you never get a physical exam. This further exacerbates the reality that doctors no longer listen to patients to gather vital info; they mostly pour over lab results and radiology and pathology reports. A quick glance at the paper, a quick script for medicine, and the patient is sent packing.

Facing cancer, this is not the type of experience you want. You need to form a healing partnership with your physician and treatment team.

In *House Calls*,[2] Dr. Patch Adams explains the import of observing a patient at home. The doctor has opportunity to see family dynamics, the normal diet and exercise routine, home-environment toxins, and other health-affecting details that would never be noted in the exam room.

Aside from resuming house calls, Adams urges doctors to spend three to four hours in the initial patient interview.[3] This allows for real bonding and formation of a friendship/partnership between doctor and patient. He believes so strongly in this relationship that he says malpractice insurance would no longer be needed. The doctor would do his absolute best to help his friend the patient. The patient would know his friend the doctor had done his best, even in the event of a mistake.

It's critical that a doctor knows his patient well.[4] In this way he can discover the patient's health beliefs and then build a treatment program the patient will readily embrace and adhere to.

Roles and Responsibilities

Dr. Bernie Siegel describes the doctor-patient relationship like a marriage,[5] wherein each has a role and responsibilities. The model of a patient passively allowing treatment is terribly inadequate; especially when facing a challenge like cancer. It takes the two working together.

The bond could also seem like a coach-player relationship, teacher-student relationship, counselor-client relationship, or trainer-olympian relationship.

The doctor has certain skills and knowledge to give; to reach the goal, the patient must be an active participant in the process.

Michele Pettit proposed a teaching model, based[6] on the movie *Patch Adams*,[7] where students would be educated about this relationship. She provides an excellent list of qualities, roles, and responsibilities to which each needs to commit. I've arranged them side by side here:

DOCTOR	PATIENT
Knowledgeable	Attentive
Understanding	Prepared
Empathetic	Responsible
Personable	Resourceful
Nonjudgmental	Assertive
Qualified	Accountable for actions
Affiliated with accredited academic institution	Skilled note taker: Record symptoms, meds, questions prior to doctor visit.
Committed to maintaining knowledge of current research by reviewing journals	Document strategies for medical self-care.
Listen to the people they serve	Seek clarity during appointments.

Good Medicine: Communication and Trust

Clear communication underscores all healthy relationships. Patients don't want their doctor to be ambiguous or confusing. Clarity and honesty are equally important. For example, if a doctor says, "We'll see what we can do about that," a statement that misuses the first-person plural, the patient may not know whether he is referring to himself, the patient, or both.[8] For the doctor to collect accurate data so that he can help the patient, it's vital that the patient is clear and honest.

It's also key that communication remains focused on the patient. Rapport must be built; the patient can perceive the doctor's insensitivity if she rambles on about personal issues. In the collaborative therapeutic relationship, a medical interview can be the means toward developing a highly personalized patient-centered treatment protocol. And this is precisely what the cancer patient needs.[9]

I'll never forget going in with a very sore throat. I waited in the exam room thirty minutes. I was so cold—why should those rooms feel like an icebox? Then the doctor stormed in and barked, "What are you here for?" I said, "My throat is sore. I think I have a throat infection." "You don't know anything," he scolded. "Let me take a look." He shoved a tongue depressor into my mouth, shined a light, grunted, and pulled out the wooden blade. He turned his back, started out, and, without turning to look, said, "The nurse will bring in your prescription and explain it." Then the door shut behind him. The whole interaction took less than three minutes; needless to say, I never went to see him again.

Did you know 40% of people don't trust their doctor?[10] Yet trust is the therapeutic agent that makes the doctor-patient relationship a healing power. This is more apparent in the realm of counseling. Carl Rogers used the trust relationship as *the* healing agent.[11] Unlike Freud, who'd psycho-analyze the trauma you experienced since birth;[12] unlike Frankl, who'd help you find meaning;[13] unlike Bowen, who'd look for the anxiety source that's stressing the family system,[14] Rogers was person-centered. He listened empathically, reflected nonjudgmentally, and parroted back what the client said so she would know she was being heard. By creating a safe, trust-based connection, the client would find her own answers to facilitate deep healing. Looking at cancer care through the lens of psychoendoneuroimmunology (see chapter 3), it's logical to conclude that a trust-based doctor-patient relationship could have positive socio-physiological influence on the patient's health.

Conclusion

Our center's founder, Dr. Ernesto Contreras, Sr., practiced the art of medicine. He modeled the power of loving his patient as himself and refused to prescribe any treatment he wouldn't take if facing the same illness. He'd make a friendship with his patient for life, which led to one of our slogans: we are "Your Healing Partner for Life." The dual meaning is intended: (1) For life—meaning now and forever; (2) For life—meaning we're focused on extending the duration and improving the quality of life.

When asked about the doctor-patient relationship, he stated, "A doctor always has something of benefit he can offer a patient. Even when there is no medicine that can help, he can always sit by his patient's beside and hold his hand to be a comfort. There is healing in that." Fifty years after he founded Oasis of Hope with those principles, we continue to promote the therapeutic value of the doctor-patient relationship.

ACTION STEPS

1. Find a doctor who gives personalized, patient-centered treatment.
2. Fulfill your patient roles and responsibilities as outlined in this chapter's table (above).
3. Let your physician know what you believe about cancer and the available treatment options.

CANCER VICTOR TIPS

S. K., Japan
Breast Cancer
Victor Since 2000

1. Reflect on your past to identify what led to being diagnosed. Then make the changes necessary to be free of cancer in the future.
2. Change your diet. For example, substitute whole grains for white rice.
3. Change your lifestyle to nurture peace and minimize stress.
4. Change the way you think to develop a healthy outlook.
5. Find out how to overcome the fear of cancer. Get informed, read books, talk to others. Choose a doctor who will work with you and not pressure you to do treatments you don't believe are in your best interest.

The Healing Power of the Doctor-Patient Relationship
https://vimeo.com/62385195

Chapter 44

Hormone Replacement Therapy

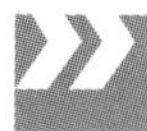 **Q:** *What are the risks of hormonal imbalance?*

 **A:** Estrogen dominance is a major contributing factor for the development of breast and other gynecological cancers. All efforts should be made to abolish estrogen dominance and balance your hormonal environment.

Hippocrates, "father of western medicine," defined disease as the imbalance of our four "humors" (bodily fluids): black bile, yellow bile, phlegm, and blood.[1] Greek, Roman, Islamic, and European physicians adopted humoral theory, which held sway up to the advent of modern medical research. The model isn't far from the truth–it just lacked the tools to more extensively reveal our complicated physiology. Had Hippocrates known, he could have called it *hormonal* theory; he described breast cancer as a black-bile-caused humoral disease and labeled cancer *karkinos* ("crab") for the tumors' crab-leg-like tentacles.[2]

Our health does in fact depend on the balance of the contents of all fluids within our bodies, and for maintaining and sustaining health no components are more important than hormones. We depend on them to enjoy life, but as the female hormonal system is vastly more intricate than the male's, I'll address hormonal balance from a female vantage. I'm uniquely qualified on this subject, for on top of scientific qualifications I have stronger related credentials: a blessed ninety-four-year-old mother, four incredible sisters (three still living), a beautiful wife, four wonderful daughters, and two delightful granddaughters. Everything I discuss in this chapter I've "experienced" in every way, shape, and form!

• • • • • • • • • • • • •

Hormones—chemical messengers (proteins) produced by organs called glands (ovaries, pancreas, liver, etc.)—travel in the bloodstream to reach and instruct organs and tissues to do specific tasks. They are powerful; only minute hormone amounts are needed for the job, and tiny up or down changes in production can cause havoc, or hormonal imbalance, in our organisms. One example is diabetes: the pancreas produces less insulin than needed, sugar levels are elevated, and vital organs are damaged. Many diseases, like hypo- and hyperthyroidism, are caused solely by hormonal imbalance, and in such conditions if the broken balance is reestablished, the disease is cured or controlled.

What makes the female hormonal system intricate and sophisticated is that women are naturally, by design, unbalanced. That didn't come out right . . . what I mean is that not all imbalances are pathological. For instance, during pregnancy, the hormonal environment is completely out of whack, yet the imbalance, necessary and healthy for both mother and child, promotes the changes that will enable a girl to become a woman, establishing then a new hormonal (im)balance.

"Hormonal balance" in women is an ultra-fluid competition—the menstrual cycle—that sees many lead changes. During the follicular and luteal phases, estrogen or progesterone dominates, respectively. In an *actual* imbalance, either dominates longer than designed. Consequences will depend on the intensity and duration of this dominance, from mild physical or emotional disruptions to serious medical conditions.

Estrogen Dominance

We all produce estrogen; women produce it in significantly higher amounts. Estrogen dominance is the culprit of many ills, the scariest being breast cancer. How can an ovaries-yielded hormone be a cancer-causing agent? In normal conditions, women are protected from malignant action by this wondrous hormone. Yet strong epidemiological evidence associates it with breast, endometrial, and uterine cancers. For that reason, the 2012 *Report on Carcinogens* from the National Toxicology Program lists estrogen as "a 'known' human carcinogen."[3]

While this may seem disconcerting, there's a simple explanation. God fashioned a safe window of estrogen exposure during the female lifespan, opening at menarche and closing at menopause (first and last menstruations) with some periods of rest during childbearing time. Before the industrial revolution, this by-design window started at around age fifteen or sixteen and ended between forty-five and fifty, usually with a number of pregnancies along the way. Now, though, the exposure span has been unnaturally hyper-stretched from side to side *and* from top to bottom. Why? First, girls start menstrual cycles six to seven years earlier; second, for many women menopause never arrives; third, most women have one or two children and many have none; fourth, certain facets of progress have come at a stratospherically high price for women.

Girls today start menstruating much earlier because of high consumption of estrogen-rich products. Our environment literally is flooded with estrogen and estrogen-like substances. The animals we feed on have been over-fattened by pharmacological estrogen. Estrogen-aided milk cows produce humongous quantities compared to those that aren't so treated. Most of our fruits and vegetables are sprayed with pesticides, chemicals almost identical structurally to estrogen so that our bodies don't acknowledge the difference. Xenoestrogens (*xeno*, Greek "foreign") are endocrine-disrupting chemical compounds—pesticides, plastics—that imitate estrogen and leach into the contents of plastic bottles and plastic wrappings. Combined with all the estrogen in meats and dairy products, this promotes the over-dominance of estrogen, which is unaffected by any processing or cooking of the food. All this estrogen is a major reason two-thirds of the US population is overweight or obese. Furthermore, it's well known that fatty tissue directly produces estrogen.[4]

Also, by having very few (or no) children, women have no rest from their normal estrogen production. The more uninterrupted menstrual cycles, the higher the incidence of breast and other female cancers; the first term for breast cancer in the fourteenth century was "nun's disease" because of its high incidence in nuns.[5] A National Cancer Institute study that analyzed the cancer mortality of 31,658 white Catholic nuns from forty-one religious orders showed they displayed a striking excess in breast cancer mortality and had consistently higher rates than women with children.[6] The increased risks of breast, uterine, and ovarian cancer in nuns were associated with infertility.

Consider this: *to avoid pregnancies, women take estrogen*, the active ingredient of oral contraceptives. The "pill," age fifty-three in 2013, has long been touted as the invention that liberated and projected women into a new age. Despite red flags elevated by epidemiological evidence of risk, the only change was in lowering the estrogen dose in contraceptives, a small and inadequate step. Lynn Rosenberg, analyzing 53,848 Black Women's Health Study participants, found that those taking birth control pills increased the incidence of hyper-aggressive triple-negative breast cancer by 65%; those who'd used the contraceptive within the past five years and had taken it for longer than ten had risk doubled to 130%.[7]

Dr. Rosenberg wanted to study black women because (1) their incidence of that cancer is higher and (2) they've been underrepresented in cancer research. But women of other races and ethnicities are affected also. An NIH-sanctioned, federally sponsored study showed a solid link to aggressive breast cancer, and while some researchers have warned of this risk for at least a decade, this data has been swept under the rug. Jessica Dolle, reporting a strong tie between use of oral contraceptives and triple-negative breast cancer,[8] found the connection highest among women who began using them as teenagers. Those who start taking the pill before age eighteen had an aggressive breast cancer risk almost 370% higher, and if they continue taking it more than a year, up to five years, it jumped to 420%.[9] And the study showed a 40% risk increase for those who've had abortions, a stoutly contested and widely denied factor.

Asleep at the Wheel

Though several published studies in multiple countries corroborate these results, many researchers aren't impressed with increased risk of between 100% and 400%. Smoking increases lung cancer risk by 2000%, and yet for years medical authorities refrained from speaking against cigarettes! The same is happening with the pill. For many women around the world, benefits are perceived to outweigh risks—but that doesn't excuse underplaying the risks. The American Cancer Society, the NCI, and other influential institutions make no effort to warn women to reduce breast-cancer rates with estrogen-free contraceptive methods. By underreporting or distorting, the media aids and abets the medical establishment as a "liberation" agenda supersedes women's health. Through societal indolence, lack of data dissemination, and poor or incorrect education, many women will be diagnosed with cancers that keep them from lasting as long as the half-century-plus that the pill has thrived. Again and again and again, girls and women are prescribed temporary hormonal manipulation that increases their estrogen dominance and can disrupt, decrease, or destroy their quality of life.

Among the consequences of hormonal imbalance in menstruating women are premenstrual syndrome (PMS), with symptoms including painful and prolonged or irregular cycles with heavy bleeding, weight gain or abdominal bloating, breast tenderness or swelling, heart palpitations, headaches, joint and/or muscle pain, swollen limbs, and mood swings during certain times of every month (from crying for no reason to intense sadness or panic attacks). Other serious side effects of prolonged estrogen dominance are fibrocystic breast disease, ovarian cysts, endometriosis, and infertility. *All* of the above have an estrogen-dominance compounding effect.

The estrogen window is further stretched when menopause is never allowed; the medical industry converted it into a disorder that must be corrected with *hormone replacement therapy* (HRT), mostly with estrogen. By design, as women mature their ripened ovaries reduce hormone amounts to where a pregnancy is impossible. But in the adjustment from a high hormonal balance to a low hormonal balance their bodies go through fire—literally. Before the age of medical interventionism, animal hormone exploitation, and chemically enhanced living, the "change of life," as it was called, was endured cold turkey and lasted a few months. Then women really were liberated from the vicissitudes of menstrual cycles and the concerns and worries of controlling the size of their family.

This has all been thrown out the (estrogen) window, because mature women initiate this change already unbalanced with tremendous estrogen dominance from the factors mentioned above. This unbalanced hormonal environment has augmented menopausal symptoms to the nth degree. Countless women suffer plaguing symptoms like hot flashes, night sweats, broken sleep patterns or insomnia, and diminished sexual drive. For some, unexplainable mood swings, lack of concentration, memory loss, fatigue, and anxiety are near to unbearable. Others endure skin problems, acne, and dryness of mouth, eyes, and genitalia; many experience loss of appetite and gain unwanted weight at the same time.

With millions of the distressed eager for any deliverance from this perdition, the medical industry, loath to pass up a lucrative opportunity, belted a grand slam. This is the logic of HRT: menopause symptoms are caused by estrogen depravation; women are estrogen junkies; restore hormone levels to premenopausal status and, voilà, problem solved, no more symptoms. This goes against the hormonal-window-of-exposure design; we shouldn't be surprised that the price tag for estrogen-based control includes increases in various cancers and other diseases.

The elevated risk had been known for decades, yet doctors assumed the high heart attack rate in menopausal women was due to estrogen deficiency, and because heart attacks kill many more women than breast cancer, HRT was ethical; benefits outweighed risks. Or did they? Many researchers criticized this assumption, unbacked by scientific data but merely "logical." In 1991 the NIH finally launched the Women's Health Initiative, a set of clinical trials and an observational study of 161,808 generally healthy postmenopausal women. The objective of one study, with more than 16,600 women between fifty and seventy-nine taking HRT, was to evaluate its health benefits and risks through a randomized controlled primary prevention trial, with planned duration of 8.5 years.[10]

Five years in, well before the planned finish, the researchers put a sudden end to it because risks far exceeded benefits in the group taking HRT. First, HRT's main indication was to prevent heart attacks, yet the study's main outcome was that HRT markedly *increased* the incidence of nonfatal and fatal attacks. Second, the HRT group had a much higher incidence of breast cancer, and HRT promotes denser breast tissue, reducing mammography's effectiveness and so hampering chances of early diagnosis. Other side effects found were substantially increased incidence of stroke, pulmonary embolism, endometrial and colorectal cancer, hip fracture, and death by other causes. The conclusion: HRT "should not be initiated or continued for primary prevention of CHD" (coronary heart disease).[11]

Another HRT study that had to be stopped was HABITS ("Hormone Replacement After Breast Cancer—Is It Safe?"), a clinical trial to evaluate HRT given to relieve breast cancer survivors of menopausal symptoms because oncologists weren't convinced it harmed them! Researchers determined without a doubt that survivors taking HRT were more likely to develop new or recurrent breast cancer than those who didn't take it.[12] Hopefully this finally will convince oncologists to stop the practice.

• • • • • • • • • • • • •

Half the American women over fifty taking HRT in the early 2000s stopped after the Women's Health Initiative results were made public. In general, while younger women have disregarded the risks to enjoy the benefits of the pill, older women have made maturity count by finding alternatives that have rapidly paid off. Breast cancer incidence had been constantly increasing for twenty years. Suddenly, just a year after HRT's risks were announced and women began dropping it, breast cancer rates likewise dropped dramatically. Fourteen thousand fewer US women were diagnosed in 2003 than in 2002.[13] A 7.2% decline hadn't been seen since statistical data has been recorded; Dr. Peter Ravdin called it "the largest single drop in breast cancer incidence within a single year I am aware of."[14] The study's authors believe the decrease in use of hormone replacement therapy caused the sharp breast-cancer-diagnosis decline.

Let me go back and quote verbatim the pronouncement of estrogen as a cancer-causing agent: "The federal government today published its biennial *Report on Carcinogens*, adding steroidal estrogens used in estrogen replacement therapy and oral contraceptives to its official list of 'known' human carcinogens."[15] While estrogen can cause cancer, they're not blaming the estrogen ovaries produce but the one doctors prescribe.

Conclusion

What's the safe alternative? If not HRT, what can women tormented by menopause do to improve their quality of life? Again, *menopausal symptoms aren't intensified or prolonged for lack of estrogen.* By design, women *need* to drastically reduce their hormone production, and their ovaries comply, but once this happens, there's still excess estrogen in comparison to progesterone. *This* imbalance causes mayhem.

Bringing estrogen back to premenopausal levels, as HRT does, is very dangerous. We can't reduce extracurricular estrogen, but I've helped thousands of menopausal women regain hormonal control by increasing their progesterone level to neutralize estrogen dominance. You'll increase your likelihood of reigning over your hormones if you adopt a healthy diet, exercise, and use natural progesterone supplements or creams.

ACTION STEPS

1. Guard against external estrogen contamination—eat organically produced food (no hormone-fattened animals, no xenoestrogens).
2. If you're young and need birth control, choose non-hormonal methods, and look for the new estrogen-free contraceptives.
3. If you're still taking HRT, seek a practitioner's help with bio-identical hormones to combat menopause symptoms as you transition.

CANCER VICTOR TIPS

Lorraine A. Weaver, Minnesota
Esophageal Cancer
Victor Since 2004

1. Ask God for guidance.
2. Change your dietary habits (less meat).
3. Find out what treatments are available.
4. Call Oasis of Hope immediately for options.
5. Don't fall for doctors telling you to have chemo and radiation.

Hormone Replacement Therapy
https://vimeo.com/62647620

Chapter 45

Stem Cell Therapy

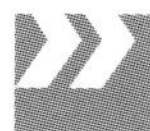

Q: *Is stem cell therapy available for cancer?*

A: Not yet. Cancer stem cells must be destroyed, or recurrence is nearly certain. While chemo and radiation don't kill them, there are natural therapies that do.

The 1850 innovation of the inverted microscope gave scientists the basis for understanding human development. For the first time they saw the building blocks of living organisms in action, witnessed cells giving rise to other cells, propagating and differentiating. A century later, European researchers saw that all blood cells (white, red, and platelets) came from a particular cell they called "mother" or "stem," which opened the door for bone marrow transplants after radiation and chemo. Then, in 1963, Ernest Armstrong McCulloch described the differentiating characteristic between normal and stem cells, with their self-renewing capability.

Embryonic Stem Cells vs. Adult Stem Cells

Biotechnological advances in the last few decades have been breathtaking. Scientists now grow human cells and even alter their genetic material. In 1998 the world's first human embryonic stem cell line (which still exists) was established by James Thomson, who removed cells from spare embryos at fertility clinics and grew them in the lab. This feat became the epicenter of the "stem cell ethics vs. progress" controversy that still worries scientists, lawmakers, theologians, and patients, for "spare embryos" are human beings in an artificially suspended state of development.

The "progress" argument is that these stem cells have potential to generate replacement cells for a broad array of tissues and organs (e.g., heart, liver, pancreas, lung, and nervous system). So, these artificially suspended humans could and, as many say, should be sacrificed for the benefit of those suffering. Yet despite tremendous progress in research (annually, over two thousand papers on embryonic and adult stem cells are published in reputable scientific journals), *embryonic* stem cell research has yet to produce any practical application for any disease. Exploiting their potential to develop replacement tissues or organs is, at best, likely to still take a long time. Conversely, uncontroversial *adult* stem cells are already being used in treatments for more than a hundred conditions, including Parkinson's and heart disease. And for more than sixty years these cells have been helping cancer patients rebuild chemo-decimated bone marrow.

Ilyas Singec said stem cell research has been validated sufficiently in animal models and that progress in cell culture conditions, long-term propagation, directed differentiation, and transplantation of both human embryonic and adult (or "somatic") stem cells have set the stage to "move this technology closer to clinical application."[1] Even so, after decades of research and a multitude of scientists enthusiastically investigating, this complex biotechnology still has not matured enough to come to the rescue of so many patients in need. Again, *adult* stem cell transplant (see below) has advanced into clinical application for a number of chronic degenerative diseases with encouraging results. As a Christian physician who defends life's sanctity for both the born and the yet to be born, I concentrate all my efforts on autologous adult stem cells.

What *Are* Stem Cells?

Stem cells are different than cells of a specific tissue or organ; every organ and type of tissue in the body contains a small number of "adult" or "tissue" stem cells. Stem cells ensure a continuous supply of new cells to replace the ones that wear out or are destroyed. These are the characteristics of stem cells that set them apart from normal cells:

1. *Plasticity.* They have the ability to differentiate to cell types different from the tissue of origin.
2. *Self-renewal.* They divide to make exact copies of themselves without differentiating.
3. *Multipotent or Pluripotent Differentiation.* They can convert into progenitor or specialized cells to form or maintain different organs and tissues.

4. *Duplication.* Their duplication is singular; when they divide they make one exact self-copy and one progenitor cell, maintaining a fusion of stem and differentiated cells. Progenitor cells divide and multiply into mature organ cells.
5. *"Immortality."* Progenitor cells divide to make self-copies, forming a cell line or "family line," but can only divide a certain number of times before the entire family dies. A stem cell line can keep dividing indefinitely; it doesn't die out.

It is stem cells' plasticity and multi- and pluripotency to become whatever type of cell needed that makes them attractive for intervention strategies. The aim: to implement regenerative stem-cell-based medicine for individuals with Parkinson's, Alzheimer's, diabetes mellitus, spinal cord injuries, osteoarthritis, heart disease, etc. Geoffrey Gurtner believes the goal of this medicine will be achieved through a multidisciplinary effort by experts in the fields of stem cell biology, genetics, materials science, bioengineering, and tissue engineering. He and his collaborators maintain that there's a foundation for developing new clinical therapies to augment and stimulate human regeneration applications that range from fetal wound healing to limb regeneration—the treatment of many if not all chronic degenerative diseases.[2]

Stem cell breakthroughs have not improved cancer treatment. The only oncological application today is the same as in the 1950s—restoring bone marrow severely damaged by high-dose chemo or radiation therapies. But I don't want to downplay the importance of this. Many of my patients have needed adult autologous stem cell transplant therapy to replace bone marrow, and it has boosted their immune systems.

There are three types of stem cell transplants:

Autologous. You are your own donor. When your oncologist knows the chemo protocol is so harsh that bone marrow destruction is quite certain, your marrow or peripheral blood stem cells are harvested, frozen, then, if/when needed, transplanted back to you.

Allogeneic. The cells are harvested from a compatible donor's marrow, with very high risk of rejection immediately or at a later time.

Syngeneic. The cells are harvested from an identical twin, and the chance of the transplant being rejected is significantly reduced.

Cancer Stem Cells

Now, some stem-cell discoveries are *promising* for cancer patients. Again, we know there are cancer stem cells, and some researchers believe the key to a cancer cure relates to inhibiting their proliferation.

Let me explain further. The fertilized egg (zygote), a single cell, is the mother of all multipotent stem cells, which have power to differentiate from all tissues and organs until a baby is fully developed. All tissues and organs have a small population of pluripotent ("adult" or "tissue") stem cells that will be available until old age; these "immortal" cells are needed to sustain replacement through the normal cell death process.

As to cancerous tissues having their own stem cell population, for years the research community was skeptical that they counted on these cells for survival, but in 1997, after a three-year search, Canadian geneticists first established conclusive evidence.[3] Dr. Dominique Bonnet isolated a subpopulation of leukemic cells that express a specific surface marker normal malignant cells lack. Normal cells are indistinguishable from stem cells under the microscope; Bonnet and colleagues developed the method to detect specific proteins on the stem cell's surface that are not present on regular cancer cells.

Another practical and less sophisticated test consists of inoculating human cancer cells into mice that are genetically engineered to lack a cancer-fighting immune system. If the mouse does not develop a tumor, the injected cells had a zero cancer stem cell population, for ordinary tumor cells will divide a few times and then die. A tumor will only develop in the presence of cancer stem cells that perpetuate the growth cycle.

Since Bonnet's study, other cancer stem cells have been discovered, and the methodology to find and isolate them has also improved. The first solid tumor stem cell was discovered in 2003 by Muhammad Al-Hajj, using malignant cells from a group of breast cancer patients.[4] Only a few of the cells had ability to form new tumors, so they identified and isolated the non-tumor-generating from the tumor-generating ones, tagged as cancer stem cells according to specific cell surface markers. Once completely separated and identified, the cells were inoculated into two groups of immune-compromised mice; even tens of thousands of normal cancer cells failed to form tumors, while as few as a hundred cancer stem cells were able to form tumors. Only 1% to 3% of the entire malignant cell population was identified as cancer stem cells.

Without doubt, malignant tumors harbor a small population of stem cells capable of self-renewal and differentiation into multiple malignant cell types; these are the main drivers of metastatic proliferation and relapse. Michael Clarke (who directed Al-Hajj's study) and his collaborators have since discovered and isolated cancer stem cells in pancreatic cancer (2007), head and neck cancer (2007) and glioblastoma (aggressive brain cancer, 2009). And they plan to find a lot more.

• • • • • • • • • • • • •

Think about this: if tumors can't sustain growth without cancer stem cells—in fact, tumors cannot survive without them—then we should develop target-specific therapies to destroy them. This is the new hope for improving survival and quality of life for cancer patients, especially those with advanced disease. For years some researchers have proposed that the reason for chemo's failure, for its inordinate recurrence rate, is that even though it effectively kills the bulk of a tumor's malignant cells to the point of remission, chemo/radiation-resistant cancer stem cells go untouched, ready for a new beginning.

What's more, it would be less toxic, and theoretically more effective, to target treatments directly at the small population of cancer stem cells instead of trying to kill all the billions of cells in a tumor. Eliminating the stem cells would ultimately kill the cancer and halt metastasis. Therefore a number of US and European pharmaceutical labs have developed drugs to selectively target cancer stem cells and are in early clinical phase trials. Results are somewhat encouraging but also are mixed, still far from being FDA-approved, and likely to be very expensive.

While we wait for wonder drugs, there's an alternative for directly and selectively attacking cancer stem cells. Incredibly, this option comes from observational studies of diabetes, a chronic disease correlated with increased risk of breast and other cancers. Metformin, extensively used for treating diabetes, obesity, and polycystic ovarian syndrome, also has been shown to inhibit growth of breast cancer cell lines and tumor growth of aggressive cancers. Dr. Heather Hirsch and colleagues said "the combination of metformin with existing chemotherapeutic drugs, which attack non-stem cancer cells, was shown to have a dramatic effect on reducing tumor mass and prolonging tumor remission."[5]

Since diabetic patients with ovarian cancer taking metformin have better outcomes than those not taking it, the Al-Hajj group designed a study to evaluate metformin's impact in ovarian cancer stem cells. Dr. Jessica Shank reported that metformin significantly restricted the growth of those cell lines in vitro and inhibited formation of cancer stem cells from patient tumors.[6] They also combined metformin with chemotherapy and found it to restrict tumor growth due to a decrease in cancer stem cell population, malignant bulk cell proliferation, and angiogenesis.

Conclusion

Because of the demonstrations that metformin can greatly improve patient outcomes with direct and selective killing effects on cancer stem cells, patients at Oasis of Hope have been receiving it since 2007 as a part of our comprehensive and integrative anti-cancer approach.

ACTION STEPS

1. Talk with your oncologist about integrating metformin into your program.
2. If he or she is not informed, ask him/her to read the literature.
3. Ensure that he or she helps you design the most comprehensive anti-cancer therapy you can have.

CANCER VICTOR TIPS

Betty Donald-Couty, Florida
Stage IV Uterine Cancer
Victor Since 1976

1. Have the right (positive) attitude.
2. Get support from family and friends.
3. Eat the foods the hospital tells you to eat.
4. Take your food supplements every day.
5. Don't listen to people who question going to Oasis of Hope.

Stem Cell Therapy
https://vimeo.com/62653215

Chapter 46

EMFT

Q: *Is Electromagnetic Field cancer therapy available today?*

A: My clinical team has tested several EMF devices that claim to kill cancer cells, but none has proved effective. I do believe we will see certain EMF technologies useful for combating cancer; one already being utilized with solid objective results is Radio Frequency Ablation, or RFA (see chapter 39).

I'm a strong believer in the potential of electromagnetic fields to treat and possibly cure cancer. Since the 1920s scientists have theorized that normal and malignant cells have electrical, magnetic, and even frequency differences that can be exploited. Dr. Royal Rife believed a cancer virus existed that could be cured with a frequency of electromagnetic energy to cause the cancer cells to self-destruct. He created the Beam Ray machine to generate this frequency, using it on mice and later on humans.[1]

There are some internet reports of a 1934 USC study with sixteen incurable and terminally ill cancer patients treated with the Beam Ray, or Rife Frequency Machine, where all experienced a complete remission.[2] There also are conspiracy theories about reasons for the Rife Machine's demise, but the fact remains that no more scientific investigations were conducted. I did several clinical trials in the 80s and 90s with electromagnetic devices, claimed by reputable outfits to be constructed with the Rife blueprints. We found zero evidence of tumor reduction.

The Electrical Human Body

Though I haven't found a "Rife"-type machine that works, I believe amazing medical breakthroughs will come in electromagnetic field therapy, for the human body is an electrical entity. An example is the nervous system, built according to an electrical design. It electrically transmits information (via impulses) neuron to neuron; through these impulses we receive info from within and without and then send it to our brains, and vice versa. Experts in neurology believe that in the brain there are between ten trillion and one hundred trillion synapses (connections between neurons), each operating through electrical pulses.

In 1983 Bjorn Nordenström, an astoundingly credentialed scientist who is author or co-author of more than 150 publications in radiology, electrobiology and pharmacology, found that our circulatory system is electrically charged and that there's a difference in the charge of arterial and venous bloods. In other words, there's an electrical flow of charge between arteries and veins. Whenever there's an electrical flow through a conduit (e.g., a wire), there's also an electromagnetic field generated around the conduit. Dr. Nordenström thus established that the "human body has an immense network of blood vessel 'cables' that are surrounded by electromagnetic fields."[3]

New research now shows that every cell in the body may have its own electromagnetic field (EMF) and that even though we still cannot measure it, proper body function depends on proper fields. Physicists have demonstrated that our cells not only communicate with each other via bioelectrical signals but also via electromagnetic fields.[4] EMFs are responsible for crucial biochemical processes and regulation of all kinds of metabolic pathways. Our health depends on cellular electromagnetic fields; any disruption of their balance opens the door to trouble.

EMFs Defined and Illustrated

Let me briefly explain the gist of fields encompassed in EMFs and later their application in cancer. An electric field is created by differences in voltage: the higher the voltage, the stronger the field. A magnetic field is created when electric current flows; the greater the current, the stronger the field. A table lamp is a simplistic example: when it's off, it has an electric field, but when on it creates a magnetic field. Together they're an electromagnetic field. There are natural EMFs produced by thunderstorms; birds and fish use earth's magnetic field as a compass for navigation. We're surrounded by EMFs in our environment, and while some can be harmful to us, others can be harnessed to fight disease.

X-rays and radiation for cancer can be harmful because their electromagnetic field's frequency is so high that it can break and damage molecular bonds like those found in our DNA, these types of EMFs are called ionizing. Non-ionizing EMFs—e.g., electricity, microwaves, and radiofrequencies (mobile phones, TVs, radio transmitters, radars) do not affect molecular bonds and are non-carcinogenic but still can be deadly.

It's difficult to evaluate and establish standards for public safety on many of these devices, and there's much conflicting data on their safety. For instance, some researchers believe the cell phone is a huge threat; other studies demonstrate their harmlessness. To try to standardize, a group of scientists, researchers, and public health policy professionals from ten countries produced *The BioInitiative Report*, an examination of the health risks of electromagnetic fields and radiofrequency radiation.[5] The authors believe existing public policies are completely inadequate to protect our health. While it may be true that we're abusing EMF devices and could pay a future price, there also are applications that may help us better help cancer patients in the near future.

Effective EMF Devices

Radio Frequency Ablation (RFA, see chapter 39) is an EMF-based therapy that elevates temperature to kill cancer. Other devices utilize electricity to open the pores of cell membranes to allow the introduction of drugs or DNA. There is now a purely electrical medical device that uses ultrashort electrical pulses to kill tumors without hyperthermia or drugs. Dr. Richard Nuccitelli has treated over 300 murine melanomas in 120 mice with these pulses (also called nanosecond-pulsed electric fields, they last 300 billionths of a second) with dramatic results. Every tumor exposed to a treatment falls into rapid cell death and destruction of the tumor's vessel network and shrinks by an average of 90% within two weeks. A second treatment completely eliminates the tumor. This stimulates melanomas to self-destruct not only without drugs but also without significant side effects; the technique "provides a highly localized targeting of tumor cells with only minor effects on overlying skin."[6]

I've also mentioned that nanoparticles can be used to generate heat destructive to tumors (see chapters 37, 39). South Korean researchers have figured out how to slay cancer cells with purely magnetic field therapy;[7]

they've developed metal nanoparticles that trigger cancer cells' own death machinery. In this revolutionary approach, a protein guides each nanoparticle to a cell membrane receptor, appropriately called death receptor 4, on the surface of certain cancer cells. Once the nanoparticles are in place, they're remotely activated by a magnetic field device that causes them to clump together, turning on a molecular self-destruction switch. The experiment was conducted in vitro; within twenty-four hours, more than half the cells exposed to the magnetic field were dead. This team is now working to extend the "remote control switch" concept on other cell receptors, such as the vasculoendothelial growth factor (VEGF) that controls blood vessel growth. This technology is still in its infancy and has many hurdles to overcome, but it clearly represents a major opportunity for truly targeted cancer therapy.

Another new weapon for arresting cancer's progression has been developed by Yoram Palti, with low-intensity electric fields that disrupt cancer cell division and slow tumor growth. This non-invasive treatment uses what Dr. Palti calls Tumor Treating Fields (TTF), which disrupt cell division at the nuclear level by hampering the mitotic spindle structure, also called microtubules. Their positive and negative charges maintain them together but are polarized during chromosome division to form daughter cells. The electric field interferes with this process, impeding division specifically in cancer cells. If the mother cell gets to divide, then the TTFs sometimes disintegrate the daughter cells just before they split from their partners.[8]

After the theory was proved in the lab and in animals, Dr. Eilon Kirson conducted a human trial with patients with glioblastoma multiforme, an aggressive brain cancer with very poor prognosis that had received conventional treatments without success. In light of the trial's remarkable results,[9] the FDA approved this non-invasive treatment as a chemo alternative. The device has a power source that weighs about six pounds, and because the treatment should be uninterrupted for days, the patient carries it in a backpack. The TTFs are transferred via cables to electrodes attached to an adhesive patch applied to an area of hair-free skin—in the case of brain tumors, the scalp. Researchers are now doing clinical TTF trials on lung cancer with encouraging results.[10]

Conclusion

A number of EMFTs are under development, and a few are in use, but access is very limited. If you're a candidate for either RFA or TTF and can gain access to the treatments, they stand to benefit you greatly. I'll be keeping my eye on further developments because I believe some of the greatest cancer breakthroughs will come from EMF technology.

ACTION STEPS

1. Practical EMF applications are still in infancy, but soon we should have effective devices.
2. Become and remain informed regarding EMFT advancements.
3. Meanwhile, take advantage of all other practical therapies available.

CANCER VICTOR TIPS

Susan Novak, Alaska
Breast Cancer
Victor Since 2003

1. Contact Oasis of Hope to schedule a consultation with a doctor.
2. Gather all your records to send and to refer to in the consultation.
3. Be aware that conventional doctors may try scare tactics to sway you toward conventional treatment.
4. Arm yourself with knowledge about Oasis of Hope treatments and with testimonials from real patients.
5. Change your diet immediately to vegan (or at least Mediterranean).

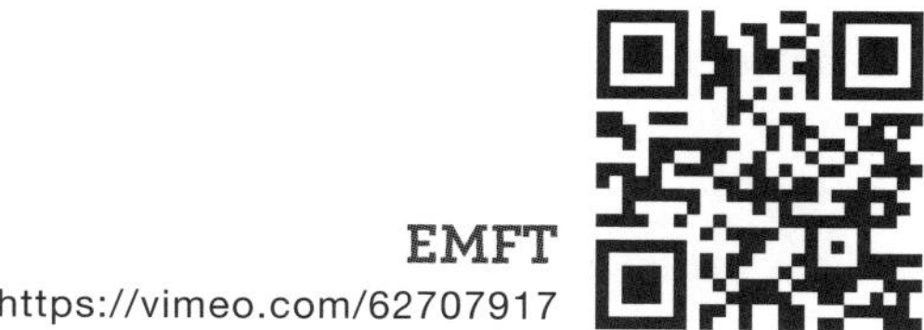

Chapter 47

Believe

Q: *How could my perceptions and beliefs impact my treatment outcome?*

A: The mind's power is great. Hope is a vital healing force in the fight against cancer. Perception of life and death is defined by beliefs. If you know God loves you and Jesus has saved you, your spiritual eternity is resolved. You can stand firm on God's promise that all things work together for good and dismiss the fear of dying. This fortifies your immune system and sets you up for a miracle.

One Monday morning I got an urgent call. The receptionist said, "Come quickly, a new arrival is very upset and won't talk to anybody."

I rushed down three flights of stairs. As I approached, the woman pointed her finger and growled, "*Stop right there.* If you don't get me a hamburger and a cigarette, I won't talk to you. I don't think this is the right place for me."

"I think you're right," I said. "This isn't the place for you. Let me call the driver, then I'll help you change your flight so you can leave today."

"Wait, are you kicking me out?" She looked puzzled.

"Of course not. You are welcome to stay. But here you won't get a hamburger or a cigarette, because those won't help you beat cancer. We offer organic foods and natural therapy. If you believe you need unhealthy things, you better find a different treatment center."

A peace came over her face, and she said, "I was angry because my family forced me to come. But I know I need healthy foods to help me get better. And I want to get better. May I stay?"

I said we had a great room ready for her, and I helped her with her bags. She stayed for the full course of treatment and did very well.

My staff asked if I'd used reverse psychology to convince her to stay. I said I'd never do that, out of respect. Mainly I'd just listened and assessed her beliefs before replying. This chart explains my assessment:

STATEMENT	BELIEF
Stop right there!	People aren't listening. I don't want another person telling me what to do.
If you don't get me a hamburger and a cigarette, I won't talk to you.	I need comfort food and nicotine to stay calm and manage my anxiety.
I don't think this is the right place for me.	I don't feel comfortable here, so I'd feel safer leaving.

I validated the woman's feelings. I also gently offered some info to process and see if her beliefs would allow her to be open to the care we offer. By affirming that I thought she was in the wrong place because we offer healthy foods as part of treatment, she had a chance to decide what was most important to her. She decided getting well was her priority, and her anxiety dissipated because she felt heard and supported. She felt in control. No one was forcing her to stay.

Belief, more powerful than medicine, is one of the key indicators of whether or not a person will beat cancer. People often ask if Oasis of Hope is the best treatment option for anyone facing cancer. I always answer that it's the best option for patients who believe it is. Do *you* believe my last answer is true? Consider the placebo effect.

Placebo Effect

Take a look at the following definitions:

Pla·ce·bo [pluh-*see*-boh][1] ***noun;*** **plural: pla·ce·bos, pla·ce·boes.** A substance having no pharmacological effect but given merely to satisfy a patient who supposes it to be a medicine.

Pla·ce·bo effect [pluh-*see*-boh][2] *noun*
A reaction to a placebo manifested by a lessening of symptoms or the production of anticipated side effects.

A placebo (a sugar pill) has no medicinal value, but studies show that if a person believes the placebo is really a medicine, it will have a physiological effect in their body. Clinical studies have demonstrated that messages are transmitted through neural pathways, inciting biochemical responses.[3] For example, a patient taking a placebo for pain believes he took a painkiller and experiences relief. Belief that he took an analgesic stimulates an opioid release in his brain, which naturally alleviates pain. In the same way, a placebo for depression will, through a patient's belief, release natural serotonin, and symptoms will subside. In chapter 3 I explain how fear causes a blood-level increase of the hormone cortisol via the hypothalamus-pituitary-adrenal axis.

Your beliefs *will* bring about placebo responses, favorable or unfavorable. You may be unaware of all the beliefs you have. You have a belief about every aspect of cancer and its treatment. Learn your beliefs, and modify those that don't embrace the probability that you will beat cancer. The Bible stresses this: "As he thinks in his heart, so *is* he."[4]

• • • • • • • • • • • • •

From the moment you received a diagnosis, you were thrown into a decision-making whirlpool. Whether it's conscious or subconscious, you have a belief about everything you're dealing with. Here are just a few of the issues about which you're probably forming beliefs:

1. I have sufficient family support.
2. My doctors/nurses know what they're doing and can help me.
3. The treatment I'm taking can help me.
4. I have sufficient insurance and finances to pay for treatments.
5. God will help me stand up under this and be victorious.
6. I have a greater purpose to accomplish, and this experience is preparing me for my mission.
7. I can tolerate the negative side effects.
8. Cancer is not a death sentence.

Even if you believe the opposite of everything listed (all positive), my goal is to help you transform your beliefs toward your goal of beating cancer.

"I Will Beat Cancer"

Your body will follow what you believe. One study found that only 27% of patients believed the cancer they had was curable; 42% were unsure if it was curable; 31% believed it was uncurable.[5] Statistics rarely inspire hope. If the doctor says there's a 90% cure rate, most people worry about being in the 10% that won't make it. You must make the decision to see yourself as a part of the group that beats cancer, even if the doctor say you only have a 5% chance of survival. Somebody will make up a part of the percentage that does survive. Choose to believe you are one of those who will survive and thrive!

"I Have Cancer Because . . ."

Whether consciously or unconsciously, everybody has a belief about why they have cancer.[6] I remember a patient telling me he'd stopped loving life three years before he'd been diagnosed. He said, "I brought it on myself. I told myself I didn't want to live anymore, and the result was cancer." Another patient shared that as a child he'd been sexually molested. "I must have done something wrong as a child," he said, "Now I am being punished." Your story may not be so dramatic, but you do have an explanation of why you have cancer. You may think it's because you were a smoker, a drinker, a donut eater, or a promiscuous person. There may be some truth to your belief, or it may be entirely untrue. Living in a toxic world is a sufficient explanation of why you got cancer.

I want to encourage you to get past whatever is your belief about the reason for the cancer. Let it go. Don't beat yourself up. Instead, develop positive resolve to beat cancer. (And please read chapter 20.)

"I Have the Right Stuff"

It's very important that you realize you don't have to beat cancer alone. Those who believe they have the skills and strength to tolerate treatments and deal with pain issues manage their stress better and do have a higher probability of getting better. There's empirical evidence that a person's belief about self-efficacy helps repel negative psychological outcomes like anxiety, fear, and anger.[7]

You may wonder, "But what happens if I don't believe I have what it takes to get through this?" *Nobody has the skills and strength to get through cancer alone.* But, with the help of doctors, nurses, counselors, nutritionists, physical therapists, and caregivers, you *can* make it!

Conclusion

It is common for people to believe that cancer is untreatable and ultimately causes death.[8] That's not true for everyone. It doesn't have to be true for you. But if you're like most people, you don't want others to tell you what to do; you believe they cannot possibly give advice because they don't know what it's like to have cancer. Instead of closing everyone out, choose who you will listen to. It may be more effective to continue putting together your own cancer battle plan by gathering information, just like you're doing by reading this book. Thank you for allowing me to share knowledge and experience with you.

Even though I don't know you, I'd still like to help. That's why I wrote this book. If there were one gift I could give you, I would impart the belief that you have a bright future. People who believe they have the help of God, family members, and their medical team fare better. Optimism and spiritual fortitude overcome hopelessness.[9] When it comes to cancer, hope is most powerful of all.

ACTION STEPS

1. Believe you will beat cancer.
2. Believe you and your team can overcome all challenges.
3. Believe God is helping you.

CANCER VICTOR TIPS

Patrick Clements, Australia
Stage IV Prostate Cancer
Victor Since 2009

1. *Do not* take chemo and/or radiation therapies. My specialist wanted me to have a biopsy, chemo, and radiation; I refused, having a foreknowledge of alternative treatments from reading *World Without Cancer* by G. Edwin Griffin. Read it if you have time; otherwise, trust me.
2. Get online and seek out a hospital that uses laetrile (Vitamin B17) in their treatments. My brother researched and picked Oasis of Hope as they have the best credentials and have been operating for decades.
3. I'm now a firm believer that what you eat can both cause cancer and cure cancer.
4. It's very important to believe that you will be cured.
5. Make sure you get testimonials from people treated and cured at the Oasis of Hope hospital.

Believe
https://vimeo.com/61059341

Chapter 48

Noetic Therapies

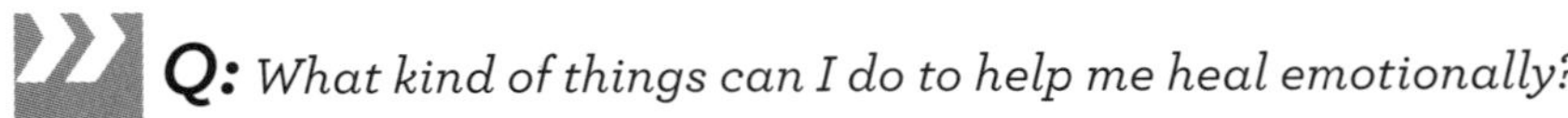

Q: *What kind of things can I do to help me heal emotionally?*

A: Emotional and spiritual healing enables patients to release heavy immune destructive baggage. Noetic therapies can help a person generate and maintain a positive attitude toward the illness and treatment. This will help a person fare much better.

Saul, Israel's first king,[1] was handsome and strong; he had all a man could want, with one exception. Lacking inner peace, he was a tormented soul, consumed with anxiety, fear, and depression. The terror that filled his waking moments was that his reign would be overturned. All that calmed his panic was music. Ironically, David, the shepherd boy whose peaceful harp soothed his soul, would succeed him on the throne.

Remedies and interventions that help bring peace to the mind are called *noetic therapies*. In "Toward a Noetic Model of Medicine,"[2] Marilyn Schlitz wrote, "A guiding premise of the noetic sciences is that the interface of inner experience and the outer world may provide the greatest opportunity for breakthroughs in our understanding of health and healing." Many different interventions, from talk therapy to touch therapy, fall under the noetic umbrella. One dimension of such therapies focuses on philosophical and existential issues;[3] this chapter gives an overview of *emotion*-directed therapies that function to manage stress and promote calmness, a sense of well-being, and rationality in the mind.

A Few Suggestions

I believe that this field is essential and that you will truly benefit by integrating some of the therapies outlined here. I've seen them benefit countless patients, and I have benefitted personally. I'll never forget a night I was hospitalized with pneumonia. I was having much difficulty breathing and not responding well to respiration therapy. Around 3:00 am, my bronchioles began to spasm; I couldn't calm down. A nurse dimmed the lights and began gently rubbing my arm while humming. She transmitted to me a confidence that the cough attack would pass. Soon I felt relief in my lungs and began to breathe easier. Sleep ensued.

Pills, inhalers, shots, and infusions came up short. Caring pulled me through. That is the worth and the power of noetic therapies.

Music Therapy

Dr. Ernesto Contreras, Sr. may be the only oncologist in history who played his guitar with his patients. He made up funny songs with their help, putting original lyrics to well-known songs. He'd play the music to "Deep in the Heart of Texas" while singing, "Contreras is, the best there is," (clap clap clap clap) "Deep in the heart of Playas" (the Mexico beach city where our hospital is). He intuitively knew the power of music.

Clinical studies now confirm that music is therapeutic.[4] We even know when to use music, when silence is preferred, and what type of music facilitates desired outcomes. For instance, one study concluded that music for people taking long-term chemo would lower their anxiety levels; classical is the music of choice for its calming effect. Participants explained that during the movements of a classical piece, they would be inspired to keep fighting cancer. Patients with a high fever prefer silence and tend to return to music listening once the fever subsides.

At Oasis of Hope, we sing worship songs focused on healing during daily devotions. I believe that God inhabits the praise of His children,[5] and our patients comment how they feel His presence when we worship together. In our treatment rooms, we often play DVDs with scenes of nature, Scripture verses, and gentle music.

Art Therapy

There is evidence that art can help manage adjustments to the changes, uncertainties, and losses associated with cancer.[6] By drawing, painting, and sculpting, people can process and express feelings that words fail to communicate. I'm frequently surprised to see how a patient's soul can bypass cognition and go straight to the canvas.

It's been my experience that patients often resist at first and say, "I can't draw." I use booklets with crayons and start each session stating, "If you graduated from kindergarten, you have the skills to participate here. We'll draw, scribble, and doodle." Almost everyone smiles, and consistently we have at least 90% participation. My normal exercise is to have people draw how they felt when they first received a cancer diagnosis. I tell them not to think about it but to draw the first thing that comes to mind. Most grab red and black crayons and start to draw things like storms and sinking ships. I often see stick figures trapped in a box. Red often represents danger or a warning of an imminent threat.[7] Black usually refers to being scared, to feeling depressed, and death.

Then I ask them to draw how they're feeling since they started at Oasis of Hope. Across the board, people use colors like green, for life, purple, for spirituality, and yellow, for happiness and increased energy.

The best benefit I've found with art is how it facilitates conversations between patients and caregivers. I've even seen couples with strained marriages start to hug after looking at each other's drawings. Sometimes they say "I didn't know you felt that way" or "I want to understand that."

Laughter Therapy

The use of humor in medical settings has been shown in numerous studies to provide psychological *and* physiological health benefits like lowered blood pressure, stress management, increased oxygenation, and coping with pain.[8] In the 70s, Norman Cousins emerged as an advocate for laughter therapy, explaining his cure from a degenerative disease by watching comedies and reading funny books.[9] Though no studies corroborate the curative power of humor such as he described, there's no disputing its therapeutic value for palliative care. Some hospitals provide "mobile laughter carts" that bring books and videos and more for patients.[10] Manuel Borod outlined another benefit by concluding that humor could aid and enable improved communication between doctors and patients as well as elevate the mood of family members who find it difficult to see their loved ones facing advanced illnesses.[11]

We use joke telling and videos with Christian comedians. We even have a comic who provides belly-busting laughter with impersonations and parodies. Informally, we've monitored blood pressure and noted that all patients experience a lowering after just a few minutes of this. And everyone's heart is warmed to see people who've been quieted by cancer-related anxiety and suffering perk back up and laugh to their heart's content. Laughter has a way of bringing us back to the art of living.

Visualization

Also called guided imagery, visualization is another effective stress management technique, wherein a patient closes her eyes as a counselor uses narration to guide her through an experience. Though it hasn't been shown to help with treatment-related physical symptoms (e.g., nausea), studies do conclude that visualization brings comfort and emotional support.[12] I find that it's so effective it often puts people to sleep.

I guide people through an imagined day on a private beach in the Caribbean. I describe the water, beaches, and trees. I have them imagine how the warm white sand feels under their feet, how the hot sun feels on their skin, how the cool breeze feels in their hair. I ask them to envision dipping their feet in the water and sipping cold lemonade. Most patients report that, for a brief time, they really felt they were on the island and they truly could see, taste, feel, and smell what I described.

Progressive Muscle Relaxation

It can be common to feel anxiety before a medical procedure or just before going to sleep. Progressive muscle relaxation (PMR) can assist the body in releasing tension and bring the mind to feel that it's back in control. Some nurses teaching patients in treatment note that PMR helps alleviate chemo-related fatigue and allows patients to sleep better.[13]

The technique I use is a tensing and then relaxing of the muscles. We start with the feet only; I ask them to tense up their feet as hard as they can and hold the tension for five seconds. I count down to one and tell them to release. Then I have them tense their feet and calf muscles and repeat the tensing, holding, and releasing. Each time we repeat the cycle, we add a muscle group (hence, "progressive"): feet, then calves, thighs, abdomen, chest and shoulders, and arms. Patients say it relaxes them quite a bit (though not as much as laughter therapy!).

Massage

The documented benefits of massage include reduction in anxiety, decrease in cancer-related nausea, and improvement of pain control.[14] More and more practitioners are accepting that emotional stress and trauma is not only remembered in the brain cells but also in other types of cells. No study has proved this theory, but it could be that through massaging tender muscles until they're no longer tense, some of the stored emotional stress in those muscles is relieved as well.

I have my own personal experience with muscle memory of trauma. Years ago I spent six days in agonizing pain from kidney stones. To this day, when I tell people about it, I suddenly feel sharp pain in my left kidney region. When I change the subject, the pain goes away.

Another facet of massage therapy is the power of touch. Gentle human touch can often bring about a feeling of security. This innate response may be triggered because the subconscious travels back to infancy to the experience of feeling safely enveloped in a mother's arms.

Conclusion

Many different types of interventions could fall under the large noetic-therapy umbrella; here I've shared a few with which my patients have had good results, and I talk about other techniques in chapters 6 and 9. One study involving 120 heart patients found that people with a high anxiety level experienced fewer in-patient hospital complications if they included noetic therapies.[15] Though I haven't conducted a related clinical study at Oasis of Hope, hundreds of patients have told me how much better they've been able to cope with the stresses of cancer and treatment because of our group sessions. Please do integrate some noetic therapies into your own healing plan.

ACTION STEPS

1. Watch one funny movie per day.
2. Listen to classical music throughout the day.
3. Look for an art therapy group or class in your area.

CANCER VICTOR TIPS

Roy Tirtaji, Indonesia
Stage IV Colon Cancer
Victor Since 2013

1. Do not grumble!
2. Do not ask why God allowed you to experience cancer.
3. Rejoice, pray, and give thanks! (1 Thessalonians 5:16–18).
4. Trust God! All things work together for good (Romans 8:28).
5. Ask God what He wants you to do for *Him* at any stage (Acts 22:10).

Noetic Therapies
https://vimeo.com/61658853

Chapter 49

Spiritual Care

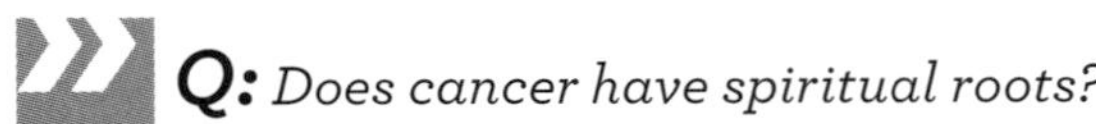

Q: *Does cancer have spiritual roots?*

A: I don't believe cancer happens as a result of sin, but it has been established that catastrophic events promote dysfunctional emotions that promote cancer. Since emotional response is directly related to spiritual fortitude, cancer does have spiritual roots.

A few years ago, I took my family to Legoland. Fortunately for my wife there are outlets nearby, so I dropped her off and made my way to the theme park with the children. When we parked, drizzle started to fall, and for some reason my window wouldn't raise. I said that if I couldn't get it to close, we wouldn't be able to go into the park; the kids looked so disappointed, and I quickly asked, "What should we do when we have a problem but don't see the answer?" They said we should pray.

And we did. I began by giving thanks to God and recognizing Him as sovereign and good all the time. I explained the problem and asked for a solution. Instantly I remembered we'd driven by a Honda dealership between the outlets and Legoland. I gave thanks again for the solution and said, "Let's see how quickly we can get the window fixed; maybe we can come back and still enjoy a few hours here."

At the dealership I explained the issue. The attendant said they wouldn't get to it for a few hours. Then unexpected blessings started to unfold. He said he could loan me a car. We took it and spent the whole day at Legoland, using the same parking stub I'd already paid for. When we got back, the window had been fixed. The attendant said the repair was covered under warranty and he wouldn't charge for the loaner. We had a story of God's faithfulness to share when we picked up my wife!

Some people might pick apart my tale and say that by calming myself and centering my thoughts I fixed the matter. But where did the calm and the centering come from? How was I able to tap into the clarity and power to resolve the problem? For me, the answer is simple—faith.

• • • • • • • • • • • •

In fifty years at Oasis of Hope we've been honored to treat patients from all over the world, from many cultures and spiritual orientations. I will never forget the day I walked around to meet patients in our dining room and nineteen nations were represented. All the different apparel was fascinating. Orthodox Jews from Israel wore long coats and hats. A man from India wore his Sikh turban. A number of Mennonite families wore black clothes with blue shirts. A Muslim woman wore an abaya and scarf. Many others in plain clothes also professed to be people of faith.

I'm often asked how I relate to people of other religions. My answer is that I don't change who I am to embrace who other people are: I share God's love with everyone. When a Muslim man asked me to pray for his back, I said I prayed in the name of Jesus, and he said only Jesus has the power to heal. A member of Jehovah's Witnesses told me I was the only person outside her church she trusted to pray. After devotions, one woman came up and said, "I am a Russian Orthodox Jew, but your ministry is so beautiful, I allow you to pray for me." Love builds bridges.

Through this privilege of supporting people from different faith walks while they face cancer, I've discovered aspects of spirituality that are nearly universal. Most people believe there is a God. And they believe that, with God, there is hope.

Prayer and Faith

Prayer is a powerful strategy on which many cancer patients rely.[1] Among Americans, 90% pray; one study indicates that upwards of 66% of oncology nurses privately pray with their patients.[2] *Prayer is faith in action.* Faith in a God of goodness helps people deal with the spiritual and emotional distress cancer puts upon them. There's no doubt that spiritual care is critical in the treatment of cancer.

Praying for healing is biblical. For a believer it's not only an option—it's a directive from God himself. James, the brother of Jesus, says,

> Is anyone among you sick? Let them call the elders of the church to pray over them and anoint them with oil in the name of the Lord. And the prayer offered in faith will make the sick person well; the Lord will raise them up. If they have sinned, they will be forgiven. Therefore confess your sins to each other and pray for each other so that you may be healed. The prayer of a righteous person is powerful and effective.[3]

Jesus told the disciples, "I will do whatever you ask in my name, so that the Father may be glorified in the Son,"[4] and "Where two or three gather in my name, there am I with them."[5] From his instructions, it's clear there is power in prayer together, in groups, and that we are to pray in the name of Jesus. These are critical if we're to claim healing through His fulfillment of Isaiah's prophecy that Messiah would take all our infirmities upon himself and that by His wounds we are healed.[6]

Science supports prayer's healing power. Many books have been written about it, and many clinical trials have been conducted. One compelling study published by Ruth Stanley found that prayer may bring balance to the autonomic nervous system:

> My observations suggest that prayer types indicative of a more integrated, deeper relational spirituality have the potential to draw the body toward stronger levels of innate healing through more effective restoration of autonomic nervous system balance and adaptability. In these uncontrolled observations, the greatest physiological benefit was associated with prayers of gratefulness and contemplative prayer.[7]

The idea presented here is that focusing your prayer on your relationship with God brings deeper peace than lifting up prayers of supplication.

A 2012 study on prayer brought to light a crucial aspect that most people face when asking God for a specific outcome.[8] Many struggle when their prayers are not answered as they'd hoped. The author found that it's important for prayer to be more about the relationship with God than about the petition and the answer. Throughout decades of praying with our patients, I can tell you that peace comes through prayers of gratitude more than anything else. This peace shifts the neuroendocrine signals in the body that allow the immune system to recover.

My recommendation is that when you pray, do not put a condition on God that He must answer according to your will. Instead, be open to the many good things He will reveal to you through prayer.

Cancer Concerns

Many people believe cancer has a spiritual root. As a pastor, I have yet to identify a specific spiritual root in patients that explains why they get cancer. What's important to me is helping people break free of any spiritual concerns and emotional issues to aid the total healing process. I have not found it helpful to try casting out cancer like a demon. My belief is that being diagnosed doesn't indicate your sinfulness; it only confirms that you live in a toxic, broken world. Cancer is an opportunity for the power of God to be made manifest in your life (see John 9).

It's common in the face of a life-threatening situation to take a hard look at things and get realigned. A diagnosis can make clear what truly matters. Many people realize life is all about God and family; material things shrivel quickly. Patients often cope with cancer through spiritual support, deepening their connection with God and finding forgiveness through faith.[9] They pray for strength to deal with the illness, distress, side effects, financial burdens, and chronic pain, and for help living with the disease.[10] Those who do report a positive sense of well being.[11]

Guilt and Forgiveness

Unaddressed guilt is a poison to the human spirit, and lack of forgiveness can keep us in a prison. Focusing on being forgiven or on forgiving others is a common theme for those facing cancer.[12] I routinely address these topics in group sessions, and it's so rewarding when people open up to talk about what's been eating them up for years, then courageously forgive others and themselves.

It seems self-forgiveness is one of the most difficult things for us. But forgiveness is so vital that Jesus included it in the Lord's Prayer.

John, His disciple, tells of a woman, caught in adultery, who had many accusers; certainly she felt guilty and ashamed. When she was thrown at Jesus' feet for judgment, He began to write in the sand, and then one by one the accusers walked away. He looked at the woman and asked, "Where are they? Has no one condemned you?"

"No one, sir," she answered.

"Then neither do I condemn you," He said. "Go now and leave your life of sin."[13]

Dealing with guilt is being willing to present it to God, receiving forgiveness from Him, and then going forward without it in your life.

Spiritual Hope

Most studies on faith and healing conclude that spiritual care helps people cope and improves the quality of life they experience.[14] Hope can be built by finding meaning during the experience of cancer, making amends with loved ones, and exploring spiritual themes like God's goodness and power to heal.

Through spiritual care, many people deal with fear, maintain a positive outlook, give and receive love, and live in the presence of God.[15] When a person realizes he's unable to overcome a dire challenge, he often turns to the all-powerful God. Necessity is the field where hope grows.

• • • • • • • • • • • •

To the world, the cross is an ancient instrument of death. To Christians, the cross is what Jesus used to give eternal life. As a symbol, the cross is one of the world's most recognized icons. The cross represents the most important teaching Jesus ever gave:

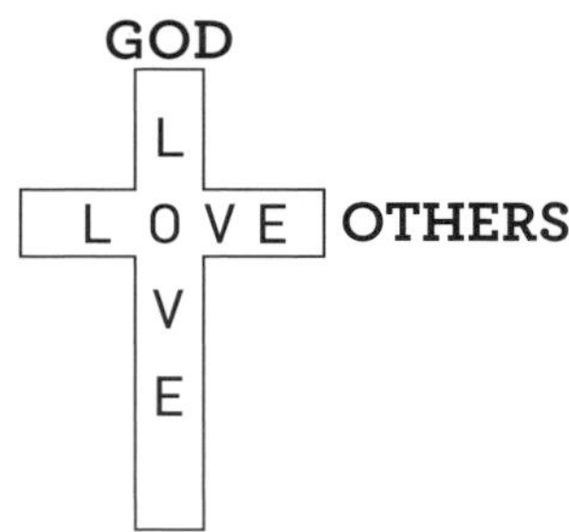

Jesus said the greatest and second-greatest commandments are, "Love the Lord your God with all your heart and with all your soul and with all your mind" and "Love your neighbor as yourself."[16] The cross is made of two wooden beams. The vertical represents our love upward, back toward God. The horizontal represents His love in us for others.

In addition to the healing power of God's love and sharing it with others, the cross is also the burdensome weight you can't stand up under that Jesus will help you carry. It represents forgiveness for yourself and others. It represents Christ's victory over disease and death. It is a reminder of the peace He purchased and offers you. It symbolizes the wounds He suffered so that you can be healed. Instead of struggling on, by yourself, take your worries and your hope to the cross.

Surrender

One of my favorite prayers ever written down is the Serenity Prayer. I believe it's useful for all of us.[17] Why not say it now?

God, grant me the serenity
to accept the things I cannot change,
courage to change the things I can,
and wisdom to know the difference.[18]

You can find peace and build up spiritual fortitude when you accept that there are things beyond your power to change. The answer to those problems is surrendering them to God. Surrender is not giving up—it's giving the issues beyond your power to resolve over to God.

At the same time, there are many things you can do to improve your quality of life. As the prayer says, be courageous, and make needed changes. Also, be wise, and invest your emotional energy in things you can change. Surrender the rest to God. Surrender is the key to peace.

Conclusion

Mark's gospel tells of Jesus and his disciples taking a boat across the Sea of Galilee. He'd been serving thousands of people, all day, healing and teaching, and the boat looked like an excellent way to step aside a while to get some rest. Exhausted, Jesus fell into deep sleep. Suddenly, a violent storm rose up; waves were crashing over the bow, and the boat was swamped. Fearing death, the disciples woke Jesus and yelled, "Don't you care if we die?" Then Jesus rebuked the wind and told the waves to be still. As quickly as the storm had hit, the seas became calm at the sound of God's voice.[19]

If you or a loved one is facing cancer, it's normal for your emotions to be tossed back and forth by the winds and waves of circumstance. It's to be expected that you may feel overwhelmed and sinking. What did the disciples do in their desperate situation? Go and talk with Jesus. They shared their fear with Him. He intervened. Peace came over them.

Pray. Share your fears. God will answer; His peace in you will follow.

Another time, on the same sea, Peter walked on the water.[20] As long as he kept his eyes on Jesus, he didn't sink. Then he saw the wind and waves. He got scared and began sinking. He cried out, "Save me!" Jesus reached out his hand and brought Peter to safety. The wind died down. Jesus told Peter not to doubt. Prayer, faith, forgiveness, hope, and surrender to God will get you through this storm.

I saw the peace that comes through faith in Christ working through all things in 1995 when my (Daniel Kennedy's) father was diagnosed with cancer. The oncologist thought he misunderstood, because he simply smiled and said thank you; he asked if he'd heard the words, then asked how he was able to take the news with a smile. My dad explained that for him to live is Christ and to die is gain.[21]

Today, he is alive and well. He's my best friend. I've been married seventeen years and have two daughters, ages fifteen and twelve; my dad has been here all along, probably because he surrendered his life to Jesus Christ. Whoever gives over his life for Jesus' sake will save it.[22]

ACTION STEPS

1. Look for spiritual meaning along your cancer journey.
2. Pray throughout the day and ask your doctors, nurses, and caregivers to pray with you too.
3. Surrender your guilt, fear, and doubts to the Lord. Accept forgiveness in exchange.

CANCER VICTOR TIPS

Shary Oden,[23] Arizona
Stage IV Small Lymphocytic Lymphoma
Victor Since 2011

1. Realize that every day is a gift from God. His Son, our Lord and Savior, is our Healer. There is absolutely nothing He cannot do.
2. Put Jesus in the driver's seat. We can ask for anything in prayer, believe we've already received it, and it will be ours (Mark 11:24).
3. Read Dodie Osteen's *Healed of Cancer.*
4. God spoke everything into being. The spoken word is powerful.
5. Never claim the cancer or call it yours. Call it, "the cancer."

Chapter 50

A New Approach to Cancer Control

Q: *What is the difference between a cancer cure and cancer control?*

A: Invasive cancer is formidable. Eliminating late-stage cancer is in most cases won't happen. But eliminating the life-threatening potential is possible in many. For fifty years Oasis of Hope physicians have successfully developed therapies to convert cancer from a "terminal" disease into a chronic ailment to manage for many years of quality living. Our work is the wave of oncology's future.

Contreras Metabolic Integrative Therapy (CMIT) is the joining of therapies with a powerful synergistic effect. Synergy is what happens when forces work together so the total effect is greater than the sum of the forces. Usually, cytotoxic therapies such as radiation or chemo represent 100% of the treatment. At Oasis of Hope, cytotoxic therapy is just one integrative facet. The nine other elements that comprise CMIT are every bit as important and compelling.

CMIT is designed to destroy cancer cells, delay their growth and mutagenesis, and impede their spread as long as possible. It is also designed to maximize the time for which the patient enjoys a high quality of life. Let me introduce a whole new world of treatment possibilities.

Oxidative Preconditioning

Oxidants, substances in the body that can damage our cells, may be normal waste, produced through normal metabolism—protein-rich meals produce many oxidants—or synthetic chemicals, heavy metals like mercury, or other toxins. Oxidants do harm through their molecular instability; they "grab" electrons, especially from cell membranes, DNA, and mitochondria.

*Anti*oxidants easily donate electrons and thus neutralize oxidants before they can harm cells. Our body produces natural ones; we can ingest them in fruits and vegetables and additionally as supplements, like vitamin C. However, if there are too many oxidants in our body, we may not be able to neutralize them all, a condition called oxidative stress.

Chemotherapeutic agents attack cancer cells, largely by acting as potent oxidants, but don't distinguish between malignant and normal cells, so they damage healthy as well as cancerous tissue. Oxidative preconditioning therapy boosts normal tissues' capacity to withstand chemo-imposed oxidative stress. Exposing cells to transient, repeated, mild oxidant stress increases the antioxidant defense system—our cells produce more antioxidants in response.

One such treatment I use is ozone autohemotherapy (*auto* means "self"; *hemo* refers to "blood)." About 200 ml of a patient's blood is drawn and exposed to ozone and ultraviolet light. Ozone and UV light affect the blood by producing oxidized compounds. The treated blood is re-infused, and the oxidized compounds it contains serve as a signal of oxidative stress to the body's normal healthy tissues, causing them to increase production of protective antioxidant enzymes. Repeated sessions prior to chemo ensure that normal tissues are in much better condition to cope with the oxidative stress imposed by the subsequent chemotherapy.

An alternative method to produce this effect is breathing pure oxygen in a pressurized chamber. This is called hyperbaric oxygen therapy, sometimes abbreviated HBO or HBOT. (*Hyper* means "over" and *baric* refers to atmospheric pressure.) Repeated HBO sessions prior to chemo may ensure that normal tissues are in much better condition to cope with oxidative stress. Thus, oxidative preconditioning therapy's intent is to make chemotherapy more tolerable while simultaneously improving the ability of the cancer treatment to destroy the tumor.

Cytotoxic Therapy

The second CMIT component is cytotoxic therapy. For years we've been able to use high-dose intravenous vitamin C as a powerful and natural cytotoxic agent. Certain cancer types, though, respond much better to a range of well-known chemo drugs. We test for chemo-sensitivity and select the most effective treatment course, be it high-dose IV vitamin C, low-dose chemotherapy, or radiation.

Cell Signal Transduction Therapy

The third component, cell signal transduction, uses nutraceuticals (pharmaceutical-grade vitamin supplements with medicinal qualities) and "safe" (nontoxic) drugs to target particular cancer-cell signaling pathways. "Signal transduction" refers to how cellular proteins undergo small, usually reversible changes in structure to induce alterations in cell behavior. The genetic material of cancer cells is typically altered in ways that over-activate intracellular signaling pathways that promote the cells' unregulated growth and spread, or that make them harder to kill with chemo- or radiotherapy. Targeting these pathways suppresses cancer cells' capacity to grow, spread to distant organs, grow new blood vessels that feed tumors, and, in general, makes them easier to destroy.

Redox Regulatory Therapy

Fourth, redox regulatory therapy selectively targets tumor sites with intense levels of oxidative stress. This means the therapy is designed to attack tumor cells only, with no harm to healthy tissue. The combination of high-dose IV vitamin C therapy, ozone autohemotherapy, and the vasodilator Trental achieves this effect. Redox can often hold tumor growth at bay while augmenting effects of concurrent cytotoxic therapy.

Immune Stimulation Therapy

The fifth component of CMIT, immune stimulation therapy, aids the immune system's ability to attack cancer by optimizing the function of NK cells and T-cells. The therapy employs a two-pronged approach. The first involves the use of natural products that boost the immune system's function. The second involves the use of substances that block the mechanisms tumors use to suppress the immune system.

Tumor Acidity Regulation

The sixth CMIT component is tumor acidity regulation. The acidic pH of tumors allows cancer cells to spread to neighboring tissue and distant organs.

Affecting the cells' pH is difficult with foods and water; we use proton pump inhibitors that regulate the H+/K+ of the stomach cells, significantly lowering gastric acid secretion while reducing extracellular tumor acidity. This slows proliferation and metastatic spread of cancer cells while promoting apoptosis.

Nutritional Therapy

Seventh, we teach patients how to successfully improve their diet to optimize their body's innate healing powers. The scientific evidence is compelling for the preventive and curative benefits of a diet low in fats, animal proteins, and sugar, while high in vegetables. Recent research shows how healing foods help to slow growth and spread of many pre-existing cancers. We have cooking classes, and classes on anti-cancer nutrition. Feel free to visit our website, then learn to cook with us!

Exercise

The eighth CMIT component is regular aerobic exercise. Its curative and preventive benefits likewise have been acknowledged for decades. I recommend walking daily, twenty to thirty minutes, as briskly as a patient's condition will allow. Our physical therapist teaches breathing and movement techniques, and one favorite session is chair aerobics. (It's amazing how much exercise can be done while sitting down!)

Emotional Healing

The ninth component is developing an emotional support structure, not only in the hospital but at home as well. The correlation between a person's positive attitude and improved immune system functioning (and physical health in general) is well-supported in peer-reviewed medical literature. Cancer management can tax the strongest person; the energy required to learn about the illness, embrace treatment, and alter lifestyle creates a need for an external emotional support system that strengthens and refreshes. We seek to provide that structure to foster emotional healing and its positive psychoendoneuro-immunological effects.

Spiritual Care

The tenth component of CMIT is development of spiritual fortitude. There's no question that fear and anxiety produced by the possibility of death, coupled by insecurity about the afterlife, can significantly impact a patient's physical and emotional state. Therefore, we seek to provide avenues for patients to develop the hope, peace, and security that stems from a healthy relationship with God. The positive impact this has on a patient's ability to engage in the whole process of disease management cannot be overestimated.

Fifty Years of Clinical Experience

Again, CMIT is named after my father, the Oasis of Hope founder. The overview I've just presented is simplistic and doesn't highlight the scientific evidence that supports our approach. (Some of that research was presented earlier in this book.) But what sets apart Oasis of Hope is more than research: it's our half century of clinical experience. While treating tens of thousands of people, we've learned critical cancer answers to help patients achieve favorable outcomes. No single agent will cure cancer—winning takes an integrative approach that intervenes simultaneously in as many ways as feasible to promote the death of cancer cells and halt the spread of tumors. CMIT represents a viable, innovative strategy to achieve this.

We call our therapy *Contreras Metabolic Integrative Therapy* because research supports the idea that cancer is primarily a metabolic (rather than a genetic) disease. Breast cancer, for example, is essentially a lifestyle disease. It's likely that only 5% to 10% of all breast cancers are related to genes, which would mean that 90% to 95% result from other factors—that is, factors a person can change.[1]

Recently, Angelina Jolie had both perfectly healthy breasts removed and reconstructed as a preventative measure. Jolie revealed that she has the "breast cancer gene" (BRCA1). Now, studies indicate that women with this mutation have a 50% to 87% probability of developing breast cancer at some point.[2] Yet the same studies also note that only 2% of all women who are diagnosed with breast cancer have the mutated gene. As we saw in chapter 12, this means that 98% of all women with breast cancer developed it not because of genes but because of lifestyle issues.

Results

The question most people want answered is, what are our survival rates with patients in a CMIT medical protocol? We have five-year survival rate stats for patients who've received this treatment for stage IV advanced metastatic breast, ovarian, lung, and colorectal cancer. This data was published in 2012 in the *Townsend Letter for Physicians*.[3]

For comparison, the table below presents our results side by side with conventional therapy results as reported by the NCI in 2007.[4]

SURVIVAL RATES FOR STAGE IV CANCERS:

TYPE OF CANCER	OASIS OF HOPE					CONVENTIONAL TREATMENT				
	SURVIVAL (%)					SURVIVAL (%)				
BREAST	93	73	60	51	45	65	44	32	25	20
BREAST*	100	90	83	78	75	65	44	32	25	20
OVARIAN	94	87	74	60	54	62	43	30	23	18
LUNG	70	43	31	18	9	20	6	3	2	1.6
COLORECTAL	68	48	32	20	16	43	22	13	10	7

* Oasis of Hope was the first treatment option.

It's clear that, in terms of survival, Oasis of Hope patients are doing considerably better than those receiving the average standard of care in the US. In fact, five-year survival in each of these cancers is at least two-to threefold higher than in patients receiving conventional therapy, and in some cases greater. Plainly, we all need to learn how to do better in long-term management of lung and colorectal cancer—these are notoriously chemo-resistant—but even with them our patients are doing considerably better than average. Note for example in lung cancer that chances of surviving two years or more are strikingly higher at Oasis of Hope. Ovarian cancer results are encouraging too—at the three-year point and beyond, our survival chances are about three times higher.

Further, it's germane to note the survival statistics for stage IV breast cancer patients who chose us as their first therapeutic option. Their survival at five years was 75%, compared to 20% in the US. These superior results in patients who came to us first likely reflects that they didn't have previous chemo and so are more likely to be responsive to it than patients who have evolved resistance during previous therapy. The relative chemosensitivity of their cancers, in conjunction with the range of nutraceutical and drug adjuvants, which Oasis of Hope employs in hospital and in home care, is paying off big in long-term survival.

Conclusion

A big part of our success is due to not underestimating the harmful effects of chemo and radiation. We concentrate on protecting our patients from those effects and providing effective alternatives that prolong their lives and secure their quality of life as well.

ACTION STEPS

1. Evaluate whether Oasis of Hope would be your best treatment option.
2. Incorporate healing foods and exercise into your battle plan.
3. Make sure God is the head of your treatment team.

CANCER VICTOR TIPS

Brenda J. Bray, North Carolina
Her2+ Breast Cancer, Left Breast, T3N1
Victor Since 2006

1. Always get at least a second opinion on your diagnosis and proposed treatment plan options. An integrative therapy approach (conventional with alternative therapies) under the guidance of a knowledgeable doctor has proven most successful for me.
2. Educate yourself so that you can take responsibility for your own body while partnering with your doctor(s) for your best treatment plan. Knowledge is power. Be open to new ideas and information. Knowing you have choices empowers you and takes away fear.
3. Implement a change in lifestyle; eat healthy, consume no sugar, take supportive supplements, work to improve your health habits, stay active, rest, drink plenty of water, and laugh as much as

possible. Never give cancer any power—it is not who you are, nor is it your identity. You have a much bigger life to enjoy outside of cancer!

4. The battle is won or lost in your mind. Refuse to allow thoughts of fear to defeat you. Draw on your faith for wisdom, courage, strength, perseverance, and especially hope. Know and believe in your heart that God is our Healer, and say what He says in His Word. Trust in Him, no matter how symptoms feel or how medical reports look.
5. Accept that this can be a difficult and sometimes long journey, but stay hopeful and determined to win. Never, ever give up!

A New Approach to Cancer Control
https://vimeo.com/67660884

About Oasis of Hope Cancer Treatment Centers

Oasis of Hope was founded in 1963 by Dr. Ernesto Contreras, Sr. on the vision of treating the whole person with physical, emotional, and spiritual resources. It's a comprehensive "all under one roof" center with a multi-disciplinary team that has garnered fifty years of clinical expertise in cancer treatment and research. His healing legacy lives on in the lives of patients and family members who have benefited from his "total care" approach at Oasis of Hope in Mexico and in the United States.

Our Mission

Oasis of Hope is:
Caring for the whole person: body, mind, and spirit;
Sharing the healing power of faith, hope, and love; and
Advancing medical science to defeat cancer one person at a time.

Five Reasons Oasis of Hope May Be Your Best Option

1. According to a recent publication, we may have better survival rates than any other cancer treatment center in the world.

In September 2012 the *Townsend Letter* published results of a five-year clinical study conducted by Dr. Francisco Contreras at Oasis of Hope with patients who had different stage IV cancer types. When comparing the rates with those published by the National Cancer Institute and other treatment facilities, it's evident that our objective clinical responses are second to none. Even so, note that no two cases of cancer are the same, and the report does not guarantee that all cancer patients at Oasis of Hope will experience favorable tumor reduction and increased survival rates. What the statistics suggest is that no other center offers a better probability of helping a patient beat cancer.

2. Dr. Contreras is recognized as one of the world's leading authorities in integrative and alternative cancer treatment.

Dr. Francisco Contreras was trained by his father, the late Dr. Ernesto Contreras, Sr. the father of alternative cancer treatment in the 1960s. He completed his specialty in oncology in Vienna and for the last thirty years has been director of Oasis of Hope Hospital. He has treated tens of thousands of patients, conducted many clinical trials, and reviewed hundreds of potential cancer therapies and treatment protocols. It would be difficult to find another oncologist with as much knowledge and experience integrating alternative and conventional therapies. He has the credentials and the compassion.

3. Oasis of Hope does not get you sick to get you better.

Most people come to wonder which is worse, treatment or the disease. Chemo and radiation frequently cause extreme illness. Oncologists ask patients to tolerate dreadful side effects in hope of a benefit. The Oasis of Hope doctors have a different philosophy; we don't believe we must make patients get sick to get them better. Instead, we utilize pre-conditioning natural therapies that diminish side effects and help preserve healthy cells and the immune system. You can witness the difference by the number of smiling faces you'll see when you visit us. Sometimes it's difficult to tell who the patients are at Oasis of Hope because of how healthy many look. Most don't experience hair loss, and instead of deteriorating, they become stronger even in treatment. This is a major contrast to what's typically seen in a cancer ward.

4. We will care for all of you: body, mind and spirit.

We intergrate natural and conventional medicine with emotional support and spiritual care. Our multi-disciplinary team will use every tool available to meet each of your needs.

5. We recognize Jesus Christ as our medical director, the Great Physician, and the Healer.

Contact Oasis of Hope

To see how you or a loved one may benefit
from Oasis of Hope,

please call
888-500-HOPE or 619-690-8410

or email
health@oasisofhope.com

or visit
www.oasisofhope.com
and
www.yourcanceranswer.org

Dr. Francisco Contreras and Daniel Kennedy would like to email you a copy of their e-book *Hope, Medicine & Healing*, along with twelve video downloads and an e-workbook, all for free! Call 888-500-HOPE.

References

Chapter 1

1. Lebel, S, S Beattie, I Arès, C Bielajew. Young and worried: age and fear of recurrence in *Breast Cancer Survivors. Health Psychology* 2012; np.
2. Horlick-Jones, T. Understanding fear of cancer recurrence in terms of damage to "everyday health competence." *Sociology of Health & Illness* 2011;33(6):884–98.
3. Rogers, SN, B Scott, D Lowe, G Ozakinci, G Humphris. Fear of recurrence following head and neck cancer in the outpatient clinic. European Archives Of Oto-Rhino-Laryngology: *Official Journal of the European Federation of Oto-Rhino-Laryngological Societies*: affiliated with the German Society for Oto-Rhino-Laryngology—Head and Neck Surgery 2010;267(12):1943–9.
4. Trinkaus, M, D Burman, N Barmala, G Rodin, J Jones, C Lo, C Zimmermann. Spirituality and complementary therapies for cure in advanced cancer. *Psycho-Oncology* 2011;20(7):746–54.
5. Yanez, B, D Edmondson, AL Stanton, CL Park, L Kwan, PA Ganz, TO Blank. Facets of spirituality as predictors of adjustment to cancer: Relative contributions of having faith and finding meaning. *Journal of Consulting and Clinical Psychology* 2009;77(4):730–41.
6. Isaiah 41:10. *Holy Bible: New Living Translation.* Wheaton, IL: Tyndale, 1996.
7. John 16:33. *Holy Bible: New Living Translation.* Wheaton, IL: Tyndale, 1996.
8. Ephesians 6:16. *Holy Bible: New Living Translation.* Wheaton, IL: Tyndale, 1996.
9. 2 Corinthians 3:17. *Holy Bible: New Living Translation.* Wheaton, IL: Tyndale, 1996.

Chapter 2

1. Junshi, et al. *Diet, Life-style, and Mortality in China: A Study of the Characteristics of 65 Chinese Counties.* Oxford Univ. Press, 1990.
2. McCarty, MF. Insulin and IGF-I as determinants of low "Western" cancer rates in the rural third world. *Int J Epidemiol* 2004 Aug;33(4):908–10.
3. Giovannucci, E. Nutrition, insulin, insulin-like growth factors and cancer. *Horm Metab Res* 2003 Nov;35(11–12):694–704.
4. Jousse, C, A Bruhat, M Ferrara, P Fafournoux. Physiological concentration of amino acids regulates insulin-like-growth-factor-binding protein 1 expression. *Biochem J* 1998 Aug 15;334 (Pt 1):147–53.
5. Allen, NE, PN Appleby, GK Davey, TJ Key. Hormones and diet: low insulin-like growth factor-I but normal bioavailable androgens in vegan men. *Br J Cancer* 2000 Jul;83(1):95–7.
6. Baserga, R. The insulin-like growth factor-I receptor as a target for cancer therapy. *Expert Opin Ther Targets* 2005 Aug;9(4):753–68.
7. Keum, YS, WS Jeong, AN Kong. Chemopreventive functions of isothiocyanates. *Drug News Perspect* 2005 Sept;18(7):445–51.
8. Munday, R, CM Munday. Induction of phase II enzymes by aliphatic sulfides derived from garlic and onions: an overview. *Methods Enzymol* 2004;382:449–56.
9. McCarty, MF, J Barroso-Aranda, F Contreras. A two-phase strategy for treatment of oxidant-dependent cancers. *Med Hypotheses* 2007 May 12; np.
10. Brar, SS, TP Kennedy, M Quinn, JR Hoidal. Redox signaling of NF-kappaB by membrane NAD(P)H oxidases in normal and malignant cells. *Protoplasma* 2003 May;221(1–2):117–27.
11. Wu, WS. The signaling mechanism of ROS in tumor progression. *Cancer Metastasis Rev* 2006 Dec;25(4):695–705.
12. Pugh, N, SA Ross, HN ElSohly, MA ElSohly, DS Pasco. Isolation of three high molecular weight polysaccharide preparations with potent immunostimulatory activity from Spirulina platensis, aphanizomenon flos-aquae and Chlorella pyrenoidosa. *Planta Med* 2001 Nov;67(8):737–42.
13. "Laxatives: Proceed with Caution." HCIC, Web 11/28/12. consumer-health.com/services/LaxativesProceedwithCaution.php

14. Schachter, MB. Integrative oncology for clinicians and cancer patients. *Journal of Orthomolecular Medicine* 2010;25(4):169–94.

Chapter 3

1. "How Cells Communicate During the Fight or Flight Response." Web 06/13/12. learn.genetics.utah.edu/content/begin/cells/fight_flight/
2. Dhabhar, FS. A hassle a day may keep the pathogens away: The fight-or-flight stress response and the augmentation of immune function. *Integrative & Comparative Biology* 2009;49(3):215–36.
3. García, A, O Martí, A Vallès, S Dal-Zotto, A Armario. Recovery of the hypothalamic-pituitary-adrenal response to stress.*Neuroendocrinology* 2000;72(2):114–25.
4. Caligiuri, MA. Human natural killer cells. *Blood* 2008;112(3):461–9.
5. Boscolo, P, A Donato, L Giampaolo, L Forcella, M Reale, V Dadorante, F Alparone, S Pagliaro, M Kouri, A Magrini, E Fattorini. Blood natural killer activity is reduced in men with occupational stress and job insecurity working in a university. *International Archives of Occupational and Environmental Health* 2009;82(6):787–94.
6. Segerstrom, SC. Resources, stress, and immunity: an ecological perspective on human psychoneuroimmunology. *Annals of Behavioral Medicine* 2010;40(1):114–25.
7. Valentinuzzi, ME. Neuroendocrinology and its quantitative development: a bioengineering view. BioMedical Engineering Online. Institute of Biomedical Engineering, University of Buenos Aires, 2010. Web 06/14/12. biomedical-engineering-online.com/content/9/1/68
8. Ein-Dor, T, M Mikulincer, PR.Shaver. Attachment insecurities and the processing of threat-related information: studying the schemas involved in insecure people's coping strategies. *Journal of Personality and Social Psychology* 2011, np.
9. Stansbury, JP, M Mathewson-Chapman, KE Grant. Gender schema and prostate cancer: veterans' cultural model of masculinity. *Medical Anthropology* 2003;22(2):175-204.
10. Carpenter, KM, BL Andersen, JM Fowler, GL Maxwell. Sexual self schema as a moderator of sexual and psychological outcomes for gynecologic cancer survivors. *Archives of Sexual Behavior* 2009;38(5):828–41.
11. Kopala-Sibley, D, D Santor. The mediating role of automatic thoughts in the personality-event-affect relationship. *Cognitive Behaviour Therapy* 2009;38(3):153–61.

Chapter 4

1. Suh, J, AB Rabson. NF-kappaB activation in human prostate cancer: important mediator or epiphenomenon? J *Cell Biochem* 2004 Jan 1;91(1):100–17.
2. Sclabas, GM, S Fujioka, C Schmidt, DB Evans, PJ Chiao. NF-kappaB in pancreatic cancer. *Int J Gastrointest Cancer* 2003;33(1):15–26.
3. Chang, AA, C Van Waes. Nuclear factor-KappaB as a common target and activator of oncogenes in head and neck squamous cell carcinoma. *Adv Otorhinolaryngol* 2005;62:92–102.
4. Wu, JT, JG Kral. The NF-kappaB/IkappaB signaling system: a molecular target in breast cancer therapy. *J Surg Res* 2005 Jan;123(1):158–69.
5. Yu, YY, Q Li, ZG Zhu. NF-kappaB as a molecular target in adjuvant therapy of gastrointestinal carcinomas. *Eur J Surg Oncol* 2005 May;31(4):386–92.
6. Takada, Y, A Murakami, BB Aggarwal. Zerumbone abolishes NF-kappaB and IkappaBalpha kinase activation leading to suppression of antiapoptotic and metastatic gene expression, upregulation of apoptosis, and downregulation of invasion. *Oncogene* 2005 Jun 27, np.
7. Bentires-Alj, M, V Barbu, M Fillet, A Chariot, B Relic, N Jacobs, J Gielen, MP Merville, V Bours. NF-kappaB transcription factor induces drug resistance through MDR1 expression in cancer cells. *Oncogene* 2003 Jan 9;22(1):90–7.
8. Arlt, A, J Vorndamm, M Breitenbroich, UR Folsch, H Kalthoff, WE Schmidt, H Schafer. Inhibition of NF-kappaB sensitizes human pancreatic carcinoma cells to apoptosis induced by etoposide (VP16) or doxorubicin. *Oncogene* 2001 Feb 15;20(7):859–68.

9. Arlt, A, H Schafer. NFkappaB-dependent chemoresistance in solid tumors. *Int J Clin Pharmacol Ther* 2002 Aug;40(8):336-47.
10. Jung, M, A Dritschilo. NF-kappa B signaling pathway as a target for human tumor radiosensitization. *Semin Radiat Oncol* 2001 Oct;11(4):346-51.
11. Nakanishi, C, M Toi. Nuclear factor-kappaB inhibitors as sensitizers to anticancer drugs. *Nat Rev Cancer* 2005 Apr;5(4):297-309.
12. Huang, S, JB Robinson, A Deguzman, CD Bucana, IJ Fidler. Blockade of nuclear factor-kappaB signaling inhibits angiogenesis and tumorigenicity of human ovarian cancer cells by suppressing expression of vascular endothelial growth factor and interleukin 8. *Cancer Res* 2000 Oct 1;60(19): 5334-9.
13. Tisdale, MJ. Cancer cachexia. *Langenbecks Arch Surg* 2004 Aug;389(4):299-305.
14. Chell, S, A Kaidi, AC Williams, C Paraskeva. Mediators of PGE2 synthesis and signalling downstream of COX-2 represent potential targets for the prevention/treatment of colorectal cancer. *Biochim Biophys Acta* 2006 Aug;1766(1):104-19.
15. Sminia, P, G Kuipers, A Geldof, V Lafleur, B Slotman. COX-2 inhibitors act as radiosensitizer in tumor treatment. *Biomed Pharmacother* 2005 Oct;59 Suppl 2:S272-5.
16. Meric, JB, S Rottey, K Olaussen, JC Soria, D Khayat, O Rixe, JP Spano. Cyclooxygenase-2 as a target for anticancer drug development. *Crit Rev Oncol Hematol* 2006 Jul;59(1):51-64.
17. Nie, D. Cyclooxygenases and lipoxygenases in prostate and breast cancers. *Front Biosci* 2007; 12:1574-85.
18. Eisinger, AL, SM Prescott, DA Jones, DM Stafforini. The role of cyclooxygenase-2 and prostaglandins in colon cancer. *Prostaglandins Other Lipid Mediat* 2007 Jan;82(1-4):147-54.
19. Liao, Z, KA Mason, L Milas. Cyclo-oxygenase-2 and its inhibition in cancer: is there a role? *Drugs* 2007;67(6):821-45.
20. Zeddou, M, R Greimers, N de Valensart, B Nayjib, K Tasken, J Boniver, M Moutschen, S Rahmouni. Prostaglandin E2 induces the expression of functional inhibitory CD94/NKG2A receptors in human CD8+ T lymphocytes by a cAMP-dependent protein kinase A type I pathway. *Biochem Pharmacol* 2005 Sept 1;70(5):714-24.
21. Klein, S, AR de Fougerolles, P Blaikie, L Khan, A Pepe, CD Green, V Koteliansky, FG Giancotti. Alpha 5 beta 1 integrin activates an NF-kappa B-dependent program of gene expression important for angiogenesis and inflammation. *Mol Cell Biol* 2002 Aug;22(16):5912-22.
22. Gately, S, WW Li. Multiple roles of COX-2 in tumor angiogenesis: a target for antiangiogenic therapy. *Semin Oncol* 2004 Apr;31(2 Suppl 7):2-11.
23. Williams, CS, M Tsujii, J Reese, SK Dey, RN DuBois. Host cyclooxygenase-2 modulates carcinoma growth. *J Clin Invest* 2000 Jun;105(11):1589-94.
24. Ghosh, J, CE Myers. Inhibition of arachidonate 5-lipoxygenase triggers massive apoptosis in human prostate cancer cells. *Proc Natl Acad Sci USA* 1998 Oct 27;95(22):13182-7.
25. Ding, XZ, WG Tong, TE Adrian. Multiple signal pathways are involved in the mitogenic effect of 5(S)-HETE in human pancreatic cancer. *Oncology* 2003;65(4):285-94.
26. Ihara, A, K Wada, M Yoneda, N Fujisawa, H Takahashi, A Nakajima. Blockade of leukotriene B4 signaling pathway induces apoptosis and suppresses cell proliferation in colon cancer. *J Pharmacol Sci* 2007 Jan;103(1):24-32.
27. Tong, WG, XZ Ding, RC Witt, TE Adrian. Lipoxygenase inhibitors attenuate growth of human pancreatic cancer xenografts and induce apoptosis through the mitochondrial pathway. *Mol Cancer Ther* 2002 Sept;1(11):929-35.
28. Tsukada, T, K Nakashima, S Shirakawa. Arachidonate 5-lipoxygenase inhibitors show potent antiproliferative effects on human leukemia cell lines. *Biochem Biophys Res Commun* 1986 Nov 14;140(3):832-36.
29. Ghosh, J, CE Myers. Arachidonic acid stimulates prostate cancer cell growth: critical role of 5-lipoxygenase. *Biochem Biophys Res Commun* 1997 Jun 18;235(2):418-23.
30. Avis, I, SH Hong, A Martinez, T Moody, YH Choi, J Trepel, R Das, M Jett, JL Mulshine. Five-lipoxygenase inhibitors can mediate apoptosis in human breast cancer cell lines through complex eicosanoid interactions. *FASEB J* 2001 Sept;15(11):2007-9.

31. Fan, XM, SP Tu, SK Lam, WP Wang, J Wu, WM Wong, MF Yuen, MC Lin, HF Kung, BC Wong. Five-lipoxygenase-activating protein inhibitor MK-886 induces apoptosis in gastric cancer through upregulation of p27kip1 and bax. *J Gastroenterol Hepatol* 2004 Jan;19(1):31–7.
32. Hoque, A, SM Lippman, TT Wu, Y Xu, ZD Liang, S Swisher, H Zhang, L Cao, JA Ajani, XC Xu. Increased 5-lipoxygenase expression and induction of apoptosis by its inhibitors in esophageal cancer: a potential target for prevention. *Carcinogenesis* 2005 Apr;26(4):785–91.
33. Matsuyama, M, R Yoshimura, M Mitsuhashi, K Tsuchida, Y Takemoto, Y Kawahito, H Sano, T Nakatani. 5-Lipoxygenase inhibitors attenuate growth of human renal cell carcinoma and induce apoptosis through arachidonic acid pathway. *Oncol Rep* 2005 Jul;14(1):73–9.
34. Hayashi, T, K Nishiyama, T Shirahama. Inhibition of 5-lipoxygenase pathway suppresses the growth of bladder cancer cells. *Int J Urol* 2006 Aug;13(8):1086–91.
35. Rose, DP. JM Connolly, XH Liu. Fatty acid regulation of breast cancer cell growth and invasion. *Adv Exp Med Biol* 1997;422:47–55.
36. Hardman, WE. (n-3) fatty acids and cancer therapy. *J Nutr 2004* Dec;134(12 Suppl):3427S-30S.
37. Wen, B, E Deutsch, P Opolon, A Auperin, V Frascogna, E Connault, J Bourhis. n-3 polyunsaturated fatty acids decrease mucosal/epidermal reactions and enhance antitumour effect of ionising radiation with inhibition of tumour angiogenesis. *Br J Cancer* 2003 Sept 15;89(6):1102–07.
38. Hardman, WE, L Sun, N Short, IL Cameron. Dietary omega-3 fatty acids and ionizing irradiation on human breast cancer xenograft growth and angiogenesis. *Cancer Cell Int* 2005 Apr 28;5(1):12.
39. McCarty, MF. Fish oil may impede tumour angiogenesis and invasiveness by down-regulating protein kinase C and modulating eicosanoid production. *Med Hypoth* 1996 Feb;46(2):107–15.
40. Rose, DP, JM Connolly. Regulation of tumor angiogenesis by dietary fatty acids and eicosanoids. *Nutr Cancer* 2000;37(2):119–27.
41. Murota, SI, M Onodera, I Morita. Regulation of angiogenesis by controlling VEGF receptor. *Ann N Y Acad Sci* 2000 May;902:208–12.
42. Shtivelband, MI, HS Juneja, S Lee, KK Wu. Aspirin and salicylate inhibit colon cancer medium- and VEGF-induced endothelial tube formation: correlation with suppression of cyclooxygenase-2 expression. *J Thromb Haemost* 2003 Oct.;1(10):2225–33.
43. Tisdale, MJ. Wasting in cancer. *J Nutr* 1999 Jan;129(1S Suppl):243S–6S.
44. Whitehouse, AS, HJ Smith, JL Drake, MJ Tisdale. Mechanism of attenuation of skeletal muscle protein catabolism in cancer cachexia by eicosapentaenoic acid. *Cancer Res* 2001 May 1;61(9):3604–9.
45. Wigmore, SJ, MD Barber, JA Ross, MJ Tisdale, KC Fearon. Effect of oral eicosapentaenoic acid on weight loss in patients with pancreatic cancer. *Nutr Cancer* 2000;36(2):177–84.
46. Fearon, KC, MF von Meyenfeldt, AG Moses, R Van Geenen, A Roy, DJ Gouma, A Giacosa, A Van Gossum, J Bauer, MD Barber, NK Aaronson, AC Voss, MJ Tisdale. Effect of a protein and energy dense N-3 fatty acid enriched oral supplement on loss of weight and lean tissue in cancer cachexia: a randomised double blind trial. *Gut* 2003 Oct;52(10):1479–86.
47. Zi, X, R Agarwal. Silibinin decreases prostate-specific antigen with cell growth inhibition via G1 arrest, leading to differentiation of prostate carcinoma cells: implications for prostate cancer intervention. *Proc Natl Acad Sci USA* 1999 Jun 22;96(13):7490–5.
48. Kang, SN, MH Lee, KM Kim, D Cho, TS Kim. Induction of human promyelocytic leukemia HL-60 cell differentiation into monocytes by silibinin: involvement of protein kinase C. *Biochem Pharmacol* 2001 Jun; 15;61(12):1487–95.
49. Sharma, G, RP Singh, DC Chan, R Agarwal. Silibinin induces growth inhibition and apoptotic cell death in human lung carcinoma cells. *Anticancer Res* 2003 May;23(3B):2649–55.
50. Qi, L, RP Singh, Y Lu, R Agarwal, GS Harrison, A Franzusoff, LM Glode. Epidermal growth factor receptor mediates silibinin-induced cytotoxicity in a rat glioma cell line. *Cancer Biol Ther* 2003 Sept;2(5):526–31.
51. Agarwal, C, RP Singh, S Dhanalakshmi, AK Tyagi, M Tecklenburg, RA Sclafani, R Agarwal. Silibinin upregulates the expression of cyclin-dependent kinase inhibitors and causes cell cycle arrest and apoptosis in human colon carcinoma HT-29 cells. *Oncogene* 2003 Nov 13;22(51):8271–82.

52. Tyagi, AK, C Agarwal, RP Singh, KR Shroyer, LM Glode, R Agarwal. Silibinin down-regulates survivin protein and mRNA expression and causes caspases activation and apoptosis in human bladder transitional-cell papilloma RT4 cells. *Biochem Biophys Res Commun* 2003 Dec 26;312(4): 1178–84.
53. Varghese, L, C Agarwal, A Tyagi, RP Singh, R Agarwal. Silibinin efficacy against human hepatocellular carcinoma. *Clin Cancer Res* 2005 Dec 1;11(23):8441–48.
54. Lee, SO, YJ Jeong, HG Im, CH Kim, YC Chang, IS Lee. Silibinin suppresses PMA-induced MMP-9 expression by blocking the AP-1 activation via MAPK signaling pathways in MCF-7 human breast carcinoma cells. *Biochem Biophys Res Commun* 2007 Mar 2;354(1):165–71.
55. Tyagi, AK, C Agarwal, DC Chan, R Agarwal. Synergistic anticancer effects of silibinin with conventional cytotoxic agents doxorubicin, cisplatin and carboplatin against human breast carcinoma MCF-7 and MDA-MB468 cells. *Oncol Rep* 2004 Feb;11(2):493–99.
56. Singh, RP, R Agarwal. A cancer chemopreventive agent, silibinin, targets mitogenic and survival signaling in prostate cancer. *Mutat Res* 2004 Nov 2;555(1–2):21–32.
57. Hannay, JA, D Yu. Silibinin: a thorny therapeutic for EGF-R expressing tumors? *Cancer Biol Ther* 2003 Sept;2(5):532–33.
58. Singh, RP, S Dhanalakshmi, AK Tyagi, DC Chan, C Agarwal, R Agarwal. Dietary feeding of silibinin inhibits advance human prostate carcinoma growth in athymic nude mice and increases plasma insulin-like growth factor-binding protein-3 levels. *Cancer Res* 2002 Jun 1;62(11):3063–69.
59. Singh, RP, G Sharma, S Dhanalakshmi, C Agarwal, R Agarwal. Suppression of advanced human prostate tumor growth in athymic mice by silibinin feeding is associated with reduced cell proliferation, increased apoptosis, and inhibition of angiogenesis. *Cancer Epidemiol Biomarkers Prev* 2003 Sept;12(9):933–39.
60. Gallo, D, S Giacomelli, C Ferlini, G Raspaglio, P Apollonio, S Prislei, A Riva, P Morazzoni, E Bombardelli, G Scambia. Antitumour activity of the silybin-phosphatidylcholine complex, IdB 1016, against human ovarian cancer. *Eur J Cancer* 2003 Nov;39(16):2403–10.
61. Singh, RP, S Dhanalakshmi, C Agarwal, R Agarwal. Silibinin strongly inhibits growth and survival of human endothelial cells via cell cycle arrest and downregulation of survivin, Akt and NF-kappaB: implications for angioprevention and antiangiogenic therapy. *Oncogene* 2005 Feb 10;24(7):1188–1202.
62. Yang, SH, JK Lin, WS Chen, JH Chiu. Anti-angiogenic effect of silymarin on colon cancer LoVo cell line. *J Surg Res* 2003 July;113(1):133–8.
63. Cao, Y, R Cao. Angiogenesis inhibited by drinking tea. *Nature* 1999 Apr 1;398(6726):381.
64. Jung, YD, MS Kim, BA Shin, KO Chay, BW Ahn, W Liu, CD Bucana, GE Gallick, LM Ellis. EGCG, a major component of green tea, inhibits tumour growth by inhibiting VEGF induction in human colon carcinoma cells. *Br J Cancer* 2001 Mar 23;84(6):844–50.
65. Pisters, KM, RA Newman, B Coldman, DM Shin, FR Khuri, WK Hong, BS Glisson, JS Lee. Phase I trial of oral green tea extract in adult patients with solid tumors. *J Clin Oncol* 2001 Mar 15;19(6):1830–8.
66. Lamy, S, D Gingras, R Beliveau. Green tea catechins inhibit vascular endothelial growth factor receptor phosphorylation. *Cancer Res* 2002 Jan 15;62(2):381–5.
67. Ammon, HP. Boswellic acids in chronic inflammatory diseases. *Planta Med* 2006 Oct;72(12):1100–16.
68. Catalano, A, P Caprari, S Soddu, A Procopio, M Romano. 5-lipoxygenase antagonizes genotoxic stress-induced apoptosis by altering p53 nuclear trafficking. *FASEB J* 2004 Nov;18(14):1740–2.
69. Wenger, FA, M Kilian, M Bisevac, C Khodadayan, M von Seebach, I Schimke, H Guski, JM Muller. Effects of Celebrex and Zyflo on liver metastasis and lipidperoxidation in pancreatic cancer in Syrian hamsters. *Clin Exp Metastasis* 2002;19(8):681–7.
70. Liu, JJ, A Nilsson, S Oredsson, V Badmaev, WZ Zhao, RD Duan. Boswellic acids trigger apoptosis via a pathway dependent on caspase-8 activation but independent on Fas/Fas ligand interaction in colon cancer HT-29 cells. *Carcinogenesis* 2002 Dec;23(12):2087–93.
71. Zhao, W, F Entschladen, H Liu, B Niggemann, Q Fang, KS Zaenker, R Han. Boswellic acid acetate induces differentiation and apoptosis in highly metastatic melanoma and fibrosarcoma cells. *Cancer Detect Prev* 2003;27(1):6775.

72. Syrovets, T, JE Gschwend, B Buchele, Y Laumonnier, W Zugmaier, F Genze, T Simmet. Inhibition of IkappaB kinase activity by acetyl-boswellic acids promotes apoptosis in androgen-independent PC-3 prostate cancer cells in vitro and in vivo. *J Biol Chem* 2005 Feb 18;280(7):6170–80.
73. Xia, L, D Chen, R Han, Q Fang, S Waxman, Y Jing. Boswellic acid acetate induces apoptosis through caspase-mediated pathways in myeloid leukemia cells. *Mol Cancer Ther* 2005 Mar;4(3):381–8.
74. Liu, JJ, B Huang, SC Hooi. Acetyl-keto-beta-boswellic acid inhibits cellular proliferation through a p21-dependent pathway in colon cancer cells. *Br J Pharmacol* 2006 Aug;148(8):1099–107.
75. Janssen, G, U Bode, H Breu, B Dohrn, V Engelbrecht, U Gobel. Boswellic acids in the palliative therapy of children with progressive or relapsed brain tumors. *Klin Padiatr* 2000 Jul;212(4):189–95.
76. Streffer, JR, M Bitzer, M Schabet, J Dichgans, M Weller. Response of radiochemotherapy-associated cerebral edema to a phytotherapeutic agent, H15. *Neurology* 2001 May 8;56(9):1219–21.
77. Winking, M, S Sarikaya, A Rahmanian, A Jodicke, DK Boker. Boswellic acids inhibit glioma growth: a new treatment option? *J Neurooncol* 2000;46(2):97–103.
78. Whittle, BJ, D Hansen, JA Salmon. Gastric ulcer formation and cyclo-oxygenase inhibition in cat antrum follows parenteral administration of aspirin but not salicylate. *Eur J Pharmacol* 1985 Oct 8;116(1–2):153–7.
79. Zambraski, EJ, DC Atkinson, J Diamond. Effects of salicylate vs. aspirin on renal prostaglandins and function in normal and sodium-depleted dogs. *J Pharmacol Exp Ther* 1988 Oct;247(1):96–103.
80. Cryer, B, M Goldschmiedt, JS Redfern, M Feldman. Comparison of salsalate and aspirin on mucosal injury and gastroduodenal mucosal prostaglandins. *Gastroenterology* 1990 Dec;99(6):1616–21.
81. Kopp, E, S Ghosh. Inhibition of NF-kappa B by sodium salicylate and aspirin. *Science* 1994 Aug 12;265(5174):956–9.
82. Yin, MJ, Y Yamamoto, RB Gaynor. The anti-inflammatory agents aspirin and salicylate inhibit the activity of I(kappa)B kinase-beta. *Nature* 1998 Nov 5;396(6706):77–80.
83. Borthwick, GM, AS Johnson, M Partington, J Burn, R Wilson, HM Arthur. Therapeutic levels of aspirin and salicylate directly inhibit a model of angiogenesis through a Cox-independent mechanism. *FASEB J* 2006 Oct;20(12):2009–16.
84. McCarty, MF, KI Block. Preadministration of high-dose salicylates, suppressors of NF-kappaB activation, may increase the chemosensitivity of many cancers: an example of proapoptotic signal modulation therapy. *Integr Cancer Ther* 2006 Sept;5(3):252–68.
85. McCarty, MF, KI Block. Toward a core nutraceutical program for cancer management. *Integr Cancer Ther* 2006 Jun;5(2):150–71.
86. McPherson, TC. Salsalate for arthritis: a clinical evaluation. *Clin Ther* 1984;6(4):388–403.
87. Boettcher, FA, RJ Salvi. Salicylate ototoxicity: review and synthesis. *Am J Otolaryngol* 1991 Jan;12(1):33–47.
88. Cryer, B, M Feldman. Cyclooxygenase-1 and cyclooxygenase-2 selectivity of widely used non-steroidal anti-inflammatory drugs. *Am J Med* 1998 May;104(5):413–21.
89. Van, HA, JI Schwartz, M Depré, I de Lepeleire, A Dallob, W Tanaka, K Wynants, A Buntinx, J Arnout, PH Wong, DL Ebel, BJ Gertz, PJ De Schepper. Comparative inhibitory activity of rofecoxib, meloxicam, diclofenac, ibuprofen, and naproxen on COX-2 versus COX-1 in healthy volunteers. *J Clin Pharmacol* 2000 Oct;40(10):1109–20.
90. Jick, SS, JA Kaye, H Jick. Diclofenac and acute myocardial infarction in patients with no major risk factors. *Br J Clin Pharmacol* 2007 Nov;64(5):662–7.
91. Lovborg, H, F Oberg, L Rickardson, J Gullbo, P Nygren, R Larsson. Inhibition of proteasome activity, nuclear factor-KappaB translocation and cell survival by the antialcoholism drug disulfiram. *Int J Cancer* 2006 Mar 15;118(6):1577–80.
92. Chen, D, QC Cui, H Yang, QP Dou. Disulfiram, a clinically used anti-alcoholism drug and copper-binding agent, induces apoptotic cell death in breast cancer cultures and xenografts via inhibition of the proteasome activity. *Cancer Res* 2006 Nov 1;66(21):10425–33.
93. Zavrski, I, L Kleeberg, M Kaiser, C Fleissner, U Heider, J Sterz, C Jakob, O Sezer. Proteasome as an emerging therapeutic target in cancer. *Curr Pharm Des* 2007;13(5):471–85.
94. Mrs. Ruiz is the aunt of Dr. Francisco Contreras and the great aunt of Daniel Kennedy.

Chapter 5

1. Howes, RM. Cancer therapy: a review with scientific validation for the role of electronically modified oxygen derivatives in oncologic treatment modalities. *Internet Journal of Alternative Medicine* 2010;8(1):6.
2. Clavo, B, JL Perez, L Lopez, G Suarez, M Lloret, V Rodriguez, D Macias, M Santana, MA Hernandez, R Martin-Oliva, F Robaina. Ozone therapy for tumor oxygenation: a pilot study. *Evid Based Complement Alternat Med* 2004 Jun 1;1(1):93–8.
3. Menéndez, S, J Cepero, L Borrego. Ozone therapy in cancer treatment: state of the art. *Ozone: Science & Engineering* 2008;30(6):398–404.
4. Liu, Q, X He. Clinical evaluation of sequential medical ozone therapy for primary liver cancer patients after transarterial chemoembolization. *International Journal of Ozone Therapy* 2012; 11(1):53–5.
5. Ogawa, K, Y Yoshii, O Inoue, T Toita, A Saito, Y Kakinohana, T Ariga, G Kasuya, S Murayama. Phase II trial of radiotherapy after hyperbaric oxygenation with chemotherapy for high-grade gliomas. *British Journal of Cancer* 2006;95(7):862–68.
6. E.g., K Chong, NB Hampson, DG Bostwick, RL Vessella, JM Corman. Hyperbaric oxygen does not accelerate latentin vivoprostate cancer: implications for the treatment of radiation-induced haemorrhagic cystitis. *BJU International* 2004;94(9):1275–78.
7. Aydinoz, S, G Uzun, H Cermik, E Atasoyu, S Yildiz, B Karagoz, R Evrenkaya. (2007). Effects of different doses of hyperbaric oxygen on cisplatin-induced nephrotoxicity. *Renal Failure* 2007;29(3):257–63.
8. Ibid.
9. Bradley Palmer and his family are missionaries who coordinate an orphanage (Boys and Girls Christian Home Ministries, Chandur Bazar, Central India [bgchm.org]).

Chapter 6

1. Shadyac, T. (1998). *Patch Adams*. Universal City, CA: Universal Pictures.
2. Reiner, R. (2008). *The Bucket List*. Burbank, CA: Warner Brothers Pictures.
3. Johnston, R. Aristotle's De Anima: on why the soul is not a set of capacities. *British Journal for the History of Philosophy* 2011;19.2:185–200.
4. Greer, S. Psycho-oncology: its aims, achievements and future tasks. *Psycho-Oncology* 1994;3:87–101.
5. Deshields, TL, SK Nanna. Providing care for the "whole patient" in the cancer setting: the psycho-oncology consultation model of patient care.*Journal of Clinical Psychology in Medical Settings* 2010;17.3:249–57.
6. Breitbart, W, Y Alici. Psycho-oncology. *Harvard Review of Psychiatry* 2009;17.6:361–76.
7. Greer, JA, ER Park, HG Prigerson, SA Safren. Tailoring cognitive-behavioral therapy to treat anxiety comorbid with advanced cancer. *Journal of Cognitive Psychotherapy* 2010;4.4:294–313.
8. Mehnert, A, U Koch. Prevalence of acute and post-traumatic stress disorder and comorbid mental disorders in breast cancer patients during primary cancer care: a prospective study. *Psycho-Oncology* 2007;16.3:181–88.
9. Tavoli, A, A Montazeri, R Roshan, Z Tavoli, M Melyani. Depression and quality of life in cancer patients with and without pain: the role of pain beliefs. *BMC Cancer* 2008;8.1:177.
10. O'Connor, M, S Christensen, A Jensen, S Moller, R Zachariae. How traumatic is breast cancer?" *British Journal of Cancer* 2011;104.3:419–26.
11. Jacobsen, J, B Zhang, S Block, P Maciejewski, H Prigerson. Distinguishing symptoms of grief and depression in a cohort of advanced cancer patients. *Death Studies* 2010;34.3:257–73.
12. Smith, N. Cancer patients, newly-diagnosed: providing emotional support. *CINAHL Nursing Guide* (2012):5.
13. Chan, M, S Ho, R Tedeschi, C Leung. The valence of attentional bias and cancer-related rumination in postraumatic stress and posttraumatic growth among women with breast cancer. *Psycho-Oncology* 2011;20:544–52.

14. Deacon, BJ, TI Fawzy, JJ Lickel, KB Wolitzky-Taylor. Cognitive defusion versus cognitive restructuring in the treatment of negative self-referential thoughts: an investigation of process and outcome. *Journal of Cognitive Psychotherapy* 2011;25.3:218–32.
15. Dryden, W, D David. Rational emotive behavior therapy: current status. *Journal of Cognitive Psychotherapy* 2008;22.3:195–209.
16. Nekolaichuk, CL, C Cumming, J Turner, A Yushchyshyn, R Sela. Referral patterns and psychosocial distress in cancer patients accessing a psycho-oncology counseling service. *Psycho-Oncology* 2011;20.3:326–32.

Chapter 7

1. Sun, Y. Free radicals, antioxidant enzymes, and carcinogenesis. *Free Radic Biol Med* 1990;8(6):583–99.
2. Kwei, KA, JS Finch, EJ Thompson, GT Bowden. Transcriptional repression of catalase in mouse skin tumor progression. *Neoplasia* 2004 Sept;6(5):440–8.
3. Tas, F, H Hansel, A Belce, S Ilvan, A Argon, H Camlica, E Topuz. Oxidative stress in breast cancer. *Med Oncol* 2005;22(1):11–15.
4. Arnold, RS, J Shi, E Murad, AM Whalen, CQ Sun, R Polavarapu, S Parthasarathy, JA Petros, JD Lambeth. Hydrogen peroxide mediates the cell growth and transformation caused by the mitogenic oxidase Nox1. *Proc Natl Acad Sci USA* 2001 May 8;98(10):5550–5.
5. Vaquero, EC, M Edderkaoui, SJ Pandol, I Gukovsky, AS Gukovskaya. Reactive oxygen species produced by NAD(P)H oxidase inhibit apoptosis in pancreatic cancer cells. *J Biol Chem* 2004 Aug 13;279(33):34643–54.
6. Lim, SD, C Sun, JD Lambeth, F Marshall, M Amin, L Chung, JA Petros, RS Arnold. Increased Nox1 and hydrogen peroxide in prostate cancer. *Prostate* 2005 Feb 1;62(2):200–7.
7. Arnold, RS, et al. Hydrogen peroxide mediates . . . Nox1. *Proc Natl Acad Sci USA*: 5550–5.
8. Chen, Q, MG Espey, MC Krishna, JB Mitchell, CP Corpe, GR Buettner, E Shacter, M Levine. Pharmacologic ascorbic acid concentrations selectively kill cancer cells: action as a pro-drug to deliver hydrogen peroxide to tissues. *Proc Natl Acad Sci USA* 2005 Sept 20;102(38):13604–9.
9. Chen, Q, MG Espey, AY Sun, JH Lee, MC Krishna, E Shacter, PL Choyke, C Pooput, KL Kirk, GR Buettner, M Levine. Ascorbate in pharmacologic concentrations selectively generates ascorbate radical and hydrogen peroxide in extracellular fluid in vivo. *Proc Natl Acad Sci USA* 2007 May 22;104(21):8749–54.
10. Cameron, E, L Pauling. *Proc. Natl. Acad. Sci. USA* 1976; 73:3685–89; Cameron E, A Campbell. The orthomolecular treatment of cancer. II. Clinical trial of high-dose ascorbic acid supplements in advanced human cancer. *Chem Biol Interact.* 1974 Oct;9(4):285–315.
11. Moertel, CG, ET Creagan, JR O'Fallon, AJ Schutt, MJ O'Connell, J Rubin, S Frytak. Failure of high-dose vitamin C (ascorbic acid) therapy to benefit patients with advanced cancer. A controlled trial. *N Engl J Med* 1979 Sep 27;301(13):687–90.
12. Padayatty, SJ, H Sun, Y Wang, HD Riordan, SM Hewitt, A Katz, RA Wesley, M Levine. Vitamin C pharmacokinetics: implications for oral and intravenous use. *Ann Intern Med* 2004 Apr 6;140(7):533–7.
13. Padayatty, SJ, M Levine. Reevaluation of ascorbate in cancer treatment: emerging evidence, open minds and serendipity. *J Am Coll Nutr* 2000 Aug;19(4):423–5.
14. Riordan, HD, JJ Casciari, MJ Gonzalez, NH Riordan, JR Miranda-Massari, P Taylor, JA Jackson. A pilot clinical study of continuous intravenous ascorbate in terminal cancer patients. *P R Health Sci J* 2005 Dec;24(4):269–76.
15. Padayatty, SJ, HD Riordan, SM Hewitt, A Katz, LJ Hoffer, M Levine. Intravenously administered vitamin C as cancer therapy: three cases. *CMAJ* 2006 March 28;174(7):937–42.
16. Gonzalez, M. (2012). Schedule dependence in cancer therapy: intravenous vitamin C and the systemic saturation hypothesis. *J Orth Med* 2012;27(1):9–12.
17. Calderon PB, J Cadrobbi, C Marques, N Hong-Ngoc, JM Jamison, J Gilloteaux, JL Summers, HS Taper. Potential therapeutic application of the association of vitamins C and K3 in cancer treatment. *Curr Med Chem* 2002 Dec;9(24):2271–85.

18. Verrax J, J Stockis, A Tison, HS Taper, PB Calderon. Oxidative stress by ascorbate/menadione association kills K562 human chronic myelogenous leukaemia cells and inhibits its tumour growth in nude mice. *Biochem Pharmacol* 2006 Sept 14;72(6):671–80.
19. Taper HS, JM Jamison, J Gilloteaux, JL Summers, PB Calderon. Inhibition of development of metastases by dietary vitamin C:K3 combination. *Life Sci* 2004 Jul 9;75(8):955–67.
20. Tetef M, K Margolin, C Ahn, S Akman, W Chow, P Coluzzi, L Leong, RJ Morgan Jr, J Raschko, S Shibata . Mitomycin C and menadione for the treatment of advanced gastrointestinal cancers: a phase II trial. *J Cancer Res Clin Oncol* 1995;121(2):103–6.
21. Tetef M, K Margolin, C Ahn, S Akman, W Chow, L Leong, RJ Morgan Jr, J Raschko, G Somlo, JH Doroshow. Mitomycin C and menadione for the treatment of lung cancer: a phase II trial. *Invest New Drugs* 1995;13(2):157–62.
22. Smolowe, J. Neil Armstrong (cover story). *People* 2012;78(11):88.
23. Benade, L, T Howard, D Burk: Suynergistic killing of Ehrlich ascites carcinoma cells by ascorbate and 3-amino-1,2,4, -triazole. *Oncology* 1969;23:33–43.

Chapter 8

1. "Sørensen, Søren Peter Lauritz (1868–1939)." *100 Distinguished European Chemists*. European Association for Chemical and Molecular Sciences. Retrieved 10/14/11.
2. Gillies, RJ, N Raghunand, ML Garcia-Martin, RA Gatenby. pH imaging. A review of pH measurement methods and applications in cancers. *IEEE Eng Med Biol Mag* 2004;23:57–64
3. Moss, R. Simoncini's Bicarbonate Treatment for Cancer. *Townsend Letter* 2009;(317):28–30.
4. Silva, AS, JA Yunes, RJ Gillie, RA Gatenby. The potential role of systemic buffers in reducing intratumoral extracellular pH and acid-mediated invasion, *Cancer Res* 2009;69(6):2677–84.
5. Ibid.
6. McCarty, MF, J Whitaker. Manipulating tumor acidification as a cancer treatment strategy. *Alternative Medicine Review* 2010;15(3):264–72.
7. Udelnow, A, A Kreyes, S Ellinger, K Landfester, P Walther, T Klapperstueck, J Wohlrab, D Henne-Bruns, U Knippschild, P Würl. Omeprazole inhibits proliferation and modulates autophagy in pancreatic cancer cells. *Plos ONE* 2011;6(5):1–17.
8. Gerweck LE, S Vijayappa, S Kozin. Tumor pH controls the in vivo efficacy of weak acid and base chemotherapeutics. *Molecular Cancer Therapies* 2006;5(5):1275–9.

Chapter 9

1. Unknown. *The Two Wolves Within*. Cherokee Nation folklore story.
2. Silver-Hassell, D. (1995). Food is essential but not sufficient: emotional issues in macrobiotic healing. *Macrobiotics Today* 1995;35(4):7.
3. Smith, WR, HH Sebastian. Emotional history and pathogenesis of cancer. *Journal of Clinical Psychology* 1976;32(4):863–866.
4. Hamer, RG. Changes of the skin: part 2. *Total Health* 2001;2(1):1.
5. Bergner, S. Seductive symbolism: psychoanalysis in the context of oncology. *Psychoanalytic Psychology* 2011;2:267–92.
6. Kübler-Ross, E. *On Death and Dying*. New York: Macmillan, np, 1969.
7. Grief negatively impacts physical health among soldiers post-deployment. (2012). San Diego: US Navy, Bureau of Medicine and Surgery (BUMED).
8. John 11:35. *The Holy Bible: New International Version*. Colorado Springs, CO: International Bible Society, 1984.
9. Kissen, DM, HG Hysenk. Personality in male lung cancer patients. *J Psychoso Res* (1962).
10. Gossarth-Maticek, R. Psychosocial factors as strong predictors of mortality from cancer: ischaemic heart disease and stroke. The Yugoslav prospective study. *J Psychoso Res*. 1985;29(2).
11. De La Mora, Sergio. *The Heart Revolution*. Grand Rapids, MI: Baker, 2011. Print.

12. Greene, WA Jr. Psychological factors & reticuloendothelial disease. Preliminary observations on a group of males with lymphomas and leukemias. *Pschoso Med* 1954;16:220–230.
13. Russek, L, G Schwartz. Narrative descriptions of parental love and caring predict health status in midlife: a 35-year follow-up of the Harvard Mastery of Stress Study. *Alternative Therapies in Health and Medicine* 1996;2(6):55–62.
14. Harris, GA. Early childhood emotional trauma: an important factor in the aetiology of cancer and other diseases. *European Journal of Clinical Hypnosis* 2006;7(2):2–10.
15. Johnson, G. The BLAME game. *Alive: Canada's Natural Health & Wellness Magazine* 2012;(354):35–39.
16. Luskin, F. *Forgive for Good: A Proven Prescription for Health and Happiness.* San Francisco: Harper-SanFrancisco, 2002.
17. See Matthew 6:9–13.
18. Jacinto, GA, BL Edwards. Therapeutic stages of forgiveness and self-forgiveness. *Journal of Human Behavior in the Social Environment* 2011;21(4):423–37.
19. Hong, Y, G Jacinto. Six-step therapeutic process to facilitate forgiveness of self and others. *Clinical Social Work Journal* 2012;40(3):366–75.
20. "Virginia Satir." *Virginia Satir.* np, nd. Web. 12/12/12.
21. Hart, LK, MI Freel, PJ Haylock, SK Lutgendorf. The use of healing touch in integrative oncology. *Clinical Journal of Oncology Nursing* 2011;15(5):519–25.
22. Galatians 5:22-23. *Holy Bible: New Living Translation.* Wheaton, IL: Tyndale, 1996.
23. Hawks, S.. Spiritual health: definition and theory. *Wellness Perspectives* 1994;10(4):3.

Chapter 10

1. Sinclair, KD, et al. DNA methylation, insulin resistance, and blood pressure in offspring determined by maternal periconceptional B vitamin and methionine status. *Proc Natl Acad Sci USA* 2007;104:19351–6.
2. Kotsopoulos, J, et al. Postweaning dietary folate deficiency provided through childhood to puberty permanently increases genomic DNA methylation in adult rat liver. *J Nutr.* 2008;138:703–9.
3. Lillycrop, KA, et al. Feeding pregnant rats a protein-restricted diet persistently alters the methylation of specific cytosines in the hepatic PPAR alpha promoter of the offspring. *Br J Nutr.* 2008;100:278–82.
4. Jimenez-Chillaron, JC, E Isganaitis, et al. (2009). Intergenerational transmission of glucose intolerance and obesity by in utero undernutrition in mice. *Diabetes* 2009 Feb;58(2):460–8.
5. Waterland, RA, RL Jirtle. Maternal dietary methyl donor supplementation affects offspring phenotype by increasing cytosine methylation at the agouti locus in Avy mice. *FASEB Journal* 2002;16(4):A228.
6. Dolinoy DC, JR Weidman, RA Waterland, RL Jirtle. Maternal genistein alters coat color and protects Avy mouse offspring from obesity by modifying the fetal epigenome. *Environmental Health Perspectives* 2006;114:567–72.
7. Bygren, LO, et al. Longevity determined by paternal ancestors' nutrition during their slow growth period. *Acta Biotheoretica*; 2001;49(1):53–9.
8. Kaati, G, LO Bygren, M Pembrey, M Sjostrom. Transgenerational response to nutrition, early life circumstances and longevity. *European Journal of Human Genetics*, 2007;15:784–90.
9. Contreras, F. *The Hope of Living Long and Well.* Lake Mary, FL: Siloam, 2000.

Chapter 11

1. Levy, S, G Sutton, P Ng, L Feuk, A Halpern, B Walenz, . . . J Venter. The diploid genome sequence of an individual human. *Plos Biology* 2007;5(10):e254.
2. McLendon, R, A Friedman, D Bigner, EG Van Meir, DJ Brat, GM Mastrogianakis, . . . A Sabo. (2008). Comprehensive genomic characterization defines human glioblastoma genes and core pathways. *Nature* 2008;455(7216):1061–8
3. Li, L, P Goedegebuure, ER Mardis, MC Ellis, Z Xiuli, JM Herndon, . . . WE Gillanders. Cancer genome sequencing and its implications for personalized cancer vaccines. *Cancers* 2011;3(4):4191–211.

4. Wood, L.D., *et al.* (2007). The genomic landscapes of human breast and colorectal cancers. *Science* 318 (5853): 8–9.
5. International consortium to tackle cancer genomes. *Nature* 2008;453(7191).
6. Kaiser, J. A skeptic questions cancer genome projects. *Science Insider* 2010 Apr 23.

Chapter 12

1. "Cancer Facts & Figures 2013." Cancer.org. American Cancer Society, nd. Web. 02/11/13.
2. "Genetics." Breastcancer.org. np, nd. Web. 02/11/13.
3. Rosenthal, T, S Puck. Screening for genetic risk of breast cancer. *American Family Physician* 1999;59(1):99–104.
4. Hartmann, L, D Schaid, J Woods, T Crotty, J Myers, P Arnold, . . . R Jenkins. Efficacy of bilateral prophylactic mastectomy in women with a family history of breast cancer. *The New England Journal of Medicine* 1999;340(2):77–84.
5. Eisen A, BL Weber. Prophylactic mastectomy—the price of fear. *The New England Journal of Medicine* 1999 Jan 14;340(2).
6. Healy, B. BRCA genes—bookmaking, fortunetelling, and medical care. *The New England Journal of Medicine* 1997;336(20):1448–9.
7. Ibid., 1449.
8. Fuller, S, F Liebens, B Carly, A Pastijn, S Rozenberg. Breast cancer prevention in BRCA1/2 mutation carriers: a qualitative review. *The Breast Journal* 2008;14(6):603–4.
9. Rossouw JE, GL Anderson, RL Prentice, et al. Risks and benefits of estrogen plus progestin in healthy postmenopausal women. Principal results from the Women's Health Initiative randomized controlled trial. *JAMA* 2002;288:321–33.
10. Jarvinen HJ, et al. Controlled 15-year trial on screening for colorectal cancer in families with hereditary nonpolyposis colorectal cancer. *Gastroenterology* 2000;118:829–34.
11. Hugues, Aschard. Inclusion of gene-gene and gene-environment interactions unlikely to dramatically improve risk prediction for complex diseases. *The American Journal of Human Genetics* 2012;90.6:1116.

Chapter 13

1. Early Breast Cancer Trialists' Collaborative Group. Polychemotherapy for early breast cancer: an overview of the randomised trials. *Lancet*;1998;352(9132):930–42.
2. Brennan, DJ, SL O'Brien, A Fagan, AC Culhane, DG Higgins, MJ Duffy, WM Gallagher. Application of DNA microarray technology in determining breast cancer prognosis and therapeutic response. *Expert Opinion on Biological Therapy* 2005;5(8):1069–83.
3. Staunton, JE. Chemosensitivity prediction by transcriptional profiling. *Proceedings of the National Academy of Sciences* 2001;98(19):10787–92.
4. Tuma, Rabiya S. TUMA RS: trial and error: prognostic gene signature study design altered. *Journal of the National Cancer Institute* 2005;97: 331–3.

Chapter 14

1. Kucharski, R, J Foret, R Maleszka. Nutritional control of reproductive status in honeybees via DNA methylation.*Science* 2008;319:1827-30.
2. Cloud, John. Your DNA is not your destiny. *Time Magazine* (2010): np.

Chapter 15

1. Teen who fled chemo may be heading to Mexico. AP; 2009. Web. Retr. 07/04/12. msnbc.msn.com/id/30824587/ns/health-childrens_health/t/teen-who-fled-chemo-may-be-heading-mexico/
2. Contreras, F. CNN interview; 2009. Retr. 07/04/12. youtube.com/watch?v=em3YDg1Gokc
3. Wyngaarden, JB, LH Smith. *Cecil Textbook of Medicine*. Vol 2. Philadelphia: Saunders, 1988.

4. Abel, U. *The Chemotherapy of Advanced Epithelial Cancers.* Stuttgart: Hippokrates Verlag, 1990.
5. Braverman, A. Medical oncology in the 90s. *Lancet*; 1991 Apr 13(337):901.
6. Bailar III, JC, EM Smith. (1986). Progress against cancer. *New England Journal of Medicine*, 314:1226–32.
7. "Cancer Facts & Figures 2007." cancer.org; American Cancer Society. Retr. 12/12/08.
8. Surveillance, Epidemiology, and End Results Program. Center for Disease Control, Division of Cancer Control and Population Sciences (2006):1975–2000.
9. Waugh, N. Health technology assessment in cancer: A personal view from public health. *European Journal of Cancer* 2006;42(17)2876–80.
10. Mead, GM. Chemotherapy for solid tumours: Routine treatment not yet justified. *British Medical Journal* 1995 Jan 28;310(6974):246–47.
11. Dickson, M. The cost of new drug discovery and development. *Discovery Medicine* 2004;4(22):177.
12. Morgan, G, R Ward, M Barton. The contribution of cytotoxic chemotherapy to 5-year survival in adult malignancies. *Clinical Oncology* 2004;16(8):549–60.
13. Feinberg, BA, AS Bruno, S Haislip, J Gilmore, J Gagan, and JL. Whyte. Hemoglobin trends and anemia treatment resulting from concomitant chemotherapy in community oncology clinics. *Journal of Oncology Practice* 2012;8.1:18–24.
14. Contreras, F, and LE. Connealy. Patients with metastatic cancer treated with integrative regulatory therapy. *Townsend Letter* Aug/Sep 2012;(349–50):51–6.
15. Swain, S. Chemotherapy: updates and new perspectives. *The Oncologist* 2011;16:1:30–39.
16. Coghlan, A. Multitasking drug keeps cancer at bay. *New Scientist* 2012;213(2854):14.
17. Palumbo, A, SV Rajkumar. Multiple myeloma: chemotherapy or transplantation in the era of new drugs. *European Journal of Haematology* 2010;84.5:379–90.
18. Vermorken, J. A new look at induction chemotherapy in locally advanced head and neck cancer. *The Oncologist* 2010;15 Suppl:31–2.
19. Coleman, M, G Ruan, R Elstrom, P Martin, J Leonard. Metronomic therapy for refractory/relapsed lymphoma: the PEP-C low-dose oral combination chemotherapy regimen. *Hematology* 2012;17 Suppl:1S90–S92.
20. Beniwal, SK, KM Patel, SS Shukla, BJ Parikh, SS Shah, AA Patel. Gemcitabine in brief versus prolonged low-dose infusion, both combined with carboplatin for advanced non-small cell lung cancer. *Indian Journal of Cancer* 2012 49(2):202–08.

Chapter 16

1. New IMV research study shows increased implementation of EMR by radiation therapy providers. IMV Medical Information Division. nd. Web. 02/12/13.
2. Warren, JL, KR Yabroff, A Meekins, M Topor, EB Lamont, ML Brown. Evaluation of trends in the cost of initial cancer treatment." *Journ NCI* 2008;100.12:888–97.
3. Delaney, G, S Jacob, C Featherstone, M Barton. The role of radiotherapy in cancer treatment: estimating optimal utilization from a review of evidence-based clinical guidelines. *Erratum: Cancer Journal* 2006;107.3:660.
4. "Cancer Facts & Figures 2013." cancer.org. American Cancer Society, nd. Web. 02/12/13.
5. Bogdanich W, reporting; S Akam, A Lehren, D Lieberman, K Rebelo, RR. Ruiz, contributing. The radiation boom: a lifesaving tool turned deadly. *New York Times*, 01/24/10. Web. 02/12/13.
6. Lundeen, R, S Abraham. (2006). Developing business ventures for radiation therapy services: understanding the key issues. *Journal of Health Care Finance* 2006;32(4):39–45.
7. Larson DB, LW Johnson, BM Schnell, MJ Goske, SR Salisbury, HP Forman. Rising use of CT in child visits to the emergency department in the US, 1995–2008. *Radiology* 2011;259(3):793–801.
8. Hughes, JS, MC O'Riordan. Radiation exposure of the UK population—1993 review. *NRPB-R263* 1993: np.
9. Andersen, A, L Barlow, A Engeland, K Kjaerheim, E Lynge, E Pukkala. Work-related cancer in the Nordic countries. *Scandinavian Journal of Work Environmental Health* 1999;25.2:1–116.
10. Weiss, JF, MR Landauer. History and development of radiation-protective agents. *International Journal of Radiation Biology* 2009;85(7):539–73.

Chapter 17

1. Porter, R. *The Greatest Benefit to Mankind: A Medical History of Humanity.* New York: WW Norton and CO., 1999. p.188
2. "The Avalon Project : Code of Hammurabi." Trans. L. W. King. N.p., n.d. Web. 08 June 2013. <http://avalon.law.yale.edu/ancient/hamframe.asp>
3. Sherer, A, F Epstein, S Constantini. Hua Tuo, patron of surgeons, or how the surgeon lost his head! *Surgical Neurology.* 2004;61.5:497–8.
4. Lucena, SM. America 1492: retrato de un continente hace quinientos años. *Anaya Editores Milano* (1990).
5. Silverman, M. (1951). Broken Legs Mended Quick. Saturday Evening Post, 223 (49), 30.
6. Goleria, K, RE Rana. The history of the plastic surgery department, K.E.M. Hospital, Mumbai, India. *Indian Journal of Plastic Surgery* 2004;37(2):136–42.
7. Gawande, A. Two hundred years of surgery. *The New England Journal of Medicine.* 2012;366(18):1716–23.
8. Ibid.
9. National Hospital Discharge Survey: procedures by selected patient characteristics; number by procedure category and age (2010). Web. cdc.gov/nchs/fastats/insurg.htm
10. Partridge, E, AR Kreimer, RT Greenlee, C Williams, JL Xu, TR Church, et al. Results from four rounds of ovarian cancer screening in a randomized trial. *Obstetrics and Gynecology* 2009;113(4):775–82.

Chapter 18

1. Bann, C, F Sirois, E Walsh. Provider support in complementary and alternative medicine: exploring the role of patient empowerment. *Journal of Alternative & Complementary Medicine* 2010;16(7):745–52.
2. Stang, I, M Mittelmark. Intervention to enhance empowerment in breast cancer self-help groups. *Nursing Inquiry* 2010;17(1):46–56.
3. Siegel, BS. *101 Exercises for the Soul: A Divine Workout Plan for Body, Mind, and Spirit.* Novato, CA: New World Library, 2005.
4. Ibid.
5. Interview with Dr. Bernie Siegel. *Townsend Letter* 2006 (270):96–8.

Chapter 19

1. Frankl, VE. *Man's Search for Meaning.* Boston: Beacon, 2006.
2. Schulenberg, SE, RR Hutzell, C Nassif, JM Rogina. Logotherapy for clinical practice. *Psychotherapy: Theory, Research, Practice, Training* 2008;45(4):447–63.
3. Bleger, J. (2012). Theory and practice in psychoanalysis: psychoanalytic praxis. The *International Journal of Psycho-Analysis* 2012;93(4):993–1003.
4. Del Corso, JJ, MC Rehfuss, K Galvin. Striving to adapt: addressing adler's work task in the 21st century. *Journal of Individual Psychology* 2011;67(2):88–106.
5. Ibid.
6. Nietzsche, F. *Die Götzen-Dämmerung—Twilight of the Idols.* Trans. W Kaufmann and RJ Hollingdale. Leipzig: np, 1889.
7. Sherman, AC, S Simonton, U Latif, L Bracy. Effects of global meaning and illness-specific meaning on health outcomes among breast cancer patients. *Journal of Behavioral Medicine* 2010;33.5: 364–77.
8. Mok, E, KP Lau, WM Lam, LN Chan, JS Ng, KS Chan. Healthcare professionals' perceptions of existential distress in patients with advanced cancer. *Journal of Advanced Nursing* 2010;66.7:1510–22.
9. Greenstein, M, W Breitbart. Cancer and the experience of meaning: a group psychotherapy program for people with cancer. *American Journal of Psychotherapy* 2000;54.4: 486–500.
10. "Sing Hosanna." *Hymns Old & New.* Edmunds, Suffolk: Kevin Mayhew, 2008.
11. Contreras, F. *The Hope of Living Cancer Free.* Lake Mary, FL: Siloam, 1999. Print.

Chapter 20

1. Cara, S. Redmond's looking to help torchbearer Dad over the line this time. *Mail on Sunday* (02/12/12): 17.

2. Gaining the competitive edge. *Training Journal* (2012):14.
3. Shrira, A, Y Palgi, J Wolf, Y Haber, O Goldray, E Shacham-Shmueli, M Ben-Ezra. The positivity ratio and functioning under stress. *Stress & Health: Journal of the International Society for the Investigation of Stress* 2011;27(4):265–71.
4. Tucker, J. Modification of attitudes to influence survival from breast cancer. Lancet 1999; 354(9187):1320.
5. O'Baugh, J, L Wilkes, S Luke, A George. "Being positive": perceptions of patients with cancer and their nurses. *Journal of Advanced Nursing* 2003;44(3):262–70.
6. Psalm 118:17 NIV
7. Note: David Kennedy is Daniel Kennedy's father and Dr. Contreras's brother-in-law.
8. See Daniel 3:1–30.
9. Daniel 3:16–18 NIV
10. Daniel 3:25 NIV
11. Dr. Francisco Contreras was consulted in this case for an extra opinion, but the curative surgery was performed in the US.

Chapter 21

1. "National Cancer Act of 1971." NCI. Web. 12/14/12. legislative.cancer.gov/history/phsa/1971
2. DeVita, VR. (2002). "A perspective on the war on cancer." *Cancer Journal* 2002;8(5), 352–6.
3. Ibid.
4. Sikora, K. "We're winning the war against cancer." *The Telegraph* 18 Dec 2009. Web. 12/14/12. telegraph.co.uk/health/6837951/Were-winning-the-war-on-cancer.html
5. Begley, S, A Underwood, J Interlandi, M Carmichael. "We fought cancer . . . and cancer won." *Newsweek* 2008;152(11):42–66.
6. "Cancer Survivors—United States, 2007." Centers for Disease Control and Prevention 11 Mar 2011. Web. 12/14/12.
7. Ibid.
8. "Cancer Statistics Review 1975-2009." National Cancer Institute, nd. Web. 12/14/12. seer.cancer.gov/csr/1975_2009_pops09/results_merged/sect_01_overview.pdf
9. Ibid.
10. Nearly 800,000 deaths prevented due to declines in smoking: NIH study examines the impact of tobacco control policies and programs, and the potential or further reduction in lung cancer deaths. (2012). Bethesda, MD: NIH and US Department of Health and Human Services.
11. Ibid.
12. Ibid.
13. "Cancer Facts & Figures 2013." American Cancer Society. Web. 02/07/13. cancer.org/research/cancerfactsfigures/cancerfactsfigures/cancer-facts-figures-2013

Chapter 22

1. "Joseph Vissarionovich Stalin." *Columbia Electronic Encyclopedia*, 6th ed (Nov 2011).
2. Montefiore, S. History and Biography. *History Today*, 2004;54(3):30–1.
3. "Cancer Facts & Figures 2012." American Cancer Society, nd. Web. 12/18/12. cancer.org/acs/groups/content/@epidemiologysurveilance/documents/document/acspc-031941.pdf
4. Hock, MF, DD Deshler, JB Schumaker. Enhancing student motivation through the pursuit of possible selves. *Journal of Education Research* 2011;5(3/4):197–213.
5. Miller, Mike. Understanding Cancer Statistics. *NCI Benchmarks*. nd. Web. 12/18/12.
6. Drapkin, J. (2005). An ounce of prevention. *Psychology Today* 2005;38(5):23.
7. Guidelines: exercise, healthy diet lower risk of cancer recurrence. *Urology Times* 2012;40(7):70.
8. Sasieni, PD, JJ Shelton, NN Ormiston-Smith, CS Thomson, PB Silcocks. What is the lifetime risk of developing cancer?: the effect of adjusting for multiple primaries. *British Journal of Cancer* 2011;105(3), 460–5.

9. Abraham, G, A Kowalczyk, S Loi, I Haviv, J Zobel. Prediction of breast cancer prognosis using geneset statistics provides signature stability and biological context. *BMC Bioinformatics* 2010;11277–91.
10. Lichtenberg, FR. Are increasing 5-year survival rates evidence of success against cancer? A reexamination using data from the U.S. and Australia. *Forum for Health Economics & Policy* 2010;13(2):1–18.
11. Tai, P, E Yu, G Cserni, G Vlastos, M Royce, I Kunkler, V Vinh-Hung. Minimum follow-up time required for the estimation of statistical cure of cancer patients: verification using data from 42 cancer sites in the SEER database. *BMC Cancer* 2005;548–9.
12. Bryant, H, G Lockwood, R Rahal MBA, L Ellison. Conditional survival in Canada: adjusting patient prognosis over time. *Current Oncology* 2012;19(4):222–4.
13. Binbing, Y, RC Tiwari, EJ Feuer. Estimating the personal cure rate of cancer patients using population-based grouped cancer survival data. *Statistical Methods in Medical Research* 2011;20(3):261–74.
14. Wegwarth, O, L Schwarts, S Woloshin, W Gaissmaier, G Gigerenzer. Do physicians understand cancer screening statistics? A national survey of primary care physicians in the United States. *Annals of Internal Medicine* 2012;156:340–9.
15. Clegg LX, ME Reichman, BA Miller, BF Hankey, GK Singh, YD Lin, MT Goodman, CF Lynch, SM Schwartz, VW Chen, L Bernstein, SL Gomez, JJ Graff, CC Lin, NJ Johnson, B Edwards. Impact of socioeconomic status on cancer incidence and stage at diagnosis: selected findings from the surveillance, epidemiology, and end results: National Longitudinal Mortality Study. *Cancer Causes & Control: CCC* 2009;20(4):417–35.

Chapter 23

1. Andersson, TL, PW Dickman, S Eloranta, PC Lambert. Estimating and modeling cure in population-based cancer studies within the framework of flexible parametric survival models. *BMC Medical Research Methodology* 2011;11(1):96–106.
2. Berlinger, N, A Flamm. Define "effective": the curious case of chronic cancer. *Hastings Center Report* 2009;39(6):17–20.
3. Sawyer, D. Stand Up to Cancer. *ABC News Special Report* (2010), 1.

Chapter 24

1. Quirk, WJ. Too big to fail and too risky to exist. *American Scholar* 2012;81(4):31–43.
2. Ibid.
3. Ibid.
4. Cutler, DM. Are we finally winning the war on cancer? *Journal of Economic Perspectives* 2008;22.4: 3–26.
5. "Cancer Facts & Figures 2012." American Cancer Society, nd. Web. 11/15/12. cancer.org/acs/groups/content/@epidemiologysurveilance/documents/document/acspc-031941.pdf
6. The Obama-Biden plan to combat cancer. BarackObama.com Obama for America, nd. Web. 11/15/12. obama.3cdn.net/f8a8d6b8b4b370d888_24lmvygeu.pdf
7. de Kok, IM JJ Polder, JD Habbema, LM Berkers, WJ Meerding, M Rebolj, M. van Ballegooijen. "The impact of healthcare costs in the last year of life and in all life years gained on the cost-effectiveness of cancer screening." *British Journal of Cancer* 2009;100.8:1240–4.
8. Konski, A. The war on cancer: progress at what price? *Journal of Clinical Oncology* 2011;29.12:1503–4.
9. The 2011-2016 Outlook for Cancer Therapies in The Americas & the Caribbean. (2011). Regional Outlook Reports, N.PAG.
10. Wagner, L, M Lacey. The hidden costs of cancer care: an overview with implications and referral resources for oncology nurses. *Clinical Journal of Oncology Nursing* 2004;8(3):279–87.
11. Lauzier, S, E Maunsell, M Drolet, D Coyle, N Hébert-Croteau. Validity of information obtained from a method for estimating cancer costs from the perspective of patients and caregivers. *Quality of Life Research* 2010;19(2):177–89.
12. Kendall, D. Managing the modern disease: is cancer the next frontier for employers? *Benefits Quarterly* 2012;28(1):22–5.

13. Tan, A, DH Freeman, BU Philips. Estimating the cost of cancer care for a state. *Texas Public Health Journal* 2011;63(4):18–21.
14. Kaltwasser, J. Pharma considers personalization, competition into drug costs. *Njbiz* 2012;25(6):16.
15. Dranitsaris, G, I Truter, MS Lubbe, E Amir, W Evans. Advances in cancer therapeutics and patient access to new drugs. *Pharmacoeconomics* 2011;29(3):213–24.
16. Karaca-Mandic, P, JS McCullough, AS Mustaqueem H Van Houten, ND Shah, N. D. Impact of new drugs and biologics on colorectal cancer treatment and costs. *Journal of Oncology Practice* (2011):e30s-e37s.
17. Bodenheimer, T, RA Berenson, P Rudolf. The primary care/specialty income gap: why it matters. *Annals of Internal Medicine* 2007;146(4):301–76.
18. Barkley, R.R, TU Guidi. Oncologist-hospital alignment models built to compensate oncologists Ffairly. *Journal of Oncology Practice* 2011;7(4):263–6.
19. Gilbar, PJ. (2011). Should the Pharmaceutical Industry be doing more to Reduce the Cost of Cancer Drugs?. Journal Of Pharmacy Practice & Research 2011;41(1), 4-5.
20. Gatesman, M, T Smith. The shortage of essential chemotherapy drugs in the United States. *The New England Journal of Medicine* 365(18):1653–5.
21. Ibid.
22. *The Nation's Investment in Cancer Research: An Annual Plan and Budget Proposal for Fiscal Year 2012.* National Cancer Institute, nd. Web. 11/15/12. cancer.gov/PublishedContent/Files/aboutnci/budget_planning_leg/plan-archives/nci_plan.pdf#page=58
23. Guy, GP, DU Ekwueme. Years of potential life lost and indirect costs of melanoma and non-melanoma skin cancer. *PharmacoEconomics* 2011;29.10:863–74.
24. van Lent, W, R de Beer, W van Harten. International benchmarking of specialty hospitals. A series of case studies on comprehensive cancer centres. *BMC Health Services Research* (2010):10253.
25. Schickedanz, A. Of value: A discussion of cost, communication, and evidence to improve cancer care. *The Oncologist* 2010;15 Suppl:s173-9.

Chapter 25

1. Urry, M. *The Mysteries of Dark Energy*. Yale, 2008. MP3.
2. Gamow, G. *My World Line: An Informal Autobiography*. New York: Viking, 1970.
3. Starfield, B. Is US health really the best in the world? *Journal of American Medical Association* 2000;284(4):483–5. (These deaths include from negative drug effects [non-error], from hospital infections, from miscellaneous hospital errors, from unnecessary surgery, and from medication errors in hospitals.)

Chapter 26

1. "Fleming Discovers Penicillin." PBS, nd. Web. 01/03/13.
2. "The Discovery of X-Rays." *The Discovery of X-Rays*. np, nd. 01/03/13.
3. "Evolution of Cancer Treatments: Radiation." American Cancer Society, nd. Web. 01/03/13.
4. FAQ: clinical trial phases. U.S. National Library of Medicine, 18 Apr 2008. Web. 01/03/13. ClinicalTrials.gov
5. Strauss, B. Best hope or last hope: access to phase III clinical trials of HER-2/neu for advanced stage breast cancer patients. *Journal of Advanced Nursing* 2000;31.2: 259–66.
6. Grünwald, HW. Ethical and design issues of phase I clinical trials in cancer patients. *Cancer Investigation* 2007;25.2:124–6.
7. Sargent, D, J Taylor. Current issues in oncology drug development, with a focus on phase II trials. *Journal of Biopharmaceutical Statistics* 2009;19.3:556–62.
8. Ibid.
9. Cox, K, J Mcgarry. Why patients don't take part in cancer clinical trials: an overview of the literature. *European Journal of Cancer Care* 2003;12.2:114–22.

10. Ibid.
11. Badlucco, S, KK Reed. Supporting quality and patient safety in cancer clinical trials. *Clinical Journal of Oncology Nursing* 2011;15.3:263–5.
12. Stamatakos, GS, EC Georgiadi, N Graf, EA Kolotroni, DD Dionysiou. Exploiting clinical trial data drastically narrows the window of possible solutions to the problem of clinical adaptation of a multiscale cancer model. *PLoS One* 2011;E17594 6.3:1–11.

Chapter 27

1. "Albert Einstein Quotes." Xplore, nd. Web. 01/15/13. BrainyQuote.com
2. Gever, J. Cancer deaths stay on downward path. *MedPage Today*. nd. Web. 01/24/13.
3. Trubek, LG, TR Oliver, L Chih-Ming, M Mokrohisky, T Campbell. Improving cancer outcomes through strong networks and regulatory frameworks: lessons from the United States and the European Union. *Journal of Health Care Law & Policy* 2011;14(1):119–51.
4. James, R, J Yu, N Henrikson, D Bowen, S Fullerton. Strategies and stakeholders: minority recruitment in cancer genetics research. *Community Genetics* 2008;11(4):241–9.
5. Khayat, D, D Kerr. Science and society: a new model for cancer research in France. *Nature Reviews Cancer* 2006;6(8):645–51.
6. Franklin, B. "Ounce of prevention." Web. 24 Jan 2013. USHistory.org
7. "Fruits and Vegetables." Centers for Disease Control and Prevention. Web. 18 June 2012. 05/16/13.
8. Thomson, CA, PA Thompson. Fruit and vegetable intake is associated with lower risk of ER-negative breast cancer. NCI. *Journal of the National Cancer Institute*. 24 Jan 2013. Web. 05/16/13.
9. Drapkin, J. (2005). An ounce of prevention. *Psychology Today* 2005;38(5):23.
10. Guidelines: exercise, healthy diet lower risk of cancer recurrence. *Urology Times* 2012; 40(7):70.
11. Gupta, VK, P Gupta, RK Songara. Empowering W.H.O. as a global authority and centralized pool of resources for speedy development of orphan drugs at reduced cost. *Journal of Pharmaceutical Sciences & Research* 2010;2(12):844–52.
12. Stead, M, D Cameron, N Lester, M Parmar, R Haward, R Kaplan, . . . P Selby. Strengthening clinical cancer research in the United Kingdom. *British Journal of Cancer* 2011;104(10):1529–34.
13. Bharath, EN, SN Manjula, AA Vijaychand. In Silico drug design-tool for overcoming the innovation deficit in the drug discovery process. *International Journal of Pharmacy & Pharmaceutical Sciences* 2011;3(2):8–12.

Chapter 28

1. Clark, E. His own way. *Yankee* 2005;69(1):72.
2. *Billy Best*. nd. Web. 12 Dec 2012. billybest.net
3. E.g., see quackwatch.org/search/webglimpse.cgi?ID-1&query-Burzynski
4. O'Connor, C. Steve Jobs tried to treat cancer with "magical thinking." *Biographer*. Forbes.com (2011):26.
5. London, WM. Celebrity publicizes choice of dubious cancer treatment following coverage of her liposuction. *NCAHF Newsletter* 2001;24(3):2.
6. "Alternative Medicine." NCI, nd. Web. 12 Dec 2012. cancer.gov/dictionary?CdrID-44921
7. "Complementary Medicine." NCI, nd. Web. 12 Dec 2012. cancer.gov/dictionary?CdrID-44951
8. "Integrative Medicine." NCI, nd. Web. 12 Dec 2012. cancer.gov/dictionary?CdrID-689097
9. "Complementary and Alternative Medicine." NCI, nd. Web. 12 Dec 2012. cancer.gov/dictionary?CdrID-44964
10. "Conventional Medicine." NCI, nd. Web. 12 Dec 2012. cancer.gov/dictionary?CdrID-449752
11. Kaegi, E. Unconventional therapies for cancer: 6. 714-X. Task Force on Alternative Therapeutic of the Canadian Breast Cancer Research Initiative. *CMAJ: Canadian Medical Association Journal* 1998;158(12):1621–4.
12. Consumer Health Articles: The Gerson therapy for cancer: part I. Consumer Health Organization, nd. Web. 01 June 2012.

13. Obituaries. Cancer treatment pioneers. *Journal of Alternative & Complementary Medicine*, 1998; 4(2):137–45.
14. Kulp, K, J Montgomery, D Nelson, B Cutter, E Latham, D Shattuck, . . . L Bennett. Essiac and Flor-Essence herbal tonics stimulate the in vitro growth of human breast cancer cells. *Breast Cancer Research and Treatment* 2006;98(3):249–59.
15. Saltzberg, F, G Barron, N Fenske. Deforming self-treatment with herbal "black salve." *Dermatologic Surgery* 2009;35(7):1152–4.
16. Haley, D. Ten cancer cures that worked. *Consumer Health Newsletter* 2003;26(9):1–8.
17. Ibid.
18. Hoang, B, S Levine, D Shaw, D Tran, H Tran, P Nguyen, . . . P Pham. Dimethyl sulfoxide as an excitatory modulator and its possible role in cancer pain management. *Inflammation & Allergy Drug Targets* 2010;9(4):306–12.
19. Milazzo, S. Laetrile treatment for cancer. *Cochrane Database of Systematic Reviews* (2011):11.
20. Krashen, SD. Inaccurate reporting of the effects of laetrile: mistreatment of Ellison, Byar and Newell (1978) in professional papers. *Internet Journal of Alternative Medicine* 2008;6(2):4.
21. Green, S. Shark cartilage therapy against cancer. *Nutrition & Health Forum* 1997;14(1):1.
22. Chen, K, C Hsieh, C Peng, H Hsieh-Li, H Chiang, K Huang, RY Peng. Brain derived metastatic prostate cancer DU-145 cells are effectively inhibited in vitro by guava (Psidium gujava L.) leaf extracts. *Nutrition & Cancer* 2007;58(1):93–106.
23. Sharma, M, A Sharma, A Kumar. Vital medicine asparagus racemosus willd. *Current Trends in Biotechnology & Pharmacy* 2012;6(2):210–21.
24. Ezekiel 47:12 NLT

Chapter 29

1. Christman, JK, G Sheikhnejad, M Dizik, S Abileah, E Wainfan. Reversibility of changes in nucleic acid methylation and gene expression induced in rat liver by severe dietary methyl deficiency. *Carcinogenesis* 1993;14(4):551–7.
2. Fang, M, D Chen, CS Yang. Dietary polyphenols may affect DNA methylation. *The Journal of Nutrition* 2007;137:S223–8.
3. Dashwood, R, E Ho. Dietary histone deacetylase inhibitors: from cells to mice to man. *Seminars in Cancer Biology* 2007;17.5:363–9.
4. Qin, W, W Zhu, H Shi, J Hewett, R Ruhlen, R MacDonald, G Rottinghaus, YC Chen, E Sauter. Soy isoflavones have an antiestrogenic effect and alter mammary promoter hypermethylation in healthy premenopausal women. *Nutrition and Cancer* 2009;61.2:238–44.
5. Bingham, S, E Riboli. Diet and cancer—the European Prospective Investigation into Cancer and Nutrition. *Nature Reviews Cancer* 2004;4.3:206–15.

Chapter 30

1. Llosa L. *Sniper.* Hollywood: TriStar Pictures, 1993.
2. Fuqua, A. *Shooter.* Hollywood: Paramount Pictures, 2007.
3. Afraites, L, A Atlas, A Bellouquid, M Ch-Chaoui. Modeling the complex immune system response to cancer cells. *Mathematics in Engineering, Science & Aerospace (MESA)* 2012;3(3):269–83.
4. Lissoni P. Is there a role for melatonin in supportive care? *Support Care Cancer* 2002;10(2):110–6.
5. Lee, S, S Kim, J Youn, S Hwang, C Park, Y Park. MicroRNA and gene expression analysis of melatonin-exposed human breast cancer cell lines indicating involvement of the anticancer effect. *Journal of Pineal Research* 2011;51(3):345–52.
6. Lissoni P. Biochemotherapy with standard chemotherapies plus the pineal hormone melatonin in the treatment of advanced solid neoplasms. *Pathol Biol* (Paris) 2007;55(3–4):201–4.
7. Nunnari G, L Nigro, F Palermo, D Leto, RJ Pomerantz, B Cacopardo. Reduction of serum melatonin levels in HIV-1-infected individuals' parallel disease progression: correlation with serum interleukin-12 levels. *Infection* 2003;31(6):379–82.

8. Miller G, S Lahrs, RP Dematteo. Overexpression of interleukin-12 enables dendritic cells to activate NK cells and confer systemic antitumor immunity. *FASEB J* 2003;17(6):728–30.
9. Del VM, E Bajetta, S Canova, MT Lotze, A Wesa, G Parmiani, A Anichini. Interleukin-12: biological properties and clinical application. *Clin Cancer Res* 2007;13(16):4677–85.
10. Kumar, M, A Kumar, R Nagpal, D Mohania, P Behare, V Verma, . . . H Yadav. Cancer-preventing attributes of probiotics: an update. *International Journal of Food Sciences & Nutrition* 2010; 61(5):473–96.
11. Gayathri, DD, TN Devaraja. Lactobacillus sp. as probiotics for human health with special emphasis on colorectal cancer. *Indian Journal of Science & Technology* 2011;4(8):1008–14.
12. Koizumi SI, D Wakita, T Sato, R Mitamura, T Izumo, H Shibata, Y Kiso, K Chamoto, Y Togashi, H Kitamura T Nishimura. Essential role of toll-like receptors for dendritic cell and NK1.1(+) cell-dependent activation of type 1 immunity by Lactobacillus pentosus strain S-PT84. *Immunol Lett* 2008 Jul 11.
13. Mohamadzadeh M, S Olson, WV Kalina, G Ruthel, GL Demmin, KL Warfield, S Bavari, TR Klaenhammer. Lactobacilli activate human dendritic cells that skew T cells toward T helper 1 polarization. *Proc Natl Acad Sci USA* 2005;102(8):2880–5.
14. Hoarau C, C Lagaraine, L Martin, F Velge-Roussel, Y Lebranchu. Supernatant of Bifidobacterium breve induces dendritic cell maturation, activation, and survival through a toll-like receptor 2 pathway. *J Allergy Clin Immunol* 2006;117(3):696–702.
15. Dallal, M, M Mojarrad, Z Salehipour, H Mashhad, R Raoofian, Z Rajabi. Effects of probiotic lactobacillus acidophilus and lactobacillus casei on the behavior of colorectal tumor cells. (English). *Tehran University Medical Journal* 2012;70(4):220–7.
16. Roy M, L Kiremidjian-Schumacher, HI Wishe, MW Cohen, G Stotzky. Supplementation with selenium and human immune cell functions. I. Effect on lymphocyte proliferation and interleukin 2 receptor expression. *Biol Trace Elem Res* 1994;41(1–2):103–14.
17. Kiremidjian-Schumacher L, M Roy, HI Wishe, MW Cohen, G Stotzky. Supplementation with selenium and human immune cell functions. II. Effect on cytotoxic lymphocytes and natural killer cells. *Biol Trace Elem Res* 1994;41(1–2):115–27.
18. Dennert, G. Selenium for preventing cancer. *Cochrane Database of Systematic Reviews* (2012):9.
19. Sanmartín, C, D Plano, AK Sharma, J Palop. Selenium compounds, apoptosis and other types of cell death: an overview for cancer therapy. *International Journal of Molecular Sciences* 2012;13(8):9649–72.
20. Kikuchi Y, K Oomori, I Kizawa, K Kato. Augmented natural killer activity in ovarian cancer patients treated with cimetidine. *Eur J Cancer Clin Oncol* 1986;22(9):1037–43.
21. Allen JI, HJ Syropoulos, B Grant, JC Eagon, NE Kay. Cimetidine modulates natural killer cell function of patients with chronic lymphocytic leukemia. *J Lab Clin Med* 1987;109(4):396–401.
22. Kubota T, H Fujiwara, Y Ueda, T Itoh, T Yamashita, T Yoshimura, K Okugawa, Y Yamamoto, Y Yano, H Yamagishi. Cimetidine modulates the antigen presenting capacity of dendritic cells from colorectal cancer patients. *Br J Cancer* 2002;86(8):1257–61.
23. Deva, S. Histamine type 2 receptor antagonists as adjuvant treatment for resected colorectal cancer. *Cochrane Database of Systematic Reviews* (2012):8
24. Ghiringhelli F, C Menard, PE Puig, S Ladoire, S Roux, F Martin, E Solary, CA Le, L Zitvogel, B Chauffert. Metronomic cyclophosphamide regimen selectively depletes CD4+CD25+ regulatory T cells and restores T and NK effector functions in end stage cancer patients. *Cancer Immunol Immunother* 2007;56(5):641–8.
25. Beniwal, SK, KM Patel, SS Shukla, BJ Parikh, S Shah, A Patel. Gemcitabine in brief versus prolonged low-dose infusion, both combined with carboplatin for advanced non-small cell lung cancer. *Indian Journal of Cancer* 2012;49(2):202–8.
26. Coleman, M, G Ruan, R Elstrom, P Martin, J Leonard. Metronomic therapy for refractory/relapsed lymphoma: the PEP-C low-dose oral combination chemotherapy regimen. *Hematology* (Amsterdam), 2012;17: Suppl 1S90-S92.
27. Ohta A, E Gorelik, SJ Prasad, F Ronchese, D Lukashev, MK Wong, X Huang, S Caldwell, K Liu, P Smith, JF Chen, EK Jackson, S Apasov, S Abrams, M Sitkovsky. A2A adenosine receptor protects tumors from antitumor T cells. *Proc Natl Acad Sci USA* 2006;103(35):13132–7.

28. Hill, GM, DM Moriarity, WN Setzer. Attenuation of cytotoxic natural product DNA intercalating agents by caffeine. *Scientia Pharmaceutica* 2011;79(4):729–47.
29. Sitkovsky M, D Lukashev, S Deaglio, K Dwyer, SC Robson, A Ohta. Adenosine A2A receptor antagonists: blockade of adenosinergic effects and T regulatory cells. *Br J Pharmacol* 2008;153 Suppl 1:S457-S464.
30. Takahashi A, MG Hanson, HR Norell, AM Havelka, K Kono, KJ Malmberg, RV Kiessling. Preferential cell death of CD8+ effector memory (CCR7-CD45RA-) T cells by hydrogen peroxide-induced oxidative stress. *J Immunol* 2005;174(10):6080–7.
31. Betten A, C Dahlgren, UH Mellqvist, S Hermodsson, K Hellstrand. Oxygen radical-induced natural killer cell dysfunction: role of myeloperoxidase and regulation by serotonin. *J Leukoc Biol* 2004;75(6):1111–5.
32. Thoren FB, AI Romero, K Hellstrand. Oxygen radicals induce poly(ADP-ribose) polymerase-dependent cell death in cytotoxic lymphocytes. *J Immunol* 2006;176(12):7301–7.
33. Blanchetot C, J Boonstra. The ROS-NOX connection in cancer and angiogenesis. *Crit Rev Eukaryot Gene Expr* 2008;18(1):35–45.
34. McCarty MF, J Barroso-Aranda, F Contreras. A two-phase strategy for treatment of oxidant-dependent cancers. Med Hypotheses 2007;69(3):489–96.
35. McCarty MF. Clinical potential of Spirulina as a source of phycocyanobilin. *J Med Food* 2007; 10(4):566–70.
36. Pugh N, SA Ross, HN ElSohly, MA ElSohly, DS Pasco. Isolation of three high molecular weight polysaccharide preparations with potent immunostimulatory activity from Spirulina platensis, aphanizomenon flos-aquae and Chlorella pyrenoidosa. *Planta Med* 2001;67(8):737–42.
37. Hirahashi T, M Matsumoto, K Hazeki K, Y Saeki, M Ui, T Seya. Activation of the human innate immune system by Spirulina: augmentation of interferon production and NK cytotoxicity by oral administration of hot water extract of Spirulina platensis. *Int Immunopharmacol* 2002;2(4):423–34.
38. Akao, Y, T Ebihara, H Masuda, Y Saeki, T Akazawa, K Hazeki, . . . T Seya. Enhancement of antitumor natural killer cell activation by orally administered Spirulina extract in mice. *Cancer Science* 2009;100(8):1494–1501.

Chapter 31

1. Contreras, F. *Health in the 21st Century: Will Doctors Survive?* San Diego: Interpacific, 1997.
2. Salmon, DA, SP Teret, CR MacIntyre, D Salisbury, MA Burgess, NA Halsey. Compulsory vaccination and conscientious or philosophical exemptions: past, present, and future. *The Lancet* 2006;367.9508:436–42.
3. Is military research hazardous to veterans' health? Lessons spanning half a century. US Senate, 12/08/94. Committee on Veterans' Affairs. 02/14/13. gulfweb.org/bigdoc/rockrep.cfm
4. Edlich, RF, ME Chase, CL Cross, CA Wack, CM Brock, AL Fisher, . . . RB Zura. State legislations that limit the use of thimerosal in vaccines for pregnant women and their infants. *Journal of Pediatric Infectious Diseases* 2009;4(3):229–32.
5. Grossman, L. Autism rates surge. *New Scientist* 2009;214(2859):5.
6. "Cowpox." Columbia Electronic Encyclopedia, 6th Edition (2011), 1.
7. Hansen, B. America's first medical breakthrough: How popular excitement about a French rabies cure in 1885. . . . *American Historical Review* 1998;103(2):373.
8. Biotech vaccine okayed. *Science News* 1986;130(4):52.
9. Tomljenovic, L, CA Shaw. Too fast or not too fast: the FDA's approval of Merck's HPV vaccine Gardasil. *Journal of Law, Medicine & Ethics* 2012;40(3):673–81.
10. 10 Lyseng-Williamson, KA, K McKeage. AS04-adjuvanted human papillomavirus types 16/18 vaccine (Cervarix): a guide to its use. *Drugs & Therapy Perspectives* 2012;28(3):1–6.
11. Naylor, PH, JE Egan, NL Berinstein. Peptide-based vaccine approaches for cancer—a novel approach using a WT-1 synthetic long peptide and the IRX-2 immunomodulatory regimen. *Cancers* 2011;3(4):3991–4009.

12. Li, L, P Goedegebuure, ER Mardis, MC Ellis, Z Xiuli, JM Herndon, ... WE Gillanders. Cancer genome sequencing and its implications for personalized cancer vaccines. *Cancers* 2011;3(4):4191–211.
13. Yamamoto, N. Antitumor effect of vitamin D-binding protein-derived macrophage activating factor on Ehrlich ascites tumor-bearing mice. *Proceedings of the Society for Experimental Biology and Medicine.* 1999;220(1):20–26.

Chapter 32

1. Steinman, RM. Identification of a novel cell type in peripheral lymphoid organs of mice: I. morphology, quantitation, tissue distribution. *Journal of Experimental Medicine* 1973;137.5:1142–62.
2. Gervis, A. Dendritic cells are defective in breast cancer patients: a potential role for polyamine in this immunodeficiency. *Breast Cancer Research* 2005;7:326–35.
3. Engleman, EG. The clinical use of monoclonal antibodies. *West Journal of Medicine* 1983;138.5:707.
4. Thomas, R, PE Lipsky. Dendritic cells: origin & differentiation. *Stem Cells* 1996;14.2:196–206.
5. Hsu, FJ, C Benike, F Fagnoni, TM Liles, D Czerwinski, B Taidi, EG Engleman, R Levy. Vaccination of patients with B-cell lymphoma using autologous antigen-pulsed dendritic cells. *Nature Medicine* 1996;2.1:52–8.
6. Timmerman JM, DK Czerwinski , TA Davis , FJ Hsu, C Benike, ZM Hao, B Taidi, R Rajapaksa, CB Caspar, CY Okada, A van Beckhoven, TM Liles, EG Engleman, R Levy. Idiotype-pulsed dendritic cell vaccination for B-cell lymphoma: clinical and immune responses in 35 patients. *Blood.* 2002;99(5):1517–26.
7. Using dendritic cells to create cancer vaccines. Stanford School of Medicine, Medcast Lecture Series, 17 Nov 2007. Video.
8. First cancer vaccine approved for use in people. *New Scientist* 2010;206(2759):5.
9. Dendreon Corp. *MondayMorning* 2012;20(20):1.
10. Legitimo, A, R Consolini, A Failli, S Fabiano, W Bencivelli, F Scatena, F Mosca. In vitro treatment of monocytes with 8-methoxypsolaren and ultraviolet A light induces dendritic cells with a tolerogenic phenotype. *Clinical and Experimental Immunology* 2007;148(3):564–72.
11. Spisek, R, Z Gasova, J Bartunkova. Maturation state of dendritic cells during the extracorporeal photopheresis and its relevance for the treatment of chronic graft-versus-host disease. *Transfusion* 2006;46(1):55–65.
12. Ibid.
13. Kondo, M, MF McCarty. Rationale for a novel immunotherapy of cancer with allogeneic lymphocyte infusion. *Medical Hypotheses* 1984;15.3:241–77.
14. Symons, HJ, Y Moshe, JW Levy, Z Xiaotao, Z Gang, SE Cohen, L Luznik, HI Levitsky, EJ Fuchs. The allogeneic effect revisited: exogenous help for endogenous, tumor-specific T Cells. *Biology of Blood and Marrow Transplantation* 2008;14.5: 499–509.
15. Ibid.

Chapter 33

1. Makary, M. Hospitals can kill you. *Newsweek*, 2012;160(13):44–9.
2. Davies, AR, DC Deans, II Penman, JN Plevris, JJ Fletcher, L Wall, S Paterson-Brown. The multidisciplinary team meeting improves staging accuracy and treatment selection for gastroesophageal cancer. *Diseases of the Esophagus* 2006;19(6):496–503.
3. Bunnell, CA, SN Weingart, S Swanson, HJ Mamon, LN Shulman. Models of multidisciplinary cancer care: physician and patient perceptions in a comprehensive cancer center. *Journal of Oncology Practice* 2010;6(6):283-88.
4. Ibid.
5. Chan, R, J Webster, L Bennett. Effects and feasibility of a multi-disciplinary orientation program for newly registered cancer patients: design of a randomised controlled trial. *BMC Health Services Research* (2009), 9203.

Chapter 34

1. Ancu, M. Older adults on Facebook: a survey examination of motives and use of social networking by people 50 and older. *Florida Communication Journal*, 2012;40(2):1–12.
2. Ford, A. The global network. *TIME*, 2010;176(26):58–9.
3. Chaudhry, A, M Glodé, M Gillman, RS Miller. Trends in Twitter use by physicians at the American Society of Clinical Oncology Annual Meeting, 2010 and 2011. *Journal Of Oncology Practice*, 2012;8(3):173–9.
4. Bender, JL, M Jimenez-Marroquin, AR Jadad. Seeking support on Facebook: a content analysis of breast cancer groups. *Journal of Medical Internet Research*, 2011;13(1), 221–32.
5. Yildirim, Y, S Kocabiyik. The relationship between social support and loneliness in Turkish patients with cancer. *Journal of Clinical Nursing*, 2010;19(5–6), 832–9.
6. Queenan, JA, DD Feldman-Stewart, MM Brundage, PA Groome. Social support and quality of life of prostate cancer patients after radiotherapy treatment. *European Journal of Cancer Care*, 2010;19(2):251–9.
7. De Morgan, S, S Redman, K White, B Cakir, J Boyages. "Well, have I got cancer or haven't I?" The psycho-social issues for women diagnosed with ductal carcinoma in situ. *Health Expectations* 2002;5(4), 310–8.
8. Wortman, CB, C Dunkel-Schetter. Interpersonal relationships and cancer: a theoretical analysis. *Journal of Social Issues* 1979;35(1):120–55.
9. Decker, CL. Social support and adolescent cancer survivors: a review of the literature. *Psycho-Oncology*, 2007;16(1):1–11.
10. Cicero, V, G Lo Coco, S Gullo, G Lo Verso. The role of attachment dimensions and perceived social support in predicting adjustment to cancer. *Psycho-Oncology*, 2009;18(10):1045–52.
11. Jones, SL, HD Hadjistavropoulos, SB Sherry. Health anxiety in women with early-stage breast cancer: what is the relationship to social support? *Canadian Journal of Behavioural Science*, 2012;44(2):108–16.

Chapter 35

1. Greco, M. Breast cancer patients treated without axillary surgery: clinical implications and biological analysis." *European Journal of Cancer* 1998;34:S45.
2. "Joaquín Setantí." The Quotations Page. 15 Feb 2013. quotationspage.com/quote/2177.html
3. Anderson, JB, AJ Webb. Fine-needle aspiration biopsy and the diagnosis of thyroid cancer. *British Journal of Surgery* 1987;74:29:2–6.
4. Epstein, J. Why second opinions rule. *Cancer.* 1999;86(11):2426–35.

Chapter 36

1. Exodus 20:4 NLT
2. Lennon, J. "Imagine." *Imagine*. EMI Records, 1971.
3. Laín Entralgo, P. From Galen to magnetic resonance: history of medicine in Latin America. *The Journal of Medicine and Philosophy* 1996;21(6):571–91.
4. Vesalius, A. *On the Fabric of the Human Body*. Eds. WF Richardson, JB Carman. San Francisco: Norman, 1999.
5. Natale, S. A Cosmology of invisible fluids: wireless, X-rays, and psychical research around 1900. *Canadian Journal of Communication* 2011;36(2):263–75.
6. Barley, H. (1950). Shoe-fitting with X-ray. National Safety News, 62(3): 33, 107-111.
7. Brice, J. To err is human. *Diagnostic Imaging*, nd. Web Video. diagnosticimaging.com/conference-reports/rsna2010/content/article/113619/1745046
8. Ibid.
9. Berlin, L. Errors of omission. *American Journal of Roentgenology* 2005;185.6:1416–21.
10. Bleyer, A. H Welch. Effect of three decades of screening mammography on breast cancer incidence. *Medical Benefits* 2013;30(3):9.

11. Ibid.
12. Pinto, A. Spectrum of diagnostic errors in radiology. *World Journal of Radiology* 2010;2.10:377.
13. "Russell Baker Quotes." Xplore, nd. Web. 02/15/13. BrainyQuote.com
14. "John C. Maxwell Quotes." nd. Web. 02/15/13. GoodReads.com

Chapter 37

1. Homer. *The Odyssey*. Cambridge, MA: Harvard UP, 1960.
2. Jones, T, N Saba. Nanotechnology and drug delivery: an update in oncology. *Pharmaceutics* 2011;3(2):171–85.
3. Slade, C. Public value mapping of equity in emerging nanomedicine. *Minerva: A Review Of Science, Learning & Policy* 2011;49(1):71–86.
4. Klein, S.A. (2005). For American Pharma, time is of the essence, *Crain's Chicago Business*, 28(4), 14.
5. Yallapu, MM, M Jaggi, SC Chauhan. Scope of nanotechnology in ovarian cancer therapeutics. *Journal of Ovarian Research* 2010;3(1):1–10.
6. Dhankhar, R, SP Vyas, AKJain, S Arora, G Rath, AK Goyal. Advances in novel drug delivery strategies for breast cancer therapy. *Artificial Cells, Blood Substitutes & Biotechnology* 2010;38(5):230–49.
7. Tiwari, M. Nano cancer therapy strategies. *Journal of Cancer Research & Therapeutics* 2012;8(1):19–22.
8. Siddiqui, I, V Adhami, N Ahmad, H Mukhtar, H. Nanochemoprevention: sustained release of bioactive food components for cancer prevention.*Nutrition & Cancer*, 2010;62(7):883–90.
9. Ibid.

Chapter 38

1. Breasted, JH. *The Edwin Smith Surgical Papyrus*. Chicago: University of Chicago, 1930.
2. Baronzio, GF, ED Hager. *Hyperthermia in Cancer Treatment: A Primer*. Georgetown, TX: Landes Bioscience, 2006.
3. Ibid.
4. Coley, WB. Contribution to the knowledge of sarcoma. *Annals of Surgery* 1891;14.6:199–220.
5. Coley, WB. Treatment of inoperable malignant tumors with the toxines of erysipelas and the Bacillus Prodigiosus. *The American Journal of the Medical Sciences* 1894;108.1:50–66.
6. Da Costa, JC. Modern surgery, general & operative. *Annals of* Surgery 1904;39.1: 148–60.
7. Coley-Nauts, H. Papers. Manuscripts and Archives, Yale University Library.
8. Nauts, H. Coley's toxins—the first century. *Townsend Letter* 2004;(251):107–16.
9. Maletzki, C, U Klier, W Obst, B Kreikemeyer, M Linnebacher. Reevaluating the concept of treating experimental tumors with a mixed bacterial vaccine: Coley's toxin. *Clinical & Developmental Immunology* (2012):1–16.
10. Ruckdeschel, JC, SD Codish, A Stranahan, MF McKneally. Postoperative empyema improves survival in lung cancer. *New England Journal of Medicine* 1972;287(20):1013–7.
11. Richardson, M, T Ramirez, N Russell, L Moye. Coley toxins immunotherapy: a retrospective review. *Alternative Therapies in Health and Medicine*, 1999;5(3):42–7.
12. LaVeen, HH, S Wapnick, V Piccone, G Falk, N Ahmed. Tumor eradication by radiofrequency therapy: responses in 21 patients. *JAMA*. 1976;17;235(20):2198–2200.
13. Halperin, EC, CA Perez. *Perez and Brady's Principles and Practice of Radiation Oncology*. Philadelphia: Wolters Kluwer/Lippincott Williams & Wilkins, 2013.
14. Ibid.
15. Song, CW, H Park, RJ Griffin. Improvement of tumor oxygenation by mild hyperthermia. *Radiation Research* 2001;155.4:515–28.
16. Dollinger, M. *Everyone's Guide to Cancer Therapy;* 5th rev. ed. Kansas City: Andrews McMeel, 2008, 98–100.
17. Perez, CA. *Principles and Practice of Radiation Oncology*. Philadelphia: Lippincott, 2004.
18. Van Der Zee, J., et al. Hyperthermia combined with radiotherapy: prognostic significance. *CME Journal of Gynecologic Oncology* 2001;6:364–70.

19. Ibid.
20. Bicher, H, N Al-Bussam. Thermoradiotherapy with curative intent—breast, head, neck and prostate tumors. *Deutsche Zeitschrift Für Onkologie* 2006;38.3:116-22.
21. Ibid.

Chapter 39

1. Song, CW, H Park, RJ Griffin. Improvement of tumor oxygenation by mild hyperthermia. *Radiation Research* 2001;155(4):515-28.
2. Muckle, DS. The selective effect of heat in cancer. *Annals of the Royal College of Surgeons of England.* 1974;54(2):72-7.
3. LeVeen, HH, S Wapnick, V Piccone, G Falk, A Nafis. Tumor eradication by radiofrequency therapy: responses in 21 patients. *JAMA* 1976;17.235(20):2198-200.
4. García-Jimeno, S, et al. Improved thermal ablation efficacy using magnetic nanoparticles: a study in tumor phantoms. *Progress in Electromagnetics Research* 2012;128:229-48.
5. Hilger I, et al. Thermal ablation of tumors using magnetic nanoparticles: an in vivo feasibility study. *Invest Radiol* 2002 Oct;37(10):580-6.
6. Ibid.
7. Bruners, P, M Hodenius, M Baumann, J Oversohl, R Günther, T Schmitz-Rode, A Mahnken. Magnetic thermal ablation using ferrofluids: influence of administration mode on biological effect in different porcine tissues. *Cardiovascular and Interventional Radiology*, 2008;31(6):1193-9.
8. Richter, H, M Kettering, F Wiekhorst, U Steinhoff, I Hilger, L Trahms. Magnetorelaxometry for localization and quantification of magnetic nanoparticles for thermal ablation studies. *Physics in Medicine and Biology* 2010;55.3:623-33.

Chapter 40

1. "Extreme Couponing Clips." *TLC*. 11/09/12. tlc.howstuffworks.com/tv/extreme-couponing
2. Luke 18:2-5 NLT
3. David, C, L Salo, S Redman. Evaluating the effectiveness of advocacy training for breast cancer advocates in Australia. *European Journal of Cancer Care* 2001;10:82-6.
4. Walsh-Burke, K, C Marcusen. Self-advocacy training for cancer survivors: the cancer survival toolkit. *Cancer Practice* 1999;7.6:297-301.
5. "Patient Bill of Rights." American Cancer Society, nd. Web. 11/20/12. cancer.org/search/index?QueryText-Patient+Bill+of+Rights
6. Nahuis, R, WPC Boon. The impact of patient advocacy: the case of innovative breast cancer drug reimbursement. *Sociology of Health & Illness* 2011;33.1:1-15.
7. Kahana, E, VK Cheruvu, B Kahana, J Kelley-Moore, S Sterns, JA Brown, C King, D Kulle, J Spek, KC Strange. Patient advocacy and cancer screening in late life. *Open Longevity Science* 2010;4:20-9.
8. Radley, A, S Payne. A sociological commentary on the refusal of treatment by patients with cancer. *Mortality* 2009;14.4:309-24.

Chapter 41

1. Tom, W. Giving ill children a reason to be optimistic. *USA Today* [serial online]. nd. Available from Academic Search Complete. Ipswich, MA, 05/24/13.
2. Ngo, TH, RJ Barnard, PS Leung, P Cohen, WJ Aronson. Insulin-like growth factor I (IGF-I) and IGF binding protein-1 modulate prostate cancer cell growth and apoptosis: possible mediators for the effects of diet and exercise on cancer cell survival. *Endocrinology* 2003 Jun;144(6):2319-24.
3. Barnard, RJ, TH Ngo, PS Leung, WJ Aronson, LA Golding. A low-fat diet and/or strenuous exercise alters the IGF axis in vivo and reduces prostate tumor cell growth in vitro. *Prostate* 2003 Aug 1;56(3):201-6.
4. Borugian MJ, SB Sheps, C Kim-Sing, IA Olivotto, C Van Patten, BP Dunn, AJ Coldman, JD Potter, RP Gallagher, TG Hislop. Waist-to-hip ratio and breast cancer mortality. *Am J Epidemiol* 2003 Nov 15;158(10):963-8.

5. Pasanisi P, F Berrino, M De Petris, E Venturelli, A Mastroianni, S Panico. Metabolic syndrome as a prognostic factor for breast cancer recurrences. *Int J Cancer* 2006 Jul 1;119(1):236–8.
6. Holmes MD, WY Chen, D Feskanich, CH Kroenke, GA Colditz. Physical activity and survival after breast cancer diagnosis. *JAMA* 2005 May 25;293(20):2479–86.6
7. Meyerhardt JA, D Heseltine, D Niedzwiecki, D Hollis, LB Saltz, RJ Mayer, J Thomas, H Nelson, R Whittom, A Hantel, RL Schilsky, CS Fuchs. Impact of physical activity on cancer recurrence and survival in patients with stage III colon cancer: findings from CALGB 89803. *J Clin Oncol* 2006 Aug 1;24(22):3535–41.
8. Meyerhardt JA, EL Giovannucci,MD Holmes, AT Chan, JA Chan, GA Colditz, CS Fuchs. Physical activity and survival after colorectal cancer diagnosis. *J Clin Oncol* 2006 Aug 1;24(22):3527–34.
9. Blaney, J, A Lowe-Strong, J Rankin, A Campbell, J Allen, J Gracey. The cancer rehabilitation journey: barriers to and facilitators of exercise among patients with cancer-related fatigue. *Physical Therapy* 2010;90(8):1135–47.
10. Hutnick NA, NI Williams, WJ Kraemer, E Orsega-Smith, RH Dixon, AD Bleznak, AM Mastro. Exercise and lymphocyte activation following chemotherapy for breast cancer. *Med Sci Sports Exerc* 2005 Nov;37(11):1827–35.
11. Quist M, M Rorth, M Zacho, C Andersen, T Moeller, J Midtgaard, L Adamsen. High-intensity resistance and cardiovascular training improve physical capacity in cancer patients undergoing chemotherapy. *Scand J Med Sci Sports* 2006 Oct;16(5):349–57.
12. Sander, AP, J Wilson, N Izzo, SA Mountford, KW Hayes. Factors that affect decisions about physical activity and exercise in survivors of breast cancer: a qualitative study. *Physical Therapy* 2012;92(4):525–36.
13. Lee, J, M Dodd, S Dibble, D Abrams. Nausea at the end of adjuvant cancer treatment in relation to exercise during treatment in patients with breast cancer. *Oncology Nursing Forum*, 2008;35(5):830–5.
14. Galvao, D, D Taaffe, P Cormie, N Spry, S Chambers, C Peddle-McIntyre, R Newton. Efficacy and safety of a modular multi-modal exercise program in prostate cancer patients with bone metastases: a randomized controlled trial. *BMC Cancer* (2011):11517.
15. Spence, R, K Heesch, W Brown. Colorectal cancer survivors' exercise experiences and preferences: qualitative findings from an exercise rehabilitation programme immediately after chemotherapy. *European Journal of Cancer Care*, 2011;20(2):257–66.
16. Blacklock, R, R Rhodes, C Blanchard, C Gaul. Effects of exercise intensity and self-efficacy on state anxiety with breast cancer survivors. *Oncology Nursing Forum* 2010;37(2):206–12.
17. "Key Findings." *Key Findings*. American Psychological Association, 2010. Web. 11/17/12. apa.org/news/press/releases/stress/key-findings.aspx
18. Reiss, V. Power surge. *Natural Health* 2011;41(8):64–71.
19. Maddocks, M, S Armstrong, A Wilcock. Exercise as a supportive therapy in incurable cancer: exploring patient preferences. *Psycho-Oncology* 2011;20(2):173–8.
20. 20 Peeters, CC, A Stewart, R Segal, E Wouterloot, CG Scott, T Aubry. Evaluation of a cancer exercise program: patient and physician beliefs. *Psycho-Oncology*, 2009;18(8):898–902.
21. Gjerset, G, S Fosså, K Courneya, E Skovlund, A Jacobsen, L Thorsen. Interest and preferences for exercise counseling and programming among Norwegian cancer survivors. *European Journal of Cancer Care* 2011;20(1):96–105.

Chapter 42

1. *Physician's Desk Reference*. 67th ed. Chestertown, MD: PDR Network, 2013.
2. Thall, PF. Ethical issues in oncology biostatistics. *Statistical Methods in Medical Research* 2002; 1:429–48.
3. Mehta, P, M Hester, AM Safar, R Thompson. Ethics-in-oncology forums. *Journal of Cancer Education* 2007;22.3:159–64.
4. Levy, R. Impact of "illegality" of payment arrangement under Stark Law on payment for services of referring physicians. *Journal of Health Care Compliance*, 2012;14(4):29–75.

5. Ashker, S, J Burkiewicz. Pharmacy residents' attitudes toward pharmaceutical industry promotion. *American Journal of Health-System Pharmacy (AJHP): Official Journal of the American Society of Health-System Pharmacists* 2007;64(16):1724–31.
6. Sigurdardottir, V, C Bolun, B Nilson. Quality of life and ethics: opinions about chemotherapy among patients with advanced melanoma, next of kin and care-providers." *Psycho-Oncology* 1995;4: 287–300.
7. Markman, M. Reflections on ethical concerns arising from the incorporation of results of randomized trials of antineoplastic therapy into routine clinical practice. *Cancer Investigation* 2005;23:735–40.
8. Blanke, CD, RM Goldberg, A Grothey, M Mooney, N Roach, LB Saltz, JJ Welch, WA Wood, NJ Meropol. KRAS and colorectal cancer: ethical and pragmatic issues in effecting real-time change in oncology clinical trials and practice. *The Oncologist* 2011;16.8:1061–8.
9. Ibid.
10. Levinson, W, DL Roter, JP Mullooly, et al. Physician-patient communication: the relationship with malpractice claims among primary care physicians and surgeons. *JAMA* 1997;277:553–9.
11. Biedrzycki, BA. Ethics in oncology nursing: realism and resources. *ONS* 2004;19(8):3–7.

Chapter 43

1. Kafka, F. *The Country Doctor.* Oxford: Counterpoint, 1945.
2. Adams, P. *House Calls.* San Francisco: Robert D. Reed, 1998.
3. Adams, H. The real Patch Adams. *Contemporary Pediatrics* 2008;25(12):72.
4. Street, JL, P Haidet. How well do doctors know their patients? *JGIM* 2011;26(1):21–7.
5. Siegel, BS. AHHA: the doctor and the patient: relationship, partnership or marriage? *American Holistic Health Association*, nd. Web. 11/18/12. ahha.org/articles.asp?Id-10
6. Pettit, ML. An analysis of the doctor-patient relationship using Patch Adams. *Journal of School Health* 2008;78.4:234–8.
7. Shadyac, T. (1998). *Patch Adams.* Universal City, CA: Universal Pictures.
8. Kinsman, H, D Roter, G Berkenblit, S Saha, P Korthuis, I Wilson, M Beach, M. "We'll do this together": the role of the first person plural in fostering partnership in patient-physician relationships. *JGIM* 2010;25(3):186–93.
9. Đor evi , V, M Braš, L Brajkovi . Person-centered medical interview. *Croatian Medical Journal* 2012; 53(4):310–3.
10. Banerjee, A, D Sanyal. Dynamics of doctor-patient relationship: a cross-sectional study on concordance, trust, and patient enablement. *Journal of Family & Community Medicine* 2012;19(1):12–9.
11. Kirschenbaum, H. What is "person-centered"? A posthumous conversation with Carl Rogers on the development of the person-centered approach. *Person-Centered & Experiential Psychotherapies* 2012;11(1):14–30.
12. Pizarro Obaid, F. Sigmund Freud and Otto Rank: debates and confrontations about anxiety and birth. *International Journal of Psycho-Analysis* 2012;93(3):693–715.
13. Greenstein, M, W Breitbart. Cancer and the experience of meaning: a group psychotherapy program for people with cancer. *American Journal of Psychotherapy* 2000;54(4):486–500.
14. Larson, JM. Family of origin influences on young adult career decision problems: a test of Bowenian theory. *American Journal of Family Therapy* 1998;26(1):39.

Chapter 44

1. Rosch, PJ. Stress and the body's "wisdom": friend or foe? Health & Stress, 2009(12):1–12.
2. Papavramidou, N, T Papavramidis, T Demetriou. Ancient Greek and Greco-Roman methods in modern surgical treatment of cancer. *Annals of Surgical Oncology* 2010;17.3:665–7.
3. *Report on Carcinogens.* US Dept. of Health and Human Services, National Toxicology Program, 2011.

4. Nelson, LR, SE Bulun. Estrogen production and action. *Journal of the American Academy of Dermatology* 2011;45.3:S116–24.
5. Olson, JS. *Bathsheba's Breast: Women, Cancer, & History*. Baltimore: Johns Hopkins, 2002.
6. Fraumeni Jr, JF, JW Lloyd, EM Smith, JK Wagoner. Cancer mortality among nuns: role of marital status in etiology of neoplastic disease in women. National Center for Biotechnology Information. Mar 1969. Web. 02/19/13. ncbi.nlm.nih.gov/pubmed/5777491
7. Rosenberg, L, DA Boggs, LA Wise, LL Adams-Campbell, JR Palmer. Oral contraceptive use and estrogen/progesterone receptor-negative breast cancer among African American women. *Cancer Epidemiology Biomarkers & Prevention* 2010;19(8):2073–9.
8. Dolle, JM, JR Daling, E White, LA Brinton, DR Doody, PL Porter, KE Malone. Risk factors for triple-negative breast cancer in women under the age of 45 years. *Cancer Epidemiology Biomarkers & Prevention* 2009;18(4):1157–66.
9. Ibid.
10. Gebbie, A. Risks and benefits of estrogen plus progestin in healthy postmenopausal women. Principal results from the Women's Health Initiative randomized controlled trial. Writing Group for the Women's Health Initiative Investigators. *JAMA* 2002;288(3):321–33.
11. Ibid.
12. Liotta M, PF Escobar. Hormone replacement after breast cancer: is it safe? *Clin Obstet Gynecol* 2011 Mar;54(1):173–9.
13. McNeil, C. Breast cancer decline mirrors fall in hormone use, spurs both debate and research. *Journal of the National Cancer Institute* 2007;99(4):266–7.
14. Ibid.
15. NIH Press Release—New federal "Report on Carcinogens" lists estrogen therapy, ultraviolet, wood dust—12/11/02. Web. 02/19/13. nih.gov/news/pr/dec2002/niehs-11.htm

Chapter 45

1. Singec, I, R Jandial, A Crain, G Nikkhah, EY Snyder. The leading edge of stem cell therapeutics. *Annual Review of Medicine* 2007;58.1:313–28.
2. Gurtner, GC, MJ Callaghan, MT Longaker. Progress and potential for regenerative medicine. *Annual Review of Medicine* 2007;58.1:299–312.
3. Bonnet, D, JE Dick. Human acute myeloid leukemia is organized as a hierarchy that originates from a primitive hematopoietic cell. *Nature Medicine* 1997;3(7): 730–7.
4. Al-Hajj, M, MS Wicha, A Benito-Hernandez, SJ Morrison, MF Clarke. Prospective identification of tumorigenic breast cancer cells. *Proceedings of the National Academy of Sciences of the United States of America* 2003;100:3983–8.
5. Hirsch, HA, et al. Metformin selectively targets cancer stem cells, and acts together with chemotherapy to block tumor growth and prolong remission. *Cancer Research* 2009(69):19.
6. Shank JJ, K Yang, J Ghannam, L Cabrera, CJ Johnston, RK Reynolds, RJ Buckanovich. Metformin targets ovarian cancer stem cells in vitro and in vivo. *Gynecologic Oncology* 2012;127(2):390–7.

Chapter 46

1. Niemtzow, R. Great revolutionary leaders of alternative medicine: a fascinating journey back in time. *Journal of Alternative and Complementary Medicine* 2002;8(6):699–702.
2. Lynes, B. Royal Raymond Rife & the cancer cure that worked. "Rife." *Nexus*, nd. Web. 02/20/13. whale.to/w/rife.html
3. Nordenström, B. Biologically closed electric circuits: clinical, experimental and theoretical evidence for an additional circulatory system. *Ursus Medical AB* (1983).
4. Becker, RO, G Selden. *The Body Electric: Electromagnetism and the Foundation of Life*. New York: Morrow, 1985.
5. BioInitiative Working Group. BioInitiative 2012 Report Issues New Warnings on Wireless and EMF. *Business Wire* (2001).

6. Nuccitelli, R, K Tran, S Sheikh, B Athos, M Kreis, P Nuccitelli. Optimized nanosecond pulsed electric field therapy can cause murine malignant melanomas to self-destruct with a single treatment. *International Journal of Cancer* 2010;127.7:1727–36.
7. Cho, MH, EJ Lee, M Son, J Lee, D Yoo, J Kim, SW Park, J Shin, J Cheon. A magnetic switch for the control of cell death signaling in in vitro and in vivo systems. *Nature Materials* 2012;11:1038–43.
8. Miller, J. Electric fields have potential as a cancer treatment. *Physics Today* 2007;60(8):19.
9. Kirson, ED, V Dbaly, F Tovarys, J Vymazal, JF Soustiel, A Itzhaki, D Mordechovich, S Steinberg-Shapira, Z Gurvich, R Schneiderman, Y Wasserman, M Salzberg, B Ryffel, D Goldsher, E Dekel, Y Palti. Alternating electric fields arrest cell proliferation in animal tumor models and human brain tumors. *Proceedings of the National Academy of Sciences* 2007;104(24):10152–7.
10. Schroeder, T, BL Viglianti, MW Dewhirst. Low-intensity alternating electric fields: a potentially safe and effective treatment of cancer? *Onkologie* 2008;31(7):357–8.

Chapter 47

1. "Placebo." Web. 12/06/12. Dictionary.com
2. "Placebo Effect." Ibid.
3. Pasternak, C. Placebo: no longer a phantom response. *Interdisciplinary Science Reviews* 2011; 36(1): 72–82.
4. Proverbs 23:7, NKJV
5. Kenny, S, B Roberts, B Mason, D Schlect. Beliefs and practices of patients with advanced cancer: implications for communication. *British Journal of Cancer* 2004;91:254–7.
6. Bergner, S. Seductive symbolism: psychoanalysis in the context of oncology. *Psychoanalytic Psychology* 2001;2:267–92.
7. Mystakidou, K, E Tsilika, E Parpa, P Gogou, P Theodorakis, L Vlahos. Self-efficacy beliefs and levels of anxiety in advanced cancer patients. *European Journal of Cancer Care* 2010;19(2):205–11.
8. Keeney, S, H McKenna, P Fleming, S McIlfatrick. Attitudes to cancer and cancer prevention: what do people aged 35–54 years think? *European Journal of Cancer Care* 2010;19(6):769–77.
9. Kazak, AE, KS McClure, MA Alderfer, WT Hwang, TA Crump, LT Le, J Deatrick, S Simms, MT Rourke. Cancer-related parental beliefs: the family illness beliefs inventory (FIBI). *Journal of Pediatric Psychology* 2004[29(7):531–42.

Chapter 48

1. 1 Samuel 16:6-23 NLT
2. Schlitz, M. Toward a noetic model of medicine. *Noetic Sciences Review* 1998;(47):44.
3. Zaiser, R. Working on the noetic dimension of man: philosophical practice, logotherapy, and existential analysis. *Philosophical Practice* 2005;1(2):83–8.
4. Weber, S. A pilot study on the influence of receptive music listening on cancer patients during chemotherapy. *International Journal of Arts Medicine* 1997;5(2):27–35.
5. E.g., see Psalm 22:3.
6. Wood, MJ, A Molassiotis, S Payne. What research evidence is there for the use of art therapy in the management of symptoms in adults with cancer? a systematic review. *Psycho-Oncology* 2011;20:135–45.
7. Moller, A, A Elliot, M Maier. Basic hue-meaning associations. *Emotion* 2009 Dec;9(6):898–902.
8. Berk, RA. The active ingredients in humor: psychophysiological benefits and risks for older adults. *Educational Gerontology* 2001;27(3–4): 323–39.
9. Cousins N. Anatomy of an illness (as perceived by the patient). *New England Journal of Medicine* 1976;295:1458–63.
10. Erdman, L. Laughter therapy for patients with cancer. *Journal of Psychosocial Oncology* 1994; 11(4):55–67.
11. Borod, M. Smiles—toward a better laughter life: a model for introducing humor in the palliative care setting. *Journal of Cancer Education* 2006;21(1):30–4.
12. Roffe, L, K Schmidt, E Ernst. A systematic review of guided imagery as an adjuvant cancer therapy. *Psycho-Oncology* 2005;14(8):607–17.

13. Demiralp, M, F Oflaz, S Komurcu. Effects of relaxation training on sleep quality and fatigue in patients with breast cancer undergoing adjuvant chemotherapy. *Journal of Clinical Nursing* 2010;19(7-8):1073-83.
14. Russell, NC, SS Sumler, CM Beinhorn, MA Frenkel. Role of massage therapy in cancer care. *Journal of Alternative and Complementary Medicine* 2008;14(2):209-14.
15. Krucoff, MW, SW Crater, CL Green, AC Maas, JE Seskevich, JD Land, KA Loeffler, K Morris, TM Bashore, HG Koenig. Integrative noetic therapies as adjuncts to percutaneous intervention during unstable coronary syndromes: monitoring and actualization of noetic training feasibility pilot. *American Heart Journal* 2001;142(5):760-9.

Chapter 49

1. Ross, LE, IJ Hall, TL Fairley, YJ Taylor, DL Howard. Prayer and self-reported health among cancer survivors in the United States. National Health Interview Survey, 2002. *Journal of Alternative and Complementary Medicine* 2008;14(8):931-8.
2. Taylor, EJ. FH Outlaw. Use of prayer among persons with cancer. *Holistic Nurse Practice* 2002; 16(3):46-60.
3. James 5:14-16, NIV
4. John 14:13, NIV
5. Matthew 18:20, NIV
6. Isaiah 53:4-5
7. Stanley, R. Types of prayer, heart rate variability, and innate healing. *Zygon: Journal of Religion & Science* 2009;44(4):825-46.
8. Dein, S, KI Pargament. On not praying for the return of an amputated limb: conserving a relationship with God as the primary function of prayer. *Bulletin of The Menninger Clinic* 2012; 76(3):235-59.
9. Pargament, KI, BW Smith, HG Koenig, L Perez. Patterns of positive and negative religious coping with major life stressors. *Journal of the Scientific Study of Religion* 1998;37:713-30.
10. Harvey, IS, M Silverman. The role of spirituality in the self-management of chronic illness among older Africans and Whites. *Journal of Cross-Cultural Gerontology* 2007;22(2):205-20.
11. Masters, KS, GI Spielmans. Prayer and health: review, meta-analysis, and research agenda. *Journal of Behavioral Medicine* 2007;30(4):329-38.
12. Alcorn, SR, Balboni, MJ Prigerson, HG Reynolds, AC Phelps, AA Wright, . . . TA Balboni. "If God wanted me yesterday, I wouldn't be here today": religious and spiritual themes in patients' experiences of advanced cancer. *Journal of Palliative Medicine* 2010;13(5):581-8.
13. See John 8:1-11, NIV
14. Visser, A, B Garssen, A Vingerhoets. Spirituality and well-being in cancer patients: a review. *Psycho-Oncology* 2010;19(6):565-72.
15. Ibid.
16. Matthew 22:37-39, NIV
17. Brown, J. Serenity Prayer: it's not just for addictions. *New Social Worker* 2011;18(2):27.
18. "Serenity Prayer." Widely attributed to Reinhold Niebuhr.
19. See Mark 4:35-41.
20. See Matthew 14:22-32.
21. See Philippians 1:21.
22. See Luke 17:33.
23. Shary served more than forty years as our volunteer laughter therapist at Oasis of Hope.

Chapter 50

1. Guinan, E, J Hussey, S McGarrigle, L Healy, J O'Sullivan, K Bennett, E Connolly. A prospective investigation of predictive and modifiable risk factors for breast cancer in unaffected BRCA1 and BRCA 2 gene carriers. *BMC Cancer* 2013; 13138.doi:10.1186.1471-2407-13-138.

2. Zagouri, F, D Chrysikos, T Sergentanis, G Giannakopoulou, C Zografos, C Papadimitriou, G Zografos. Prophylactic mastectomy: an appraisal. *The American Surgeon* 2013;79(2):205–12.
3. Contreras, F, LE Connealy. Patients with metastatic cancer treated with integrative regulatory therapy. *Townsend Letter* 2012 Aug/Sept;(349–50):51–56.
4. Ries LAG, JL Young, GE Keel, MP Eisner, YD Lin, MJ Horner (eds.). SEER Survival Monograph: cancer survival among adults: US SEER Program, 1988–2001, patient and tumor characteristics. NCI, SEER Program, NIH Pub. No. 07-6215, Bethesda, MD, 2007.